50.00

PSYCHOANALYSIS AND COGNITIVE SCIENCE

PSYCHOANALYSIS AND COGNITIVE SCIENCE

A Multiple Code Theory

WILMA BUCCI

THE GUILFORD PRESS
New York   London

©1997 The Guilford Press
A Division of Guilford Publications, Inc.
72 Spring Street, New York, NY 10012

Printed in the United States of America

This book is printed on acid-free paper.

Last digit is print number: 9 8 7 6 5 4 3 2

Library of Congress Cataloging-in-Publication Data
Bucci, Wilma.
    Psychoanalysis and cognitive science: a multiple code theory /
Wilma Bucci.
        p.   cm.
    Includes bibliographical references and index.
    ISBN 1-57230-213-5
    1. Psychoanalysis.   2. Cognitive science.   I. Title.
BF173.B877 1997
150.19′5—dc21   96–52825
                                                                CIP

Acknowledgments

Writing this book has been a long trip—much longer and through somewhat different terrain than I anticipated when I started out. I have been launched and accompanied on this trip by many people; I would like to take this opportunity to thank a few of them here.

Martin D. S. Braine, who died in April 1996, was my dissertation adviser and teacher in the fields of cognitive psychology and psycholinguistics, in the Experimental Psychology program at New York University. He was rigorous and demanding, also imaginative and original. He was a questioner and always open to the questioning of his students. In imagination I see him reading this book with his characteristic quizzical expression; it is a considerable loss not to know how he would actually have responded to it.

In my first professional position, at Downstate Medical Center, Norbert Freedman helped me bridge the great divide to clinical research; he also taught me ways to keep the big picture in my mind's eye, and has been an inspiring and exciting colleague for over 20 years.

This is a very collaborative field, and I feel that my colleagues have become a family for me—with many of the ups and downs of family life. Erhard Mergenthaler at the University of Ulm in Germany has been a long-time collaborator and a long-time friend; his computerized language analysis procedures have provided powerful tools for our examination of the therapeutic process. The Department of Psychotherapy in Ulm, established by Helmut Thomae and now directed by Horst Kaechele, is an international center for the field of psychoanalytic and psychotherapy research and has been a constant source of intellectual refueling for me.

I admire Horst Kaechele's dynamism and sense of realism in building and expanding the field; and I have greatly profited from theoretical and clinical discussions with Helmut Thomae, whose interest in my theoretical approach helped give me courage to write this book.

Hartvig Dahl has been a powerful force in building the field of psychoanalytic process research, including developing archives of verbatim case material and applying computer-assisted procedures to psychoanalytic sessions; we are all building on his innovative contributions today.

Richard C. Friedman and I have worked together in reconstructing the understanding of female sexuality within the framework of a new view of psychoanalytic theory; some of those ideas are represented in this book. Some years ago, Rick also suggested to me that my attempt to develop a new theory of the dreaming process would be seen as radical and that I would have to write a book to make my case; that was an empowering idea for me. Rick and I have been coinvestigators on projects funded by the Fund for Psychoanalytic Research and now share the direction of the Glass Institute for Basic Psychoanalytic Research.

I feel special gratitude and affection to Leslie Glass for her support of my research program over the past several years and for her vision in establishing the Glass Institute with its agenda of building a new psychoanalytic research culture. The Institute sounded at first like a wonderful fantasy; I feel enormously privileged to be part of the process of making it a reality. I also thank the Fund for Psychoanalytic Research of the American Psychoanalytic Association for their earlier support, which was indispensable in carrying out some of the research presented in this book.

The students in my research groups at the Derner Institute at Adelphi University have been a wonderful, joyful extended family for the past 14 years. They provide a constant flow of ideas and challenges, which have contributed greatly to the work presented here. I wish I could mention each of them individually. Some of the work of my research students is referred to in the book; here I will only mention the few students who worked directly on the production of this volume: Christine Li, whose library skills are legendary and who generated the references; Heidi Kling, the intrepid detective who solved the remaining mysteries of the reference list; and Kathryn Scrimenti, who generated the figures included here and who gracefully connects computer expertise to our clinical and research cultures. Parts of the book were developed as lectures to my Cognitive Psychology classes at Adelphi. I am glad the students in these classes have found the book useful, and I thank them for their constructive feedback and for their encouragement.

Seymour Weingarten, Kitty Moore, and Judith Grauman at The Guilford Press have been consistently encouraging and sensitive throughout this venture, and have made me feel that the book is important to them, not only to me. I thank Philip Wong for his extensive and insightful comments on an earlier version of this book, and I also thank Cecily Weintraub for many valuable comments and suggestions.

Writing this book has not been lonely because I have shared this and many other journeys, intellectual and personal, pleasant and painful, with my husband, Bernard Maskit. I cannot mention all his contributions because they are everywhere, from technological (and emotional) support to reading and commenting on the entire book, some parts of it more than once. As a research mathematician, Bernie has direct knowledge of the wide range of complex and abstract thought that goes on outside of language; he also understands the difficulties of finding words for things. He is a generative contributor of ideas, which cannot be specifically acknowledged here because our conversations and joint discoveries are a constant and ongoing process. He has also given me some perspective—from a necessary distance—on his mathematical world. We work on different sides of the same large desk, and have been together in many explorations, and that has made all the difference.

Bernie and I brought our two families together almost 20 years ago, survived the first joint camping trip, and have gone on together from there. Children are great and intense multipliers of love, joy, sorrow, and other emotion schemas, and also major providers of new worldviews. Each of our children has contributed in many ways to development of the ideas that I present here. Jocelyn Bucci Van Belle and Michael Bucci have taught me about images, emotions, and words—also about connection and autonomy—since they were born. Sidney and Jonathan Maskit and Barbara Fultner have shown me around the wilderness of modern philosophical ideas. (I also thank Jonathan for his help in translations from the French.) Bob Van Belle has shown us all around the real-world wilderness of mountains and forests. Daniel Maskit is our guide in the universe of cyberspace. I have had informative and impassioned discussions on these and many other topics with all of them. And we are now all involved in finding our way through Kyle's special world.

The theme of this book—and of these acknowledgments—is *connecting*: how one connects to other people and connects to experience within oneself, and how these two types of connections interact; how one constructs and reconstructs an inner emotional world populated with the significant other people of one's life. I learned much about all this in my own personal treatments. I thank the analysts who worked with me, particularly the third and—to date—last; and I thank the field of psychoanalysis for helping me find love and work.

Parallel Processes
of Theory Construction
PERSONAL EXPLORATION
AND A TRAIL MAP

Psychoanalysis offers its patients a way to transform themselves and to gain a second life, while remaining connected to what has gone before. That is its unique human value, differentiating it from other treatment forms. Anyone who has experienced the transforming events of psychoanalytic treatment does not need further evidence as to the efficacy of psychoanalysis—for oneself. My experience was sufficient for me to make a rational decision, in my own terms, that psychoanalysis was of immeasurable value for me.

As a psychoanalytic patient who was also a cognitive psychologist, I found myself engaged in parallel processes of discovery—applied to my own life and to the psychoanalytic process. I began treatment with the assumption that psychoanalysis had a working theory of emotion and mind. I also assumed that analysts, who appeared certain about the procedures to be followed—the basic rule, the couch, the silences, the interpretations—had a clear understanding of how these procedures worked. The discoveries I made about myself paralleled to some extent the discoveries I made about the field. Psychoanalysis—like the individuals it seeks to help—has many strengths, but is burdened with a theory that is not amenable to reality testing and assumptions that are distorted, anachronistic, and incomplete. The problems—some say failure—of

Freud's metapsychology have been widely recognized, as we will see, but the field continues to defend against this knowledge. Like other systems—individuals or families—organized around a weakness or disorder, the field of psychoanalysis has developed a set of defenses that protect against recognition and acknowledgment of its central lack. The participants in the system join in protecting one another from seeing the extent of the disability, and in maintaining structures that are maladaptive and interfere with growth.

It is not surprising that a theory that was developed a century ago, and that has not been subjected to the usual scientific assessment procedures, is no longer seen as applicable today. What is surprising, and distressing, is that the scientific processes of theory evaluation and revision, which would be expected in a scientific field, have not taken place. Psychoanalysis has become isolated from the scientific community as a result; this isolation has been seen as inevitable—in some cases, even desirable—by many writers and practitioners.

The ideas of psychoanalysis continue to engage the imaginations of many people from many perspectives—including those who dismiss or demean psychoanalysis, as well as those who love it. The vitality of the field is indicated by the recurrent discussions in the popular press about its demise. Psychoanalysis remains alive as an intellectual pursuit in disciplines such as comparative literature, political theory, continental philosophy, and rhetoric. However, psychoanalysis as a theory of mind is at best a ghost in scientific psychology or any other scientific enterprise, and the value of psychoanalysis as a treatment is increasingly under attack in the clinical and health service fields. The failure of theory affects all participants in the psychoanalytic enterprise—analyst and patient as well as researcher—and distorts the view of psychoanalysis in our intellectual zeitgeist as well, in ways that have impact on us all.

The purpose of this book is to propose a theory of psychological organization based on current work in scientific psychology, which accounts for the concepts with which psychoanalytic clinicians are concerned. Analysts, writers, and researchers in the field of psychoanalysis recognize the need for a model of psychological organization as a basis for clinical work and for research, but it must be a theory that recognizes the focus on meanings and motives that is intrinsic to this field. They also recognize that the domain of what are referred to as "ego functions" requires a model that accounts for the broad range of adaptive functions as well as the dysfunctional mechanisms of pathology. In proposing such a basic *psychoanalytic psychology*, my intention is not to map the metapsychology as such, but to provide a scientific perspective that accounts for what an analyst and patient do and what they experience, and that can be continuously evaluated and revised in empirical research.

I have written this book with a number of different audiences in mind. One group consists of clinicians and clinical researchers: practicing analysts, psychoanalytic researchers, and workers in other psychotherapy fields who draw upon the ideas of psychoanalysis. Another group would be experimental psychologists, particularly those who are interested in the interaction of language, mind, body, and emotion. A coherent psychoanalytic theory potentially provides understanding of such interactions, and the psychoanalytic situation provides a unique naturalistic context for their study. I also hope that the ideas might be of interest to the larger groups of persons who are not professionals in the areas of psychology or psychoanalysis, but who are intrigued by the ideas of psychoanalysis; and even more generally, to anyone who wonders how it might be possible to have a science that is concerned with the deep subjective meanings that define us as individuals.

Because of the diverse nature of the ideas that I cover, and because I have such a varied audience in mind, I have tried to make each section accessible to readers for whom some of these ideas might be quite new. In the Introduction, I cover general issues concerning the role of theory in psychoanalysis and also look at the factors now dividing the cognitive science and psychoanalytic fields. In Section One, I attempt to find my way through Freud's ideas about the psychical apparatus, including some of the salient areas of inconsistency in these theories, which have drawn psychoanalysis away from the scientific approach. I also review some of the discourse on the metapsychology since Freud's time. Section Two introduces current work in cognitive psychology and related research in areas of developmental psychology, neuropsychology, and emotion, which are potentially relevant to a psychoanalytic model. All of this work contributes to construction of the basic nomological network of the multiple code theory, within which psychoanalytic concepts may be defined in relation to one another and to observable events.

Section Three is the core theoretical contribution of the book. Here I present the integration of these diverse areas of theory and research in the formulation of the multiple code theory, with its central constructs of the emotion schemas and the referential process, and show how these basic concepts play out in pathology and in cure. I also examine the multiple parallel roles of the referential process, including its operation in emotional development, scientific discovery, free association, and the construction and interpretation of dreams. In addition, I show how the nomological network of multiple coding permits development of empirical methods for investigation of private mental and emotional events, which figure in the treatment process, and how the application of these measures, in turn, feeds back to support further theory development. In the final section, I present a few last words about emotional meaning and the narratives that each of us own.

Contents

Introduction

BRIDGING THE GREAT DIVIDE

During the past several decades, there has been considerable controversy within the psychoanalytic field concerning the status of its basic theory of mind—whether the metapsychology is alive or dead, and even whether psychoanalysis needs an explanatory theory at all. In the same period, a paradigm shift has occurred in scientific psychology, termed by some the "cognitive revolution," which has changed the way we conceptualize psychical—including mental and emotional—processes. The two fields have thus far remained distant: Cognitive science tries to develop a theory of language and thought, leaving emotion essentially out of account; psychoanalysis attempts to bring about change in emotion and thought, primarily through the use of language, without a general theory of mind. My thesis in this book is that a convergence of fields is needed, and this will have value for both. The paradigm shift in cognitive psychology has the potential to change the way we understand psychoanalytic concepts and are able to study them; psychoanalysis, in turn, has much to offer cognitive psychology in areas of both content and methods.

In this Introduction, I look first at issues of theory in psychoanalysis and at the question of whether and why psychoanalysis needs a basic theory of psychological organization. I then look at the great divide that now exists between psychoanalysis and cognitive psychology, and introduce the conceptual bridge that is being built—the multiple code theory—which is the subject of this book.

CHANGING VIEWS OF THEORY IN THE
PSYCHOANALYTIC DISCOURSE

Several positions concerning the need for a general theory of the mental apparatus, and concerning the status of the metapsychology, can be distinguished within the psychoanalytic discourse of the past several decades. These will be reviewed in detail in subsequent chapters, but will be outlined briefly here.

First Position

The metapsychology, the theory of the psychical apparatus as formulated by Freud, is viable; it has served as a satisfactory basis for theory development and can continue to be used in this way. Two variants of this position may be identified:

Variant 1. The concepts of the metapsychology are testable by the psychoanalytic method invented by Freud and only by that method, and have been effectively tested and developed by this means (Brenner, 1980).

Variant 2. The psychoanalytic method, as applied in the treatment situation, is not an adequate means for testing psychoanalytic propositions. However, the metapsychology, like any theoretical model, is empirically testable using modern experimental and other observational methods (Erdelyi, 1985; Grünbaum, 1984).

Second Position

The metapsychology has failed to provide a viable foundation for further theory development; a new explanatory theory is needed as a basis for clinical work and research. The physical sciences have moved far beyond the turn-of-the-century principles on which Freud's energy model was based; the application of the theory to psychological or biological systems is no longer considered seriously by scientists. We confront a "crisis of theory" in psychoanalysis today (Thomae & Kaechele, 1987). Several variants of this position can also be identified:

Variant 1. A special or clinical theory of neurosis and treatment can be distinguished from the general or metapsychological one (Rapaport, 1960). The metapsychology should be abandoned and the clinical theory, based on experience, meaning, and intentionality, should be developed as an explanatory model (Klein, 1973, 1976; Gill, 1976).

Variant 2. The clinical theory does not provide an adequate theoretical framework. The empirical interpretation of psychoanalytic propositions must be on a neurophysiological level (Rubinstein, 1965, 1976; Holt, 1967b; Reiser, 1985). The abstract constructs of the psychoanalytic theory must be reduced to concepts that are potentially translatable into neurophysiological terms.

Third Position

No scientific theory is appropriate, and no explanatory theory is required. The domain of psychoanalysis concerns private meanings rather than symptoms and behaviors. Psychoanalysis is properly viewed as a humanistic or hermeneutic rather than scientific discipline, requiring interpretive rather than explanatory theories (Home, 1966; Ricoeur, 1977; Steele, 1979). From a related perspective, Schafer (1976) has advocated abandoning the concepts of the metapsychology and has proposed his "action language" in its place.

The Position of This Book

The approach of this book takes something from these approaches but is also different from these. Psychoanalysis is in need of a basic theory of psychological organization. The metapsychology has failed; a new theoretical model is needed as a basis for research and clinical work. This cannot be a clinical, phenomenological, or neurophysiological model. It must be a model of psychological organization on the same abstract level of explanation as Freud (1900, 1916–1917, 1940) claimed but in more consistent and testable form.

The failure of psychoanalytic theory has a number of negative consequences, some manifest, some concealed. The failure of theory clearly affects the researcher, who requires a coherent framework within which the concepts of the theory can be consistently defined and propositions stated in a form that is amenable to empirical investigation. The interdependence of theory and research will be discussed throughout this book. The failure of theory affects the clinician and patient, and the analytic relationship itself, in ways that are equally pervasive but of which the participants themselves may not be aware. The theoretical vacuum in psychoanalysis also has impact on scientific psychology, and even on the general intellectual zeitgeist. I will briefly examine some of these effects, then move on to the rapprochement with cognitive psychology, through which a general psychoanalytic psychology may be developed.

THE FAILURE OF THEORY
AND THE ANALYTIC RELATIONSHIP

The analytic patient is asked to carry out a set of procedures that violate normal conversational rules (Jaffe & Feldstein, 1970)—to speak while lying down and looking away from the other, to suspend expectation of standard turn-taking procedures, to talk about deeply painful material, and also to talk about trivial and unimportant details, and irrelevant events, without monitoring the flow of ideas. He is instructed to talk without focusing intentionally or explicitly on the particular problems that have brought him to seek help. He is encouraged to talk about his relationship to the analyst rather than focusing only on the "real" relationships that are central to his life. He is expected to express feelings toward the analyst that he would rather hide, and to reveal reactions (perhaps intrusive or insulting) that might be inadmissible in normal social discourse, or even in intimate relationships. He may ask questions that the analyst does not answer; long silences may ensue; or the analyst may offer interpretations that feel unacceptable and false. When the patient denies or questions the analyst's interventions, he may be told that his negative reactions have meanings that are not accessible to him, and even that his denial itself is validation of what he denies; at other times, his agreement with the analyst's ideas may also be accepted as validation of them.

The patient needs to accept the procedures of treatment and the rules of evidence that apply in order to go on with the therapeutic work. In effect, this means that the patient must suspend independent, reasoned decision making, to some degree, in favor of trust. The authority of the analyst—or his authorities—will sometimes be invoked, however implicitly, to support the rules of treatment and the themes that are pursued. This maintains a patient role similar to that in other medical procedures; in psychoanalysis, as in any treatment, some degree of trust and compliance is necessary for treatment to work.

The problem with the standard patient stance is that the goals of psychoanalysis are unique and different from any other treatment form. Optimally, a patient's goal is to *change himself,* not to be changed. There is a conflict, which is intrinsic to the treatment, between the processes of self-directed exploration on the one hand, and the need for compliance and trust on the other. The absence of theory compounds this problem in a crucial way. It is not that the patient must work on the basis of trust in the beginning and will be able to understand the reasons for the procedures and the evidence for the analyst's formulations later. In the current state of the field, the real problem is that he must continue to work on trust throughout the treatment and even afterwards, and that the analyst must do so as well. The treatment is based on acceptance of procedures and rules whose rationale has not been and, at present, cannot be coherently explained, because they are not understood. The emotional climate supporting this treatment approach must be such that systematic evidence is not considered necessary to maintain belief in the effectiveness of the procedures that are used.

The patient's adherence to the rules in the absence of adequate explanation and evidence will depend to some extent on his own characterological issues concerning compliance and authority, as well as on the way the procedures are negotiated in the relationship. Patients may be lost or retained through these characterological issues. Some patients may be lost through unwillingness to suspend independent, rational evaluation of the treatment process, as some may be lost through unwillingness to open painful or threatening feelings. Others may be retained through ability to establish their own evaluation procedures and satisfaction with them. Still others may remain through willingness—even desire—to comply and to be controlled. In all cases, the desire for evidence and explanation will exist alongside of and interact with the gratifications or threats involved in the relationship and the general, defensive intent to avoid emotional distress. The characterological issues are perhaps less likely to be recognized and interpreted when they emerge as compliance rather than opposition; conversely, the reality underlying opposition may be ignored.

The conflict between compliance and autonomy, the need for denial of this conflict, and the consequences of the denial, are likely to exist (or to have existed at some time), not only for the patient whose own life is involved, but also for the analyst, who is responsible for the life of others, and who must believe in what she does. There is enormous diversity in clinical practice today concerning the degree to which the classical procedures are followed or abandoned. Analysts have the choice of following traditional technical principles for which there is no consistent theoretical rationale or empirical support, or turning away from classical techniques, including the "basic rule" of free association, often in favor of more interactive procedures, although there is no more theoretical or empirical support for the new procedures than for the classical ones. It is possible that the basic rule is a rigid and outmoded doctrine, that needs to be partially or completely revised; it is also possible that it is the core of the psychoanalytic process, as many analysts still hold; or all possibilities may be partially correct. At this point, without a body of relevant empirical evidence, we cannot know.

Each analyst comes to terms with the failure of theory and the lack of evidence in her own way, dependent on her own characterological issues. When the analyst recognizes that the evidence for a procedure or an interpretation is inherently problematic, she is better able to distinguish whether a patient's questioning is primarily substantive or dynamically motivated. She can also be alert to where the patient's compliance may be excessive and interpret this. Ultimately, the compliance and trust, which are given in order to go on with the treatment, need eventually to be worked through as much as opposition does—perhaps in part to become enlightened compliance, in part to be diminished. It is not clear how often or how thoroughly that kind of working through is done.

Psychoanalysis is a profoundly deep experience, offering a special and satisfying personal relationship for both participants and a unique experience of collaborative self-exploration. As the treatment proceeds, the patient who has had this experience, and who knows that she been helped, is likely to join the analyst and other analysands in being convinced of the effectiveness of the particular version of psychoanalysis in which they have been engaged. It is difficult to recognize that this conviction occurs without any valid empirical evidence having been produced; that the experiences of insight and transformation, which occur in the context of the relationship and for both participants in the relationship, do not constitute evidence in a scientific sense; that belief in an interpretation may derive from reasons other than its accuracy. Perhaps the most that can be achieved along these lines in the present state of the field is to recognize and acknowledge that scientific evidence is not present and not available; what evidence there is comes from oneself and can be used for oneself *but not beyond.*

All of this is of the deepest importance not only to the patient's life, but also to the health of the field. Regardless of the basis for an individual's beliefs concerning the efficacy of his own treatment, the conviction of an individual cannot be directly communicated to others who have not themselves experienced its effects. If we do not address the need for evidence, the field will continue to be confined to the believers and to be regarded by much of the population as somewhere between religion, cult, or fraud, or, at best, an interesting humanistic or literary enterprise and an important intellectual influence on 20th-century thought.

This point goes beyond the issues of public relations and affects our basic responsibilities as professionals and practitioners. If we recognize the possibility of long-lasting treatments that fail to help and may even harm a patient, then it is the responsibility of the field to provide means for monitoring such effects. It is also the case that in order to meet this responsibility, we need to find ways to provide evidence that is valid in psychoanalytic terms; that is, as evidence of shifts in emotional meaning, not external life changes alone; we need a coherent theory to enable such evidence to be developed.

PSYCHOANALYTIC THEORY
AND THE INTELLECTUAL ZEITGEST

There is another, more general cultural value to the enterprise of psychoanalytic theory development that may be considered here. The problems of the metapsychology reach beyond the psychoanalytic field to affect the thinking of our time. The domains of thought that are central in our current worldview, including evolution, Marxism, and relativity, along with psychoanalysis, each concern a different kind of structural transformation: changes in our understanding of the basic morphology of organisms; changes in our understanding of the economic and political structures of society; changes in our understanding of the fundamental structures of time and space. Psychoanalysis is concerned with changes in an individual's understanding of his own mental and emotional structures, and adds the unique and powerful postulate that humans have the capacity to transform themselves. The culturally interesting psychoanalytic themes of self-directed reconstruction in an interpersonal context are intrinsically related to the psychoanalytic theory of treatment. However, the ideas of psychoanalysis have been considered within literary and philosophical fields largely as independent of their psychological and therapeutic base. I suggest that a coherent psychoanalytic psychology will enrich and broaden the context within which the literary and philosophical ideas of psychoanalysis can be understood.

Psychoanalysis itself has undergone many transformations during its first century; we need to continue the scientific exploration that Freud began as we begin the second. The practitioners of psychoanalysis need to avail themselves of the fundamental psychoanalytic principles concerning self-exploration and self-direction, now applied to the discipline itself. Each individual begins life with a certain inner structure and a certain direction, developed through repeated interactions with others in his early years. Similarly, the theory of psychoanalysis has been set in a certain direction and fixed in a received theoretical structure. Optimally, in the psychoanalytic process, the individual changes direction and rebuilds internal structures, thus working toward an active and autonomous rather than passive role in the direction of his life. Like the patient, and like practitioners in any scientific enterprise, the researchers and practitioners of psychoanalysis need to carry on such a process of free and courageous examination. We can only rebuild if we are able to see the problems that we have inherited, to recognize the parts of the theory that have failed, and to acknowledge the reconstruction that is required.

THE BRIDGE TO COGNITIVE SCIENCE

To develop a coherent psychoanalytic psychology, we need to establish a scientific base that encompasses the concepts of psychoanalysis concerning inner structural change and is also amenable to empirical research. It is true, as the hermeneutic position holds, that psychoanalysis is fundamentally concerned with the meaning of events rather than their external, observable forms. The change that is sought is change in meanings and feelings as these affect symptoms and behaviors, not only in the symptoms themselves. The emphasis on meaning in no way makes it necessary to abdicate the scientific field. The scientific study of inner, subjective events—mental representations and processes—is the day-to-day work of the cognitive science field. What we need to do is essentially what Freud was attempting—to construct a theoretical framework for making inferences from external observations to subjective events, which may be conscious or unconscious. The techniques for such inferences are in place today in the field of cognitive science, in a way that was not available to Freud. In developing a psychological model for psychoanalysis, we can build on this current work. The method of studying nonobservable events through systematic inferences from observable indicators is the approach not only of cognitive science, but also of all modern science, as we shall see.

PSYCHOANALYSIS AS A COGNITIVE SCIENCE

Psychoanalysis has many features of a cognitive psychology and has had these from its beginnings, well before the so-called "cognitive revolution" with its epistemological paradigm shift (Neisser, 1967). Psychoanalysts, like cognitive scientists, infer from language and behavior, and other observable indicators, to inner representations and processes in the context of a general theory of the psychical apparatus; this is the basic nature of the work in both disciplines. It was Freud's insight to recognize the need for a theoretical model of the psychical apparatus as the necessary context for such inference, in the same sense that cognitive psychologists apply mental models today:

> We assume that mental life is the function of an apparatus to which we ascribe the characteristics of being extended in space and of being made up of several portions—which we imagine, that is, as resembling a

telescope or microscope or something of the kind. Notwithstanding some earlier attempts in the same direction, the consistent working-out of a conception such as this is a scientific novelty. (Freud, 1940, p. 145)

Freud clearly saw the general scientific power of this novel approach:

Whereas the psychology of consciousness never went beyond the broken sequences which were obviously dependent on something else, the other view, which held that the psychical is unconscious in itself, enabled psychology to take its place as a natural science like any other. The processes with which it is concerned are in themselves just as unknowable as those dealt with by other sciences, by chemistry or physics, for example, but it is possible to establish the laws which they obey and to follow their mutual relations and interdependences unbroken over long stretches—in short, to arrive at what is described as an "understanding" of the field of natural phenomena in question. (1940, p. 158)

THE VIEW FROM COGNITIVE SCIENCE

The notion of mentation that may not be accessible to awareness, the inference of such mentation from events that we can observe, and the development of abstract theoretical models based on principles borrowed from other scientific domains are all central ideas of cognitive science, which were parts of Freud's contribution. However, psychoanalysis is largely ignored in scientific psychology today. In their introductory survey of the field of cognitive science, Simon and Kaplan say:

If we are to understand cognitive science, we must know what disciplines have contributed to its formation (Norman, 1981). Among these we must certainly count experimental and cognitive psychology, artificial intelligence (within computer science), linguistics, philosophy (especially logic and epistemology), neuroscience, and some others (anthropology, economics, and social psychology will also come in for comment). (1989, p. 3)

It is striking, but not surprising, that psychoanalysis is missing from this list. In the century that has passed since Freud introduced his metapsychology, the fields of academic psychology and psychoanalysis have followed divergent paths. Psychoanalysis has been taught largely in its own institutes and in other clinical programs, insulated from general scientific scrutiny. The metapsychology has not, in the century since its introduction, been subject to the empirical evaluation and theory development that is necessary for a scientific field. Analysts rely primarily on the "psychoanalytic method"—or some version of it—as practiced in their individual clinical work, although the deficiencies of such evidence are by now well understood.

While the general enterprise of making inference from observation to underlying representations or meanings is the work of psychoanalysis, the scientific constraints that are necessary to carry out such inference are not incorporated within the metapsychology or the psychoanalytic method. The type of systematic inference that is applied in cognitive science and in all modern science requires explicit definitions that limit the meaning of the concepts, correspondence rules mapping hypothetical constructs and intervening variables onto observable events, and means of assessing reliability of observation. Each of the indicators that analysts rely on to make inferences about the conscious and unconscious states of other persons (as about one's own unconscious states) must itself be independently validated as having the implications that are assumed. The concepts of the metapsychology do not and cannot begin to meet such constraints. The scientific development of psychoanalytic theory, both as to the structure of the apparatus underlying pathology and the nature of change, has been blocked by its insulation from scientific research.

On the other face of this great divide, modern cognitive science is diminished by failure to acknowledge its psychoanalytic roots. The limitations of the mainstream cognitive field render its results open to question in far-reaching ways. Academic psychology has attempted to study human cognitive processes without recognizing their interaction with emotion and somatic processes, and the power of the interpersonal context on perception and behavior. Yuille (1986), Neisser (1976), and others have pointed to the inability of experimental paradigms to study events as they naturally occur and the distorted views of psychological processes that result. The psychoanalytic situation potentially provides a unique context for systematic study of the interaction of cognition, language, physiology, and emotion as this develops and plays out in an interpersonal setting. The psychoanalytic theory and years of observations in the psychoanalytic setting provide a rich body of knowledge that may contribute to theory development and hypothesis generating. The current isolation of fields does disservice to both. The potential of the psychoanalytic situation as a naturalistic research context remains unrealized, as does the potential of psychoanalytic theory as a component of a general theory of mind.

A SCIENCE OF EMOTIONAL INTELLIGENCE

While we need to place psychoanalysis, which began as a general theory of mind, back in the framework of modern science, we also need to recognize that cognitive science as it exists today is not sufficient to provide the theoretical framework that we seek. In their recent summary of the field, Simon and Kaplan (1989, p. 1) define cognitive science as "the study of intelligence and intelligent systems, with particular reference to intelligent behavior as computation." The field of cognitive science is concerned with two classes of intelligent systems, living organisms and computers:

> Although no really satisfactory intentional definition of intelligence has been proposed, we are ordinarily willing to judge when intelligence is being exhibited by our fellow human beings. We say that people are behaving intelligently when they choose courses of action that are relevant to achieving their goals, when they reply coherently and appropriately to questions that are put to them, when they solve problems of lesser or greater difficulty, or when they create or design something useful or beautiful or novel. We apply a single term, "intelligence," to this diverse set of activities because we expect that a common set of underlying processes is implicated in performing all of them. (Simon & Kaplan, 1989, p. 1)

From the perspective of psychoanalysis, this definition, which applies to computers as to living organisms, leaves much of what is important in human cognition and behavior out of account. To provide an adequate account of human cognitive functions and even of the functions that Simon and Kaplan cite here—the identification of "goals," and of behaviors relevant to these—the theories of cognitive science must be expanded to include the study of *emotional intelligence* and systems that possess this function.

The focus on emotional intelligence leads us to focus on the crucial ways in which living organisms and computers are not alike, as well as on the processes they share. Fodor and Pylyshyn (1988) have recognized that the differences between computer hardware and the flesh-and-blood "hardware" of human systems may have implications for the organism's mental functions: "It is obvious that its [the brain's] behavior, and hence the behavior of an organism, is determined not just by the logical machine that the mind instantiates, but also by the protoplasmic machine in which the logic is realized" (p. 59). They recognize that the protoplasmic hardware (the body), not only the operating software of the logical machine (the mind), determines mental functions and behavior. However, they do not see the hardware of protoplasm as constraining or interacting with the logical machine itself. In contrast, it is the specific goal of a psychoanalytic model to account for the effect of somatic processes on sensory, perceptual, and linguistic representations and processes, and for the converse effects as well.

The development of a model that will account for emotional intelligence becomes even more crucial when we are concerned with goals of which the individual may not be aware. Thus, we may also be able to distinguish situations of failure in the operation of human intelligence from situations where the individual is in fact successful in meeting *unacknowledged* goals. In other words, we may say that people are behaving with emotional intelligence when they choose courses of action that appear irrelevant to acknowledged goals; when they reply in a way that may appear manifestly inappropriate; when they produce something that is not beautiful; and when they repeat actions that appear maladaptive rather than producing novel solutions. In all these cases, there may be emotional intelligence at work but operating in relation to unacknowledged rather than explicit goals. Simon and Kaplan offer their general definition, although "no really satisfactory intentional definition of intelligence has been proposed" (1989, p. 1). We offer our extension of this definition, knowing that the definitions of emotion are at least as unsatisfactory, although great advances in this field have been made.

THE MULTIPLE CODE THEORY: A PSYCHOANALYTIC PSYCHOLOGY

The multiple code theory presented in this book is a psychological theory of emotional intelligence and emotional information processing. The theory concerns the interactions among diverse sensory, motoric, somatic, cognitive, and linguistic representations and processes, their integration in the organization of the self, and their adaptive or maladaptive functioning in relation to the individual's goals. In developing this model, I draw not only on experimental cognitive science and studies of computer simulation of intelligent processes, but also on related fields of infant and child development and emotion theory. The multiple code theory accounts for the ways in which maladaptive functioning may arise, the meaning of this, and the process of change toward more adaptive forms. I suggest that is the type of model that Freud was attempting to develop, although without the scientific tools that are available today.

As we now know, and as we will demonstrate in subsequent chapters, the human information-processing system is a multiple code and parallel process operator of immense complexity. Information is processed, not by a single device, but by multiple devices, processing different types of contents in different formats, operating simultaneously in parallel and in interaction. Adaptive functioning depends on adequate integration of systems. This applies for all information processing, but perhaps even more intensively for what we have characterized as emotional information processing.

Words are the medium of psychoanalytic treatment, but the changes that are sought in treatment involve perception, emotion, somatic systems, and action—how we perceive the world, what we feel, what we do, not only, or not even primarily what we say. The dual code theory that I presented in 1985, based on the work of Paivio (1971, 1986) and others, emphasized the separate processing modes of images and words, and the connections between them. There is now increasing recognition within cognitive science of a wide range of systematic human information processing beyond images and words. These would include representations and processes in which the elements are not discrete, organization is not categorical, processing occurs simultaneously in multiple parallel channels, higher level units are not generated from discrete elements, and explicit processing rules cannot be identified. It is precisely these models of *subsymbolic* processing (also called connectionist or parallel distributed processing [PDP]) that provide a basis for incorporating systematic somatic as well as motoric and perceptual functions into an emotional information-processing theory. The notion of the subsymbolic mode accounts for the type of intuitive and implicit processing, which may occur sometimes without intention and without attention, and which analysts associate with primary process thought; however, subsymbolic processes incorporate a far broader range of functions than the psychoanalytic concept of the primary process, as we shall see.

The subsymbolic system and language are essentially disjoint. The problem that the organism must solve in regulating itself and communicating with others is to connect these disjoint systems. The *referential process* is the operation that connects the multiple representational formats of the nonverbal systems to one another and to words. This is the basic symbolizing function that operates, in different ways, in the construction of new ideas and new forms in sciences and the arts, and in the construction of emotional meanings in an individual's life. In subsequent chapters, the stages of the referential process will be traced in a parallel form in emotional development, scientific discovery, the dreaming process, and the operation of free association in the context of the transference. The treatment is specifically designed to permit activation of dissociated emotion structures in a context where they can be tolerated, examined, and reconstructed. If one can activate the subsymbolic processing in the treatment situation itself, one can bring about symbolizing anew—the recategorizing of experience. The person of the analyst plays a central role in this symbolizing process, as we shall see.

CLAIMS AND CAVEATS

The purpose of this book is to develop the multiple code theory and its application to emotional information processing; to examine its roots in current research in the areas of cognitive science, emotion theory, and research in infant and child development; and then to show the application of this theory to the concepts with which clinicians are concerned. I do not claim that the theory I will propose here is a psychoanalytic model in a canonical sense. I do claim that the model accounts for a psychoanalytic view of pathology and its change in treatment, and provides a basis for empirical research in which we may study the failures as well as successes of the psychoanalytic process. We cannot expect that the constructs of multiple coding will map directly onto psychoanalytic concepts as Freud has formulated these. The role of theory is to account for data, not to account for other theories. In some cases, I will point to the relationship of multiple code constructs to psychoanalytic concepts; I will also point to instances where the new concepts lead to revision of psychoanalytic ideas. The goal here is to develop a theory that will account for the data of observations in the psychoanalytic situation, not to account for Freud's theory. The goal is also to take advantage of insights derived from psychoanalytic observations in formulating a general theory of emotional information processing that more accurately represents human information processing as it actually occurs than the models in use in cognitive science today. Thus, we attempt to place psychoanalysis, which began as a general theory of mind, back in the context of cognitive psychology and to show that an explanatory model may be developed by this means.

I hope to convince the reader to take up anew—or recover—a way of thinking about psychoanalysis as a theory of mind that has been neglected, even discredited, in recent years. The theory that I will present can be—and is being—scientifically investigated. I expect that as new questions are asked and answered, the theory will be continually reexamined and revised.

RECONSTRUCTION OF THE METAPSYCHOLOGY: THE ROOTS

In developing a new theory—a theory of an individual life or a general theory of emotion and mind—we do not start with an empty space but with a structure that is already built and has its own core identity. We need to "reconstruct" our psychoanalytic theory of mind in both senses of that term: to recall and recognize what is essential in the structure that is already present and then to rebuild where that is required.

In this section, I briefly review some of the changes in Freud's models of the psychical apparatus as these evolved over his four decades of work, focusing on his account of the role of language in organizing the psychical apparatus and in bringing about change. This brings us to a discussion of the primary and secondary processes, viewed by many in the field, including Freud himself, as the core of the psychoanalytic theory of mental functions, and by others as an indicator of the incoherence of the theory. I then turn to Freud's psychoanalytic method, which he saw as the necessary and sufficient scientific procedure for testing psychoanalytic propositions in the treatment context. Once the limitations of the psycho-analytic method have been brought to light, I will examine attempts to examine psychoanalytic concepts in experimental settings and in psycho-therapy research, and the values and limitations of these. The last chapter in this section covers some difficult issues concerning the ontological status of psychological concepts that have troubled psychoanalytic theo-rists. I will suggest a pragmatic position that can enable psychoanalytic researchers to put these issues aside so that we may go on with our work.

CHAPTER 1

Freud's Abstract Models of the Psychical Apparatus

According to Freud, in the "Outline" (1940) the scientific problem for psychoanalysis is the same as for the other sciences. Beyond the qualities that we are able to perceive lies the reality, which will always remain "unknowable." In psychoanalysis as in physics, we develop methods of making inference from the knowable (conscious) processes to the unknowable (unconscious) ones. Freud constructed his models of the psychical apparatus as the "intellectual scaffolding" for scientific knowing of this essentially unknowable internal reality. He proposed two major models of psychical structure in the course of his work.

In the "topographic model" (Freud, 1895a, 1900, 1915), the psychical apparatus is divided into "regions," or systems, based on the accessibility of mental contents to consciousness (Cs.); all psychic functions, including the distribution of mental "energy" and the characteristics of thought, are determined by this division. The systemic unconscious (Ucs.) is characterized by the primary process of thought; unconscious mental contents are nonverbal and operate according to the pleasure principle, that is, to gratify wishes, achieve pleasure, and avoid unpleasure by reducing the tension of the instinctual needs. Cathexes subject to the primary process press continuously for discharge; they are highly mobile, that is, readily displaced and also readily condensed. Mentation in the preconscious system (Pcs.) functions according to the secondary process. Thus, its energy can be bound and discharge delayed in accordance with the reality principle, and its contents are conscious, or can readily become so.

17

Conflict occurs between the forces of the two systems: the unconscious one that presses toward discharge and the conscious one that operates to delay this. Repressed excitatory processes from the libidinal instincts underlie every neurotic symptom. In development, verbalization operates to bind energy and delay discharge. In treatment, verbalization has the power to reverse the process of repression and lead to reduction of symptoms. In order for a memory trace of the system Ucs. to become preconscious, it must increase its cathexis by joining with a corresponding word trace. An interpretation or construction, which the analyst may offer to the patient, represents an attempt to fill up the breaks in what is or can be made conscious; "psychotherapy can pursue no other course than to bring the Ucs. under the domination of the Pcs." (Freud, 1900, p. 617).

Freud (1923) developed the structural theory in recognition of contradictions within the topographic model and its failure to account adequately for clinical observations. In the structural theory, the psychical apparatus is divided into agencies, determined by their relationship to internal instinctual forces and external reality, rather than into systems determined by qualities of mind (Freud, 1923). The structural theory emphasizes aggressive as well as sexual drives or instincts and focuses on the operation of the unconscious defenses and the effect of conflict among the agencies of mind. The two major agencies of the psychical apparatus, id and ego, reflect the interplay between demands of the inner world of the instinctual drives and the outer world of the environment to which the individual must adapt. The superego, a division within the ego, separates those functions that involve ideal aspirations or moral prohibitions from other ego functions.

The id contains the organic instincts or drives, the erotic and aggressive forces that represent the somatic demands upon mental life and that constitute the source of mental energy for the psychical apparatus. The operations of the id are characterized by the primary process of thought and follow the dictates of the pleasure principle, pressing toward reduction of the tension of the instinctual needs. Cathexes are mobile and push for immediate and rapid discharge; mental contents are readily displaced and condensed and are not subject to logical constraints.

The ego mediates the demands of the id, superego, and external reality. It has the task of self-preservation and uses signals of anxiety—anticipation of intense unpleasure—as warnings of dangers to its integrity. Anxiety motivates the conflict between id and ego that occurs in the course of every child's development and serves as the motive for repression and the other defenses.

The capacity to bind and neutralize mental energy increases as the child matures. The ego also has the capacity to suspend the operations of any of its functions and to regress, in a temporary and controlled manner, to a primitive level. Kris (1936, p. 290) refers to "regression in the service of the ego."

The acquisition of language is a major aspect of ego development, inherent in or even equivalent to the development of the capacity for thought, and associated with the binding of instinctual energy and the secondary process. Secondary process cathexes are bound by being attached to word representations; thus, concepts of logic and causality become possible. This aids in the achievement of realistic gratification and becomes an important element in the process of adaptation.

The structural model moves away from the topographic view of the qualities of mind as determining the modes and forms of thought, and thus eliminates the necessary correspondence of the unconscious with the primary process and nonverbal modes. From the point of view of the organization of the psychical apparatus, this is a crucial change. Treatment emphasizes analysis of the defenses that interfere with recovery of unconscious material rather than the recovery of memories per se. The goal of treatment is viewed as strengthening the patient's weakened ego and increasing its dominion, so that "where id was, there ego shall be" (Freud, 1933, p. 80). The structural model has seminal significance in marking the beginning of ego psychology; Arlow (1975) has referred to this as a paradigm shift.

RETURN OF THE SYSTEMIC UNCONSCIOUS: REGRESSION OR RECONCILIATION

In his 1940 summary statement, however, Freud appears to disregard the basic distinctions that underlie the introduction of the structural theory:

> The inside of the ego, which comprises above all the intellective processes, has the quality of being preconscious. This is characteristic of the ego and belongs to it alone. . . .
> The sole quality that rules in the id is that of being unconscious. Id and unconscious are as intimately united as ego and preconscious; indeed, the former connection is even more exclusive. (pp. 162–163)

Here he writes about the distinction between the mental qualities as entirely parallel with the division between id and ego. The assertion of a necessary correspondence between the qualities of the topographic model and the agencies of the structural theory retains the systemic aspects of the mental qualities by default. If the two systemic organizations entirely coincide, then both must be equivalent in relating to the basic characteristics of energy and its role in language and thought.

The merging of models that is represented in Freud's final position is also reflected in his description of the treatment process and the analyst's role:

> We serve the patient in various functions, as an authority and a substitute for his parents, as a teacher and educator; and we have done the best for him if, as analysts, we raise the mental processes in his ego to a normal level, transform what has become unconscious and repressed into preconscious material and thus return it once more to the possession of his ego. (1940, p. 181)

Many analysts today appear to assume this reconciliation of models and to work comfortably with it: Thus, the concept of the id is essentially tied to the unconscious and nonverbal domains; the ego is seen as preconscious or conscious and verbal. However, Arlow and Brenner (1964) have argued that the two theories are in fact incompatible, even contradictory in important respects:

> We maintain that it is actually disadvantageous to use the terms of the two theories interchangeably and to speak of the id, the ego and the superego in one breath and of the unconscious, the preconscious and the conscious in the next, a practice which . . . is so widespread among analysts as to be nearly universal. (p. 3)

According to these authors, Freud's position expressed in the "Outline" represents a step backward in his thought:

> It reverts to the *systemic* meaning of the term preconscious which was characteristic of the topographic theory. It also reverts to the topographic theory's idea that the primary and secondary processes are qualitatively distinct from each other, and that each characterizes the operations of a separate division of the mental apparatus. (p. 111, emphasis in original)

Arlow and Brenner suggest that "what Freud himself would have done with this page of the 'Outline' had he lived, no one can be sure."[1]

---

[1]While Freud's work on the "Outline" was interrupted by his surgery in September 1938, he did have a year or more to return to this work. According to Strachey, while the book "must be described as unfinished . . . , it is difficult to regard it as incomplete . . . for the programme laid down by the author in his preface seems already to be reasonably well carried out" (in Freud, 1940, p. 142).

THE ENERGY THEORY AND THE NIRVANA PRINCIPLE

While the first topographic model and the structural model (second topography) differ in many ways, both are theories of the distribution of mental energy in the psychical apparatus and share the assumptions of that system. Both assume that mental energies derive from somatic sources, that is, from the instincts or drives; that the psychical apparatus is inactive until stimulated; that the building up of instinctual energy produces unpleasure; and that mental activity is motivated toward reducing this instinctual energy by discharging or binding it. Both assume that language is associated with binding of energy, and that nonverbal functions are associated with the more primitive component of the apparatus: in the topographic model with the unconscious; in the structural model with the id; in both cases with the primary process of thought.

In his final summary statement, Freud himself recognized some of the inconsistencies and ambiguities inherent in his basic motivational system and the link between pleasure and annihilation that is implied.

> The consideration that the pleasure principle demands a reduction, at bottom the extinction, perhaps, of the tensions of instinctual needs (that is, *Nirvana*) leads to the still unassessed relations between the pleasure principle and the two primal forces, Eros and the death instinct. (1940, p. 198, emphasis in original)

Freud assumed that these problems could potentially be solved without altering the basic premises of the theory; thus, for example, he proposed that it may not be energy levels per se but the rhythmic patterns of energy flow that motivate psychical activity. While he never repudiated the energy theory, he also recognized its problems:

> We assume, as other natural sciences have led us to expect, that in mental life some kind of energy is at work; but we have nothing to go upon which enable us to come nearer to a knowledge of it by analogies with other forms of energy. We seem to recognize that nervous or psychical energy occurs in two forms, one freely mobile and another, by comparison, bound; we speak of cathexes and hypercathexes of psychical material, and even venture to suppose that a hypercathexis brings about a kind of synthesis of different processes—a synthesis in the course of which free energy is transformed into bound energy. Further than this we have not advanced. (pp. 163–164)

The basic premises of the energy theory, as a physical model applied to living systems, have been widely questioned in biological and psychobiological research. The energy model is fundamentally a theory of energy flow in a closed system, which the human organism clearly is not (von Bertalanffy, 1950). Living organisms are characterized by varying inputs of stimulation and outputs of activity, not by reverberation of a fixed quantity of energy. As Holt (1965) points out: "With the advent of open-system conceptions, the main arguments for the predominance of the economic point of view (the quantitative treatment of energies) collapse" (p. 134).

A large body of evidence disconfirming the energy model in its own terms, as applied to biological systems, has been reviewed by Holt (1989) and Eagle (1984). There is considerable evidence that organisms are constantly active, rather than becoming active only in response to external stimuli or internal needs. Intrinsic positive motives—to explore, to achieve, to be close to others—as well as negative motivations aimed at reduction of pain and tension have been established. Animals and man are motivated by curiosity; they are motivated to be close to certain members of their own species and even to seek stimulation rather than being motivated, fundamentally, to reduce tension derived from sexual and aggressive drives or tissue needs. Pleasure, distinct from tension reduction, has been shown to be an independent motivator; particular brain locations have been identified whose stimulation is rewarding (Olds, 1958).

The deeper problem with the energy theory is not that it has been disconfirmed as a theory about the operation of physical or biological systems. The deeper problems are, first, that the level of explanation that is intended by the energy model is ambiguous between the physiological and psychological level; and second, that the propositions of the theory have not been systematically evaluated on either level. If energy is defined as some actually measurable somatic quantity, then the constructs need to be defined and the propositions tested in those terms. If the metapsychology is viewed as an abstract psychological theory concerning the distribution of *psychical* energy, then we need systematic definitions of the construct of energy, the principle of constancy, the concepts of drive, need, instinct, within the psychological domain, and systematic correspondence rules that enable inference from observable data to mental constructs and changes in them. Without such definitions, every study disconfirming or confirming the notion of need reduction as a basis for motivation in biological systems can be questioned as to whether the notions of need, or tension, or drive, and the assessment of their reduction, as evaluated by the empirical studies, are equivalent to the sense in which these concepts are defined in the psychoanalytic model.

The shortcomings of the energy theory as a model of the psychical apparatus are clear. The energy model has never been systematically formulated as a coherent hypothesis concerning the functions of a psychological—not a physiological—system. The theoretical status of concepts such as instinct, libido, cathexis, and hypercathexis may in principle be equivalent to the theoretical concepts of the physical sciences such as force, mass, and attraction, as Freud claimed. However, the metapsychological concepts have never even approached the level of systematization, coherence of definition, and correspondence to observable measures that is characteristic of the concepts of the physical sciences such as force, mass, and attraction, and there is no longer any expectation that they can be. In the light of the incoherence of the metapsychology, as well as the apparent disconfirmation of energic principles, Klein (1976), Holt (1967b, 1976a), Gill (1976), and others advocated rejection of the concepts of energy and instinct, and other central concepts of the metapsychology, as we shall see in more detail throughout Section One.

THE CLUE THAT THE WITCH REVEALS: FREUD'S DUALITY OF THOUGHT

In his final summary formulation, Freud (1940) recognized the problems left unsolved in his two topographies, the problems of the energy theory, the implications of the shift from constancy to "Nirvana," and the unresolved relationship between the qualities and agencies of mind. Through all these inconsistencies and problems, one piece of solid ground, one enduring "fact" remains:

> Behind all these uncertainties, however, there lies one new fact, whose discovery we owe to psychoanalytic research. We have found that processes in the unconscious or in the id obey different laws from those in the preconscious ego. We name these laws in their totality the *primary process*, in contrast to the *secondary process* which governs the course of events in the preconscious, in the ego. In the end, therefore, the study of psychical qualities has after all proved not unfruitful. (p. 164, emphasis in original)

The solid ground that he is left with, that he holds to most firmly at the end, the result that justifies his work, is the discovery of two different modes of thought, the primary and secondary processes. These are connected most directly to the qualities rather than the agencies of mind; the mental qualities regain their central systemic role "in the end."

Freud (1937a) claims the same basic piece of solid ground when addressing the central question of how psychoanalysis can tame an instinct:

That is to say, the instinct is brought completely into the harmony of the ego, becomes accessible to all the influences of the other trends in the ego, and no longer seeks to go its independent way to satisfaction. If we are asked by what methods and means this result is achieved, it is not easy to find an answer. We can only say "So muss denn doch die Hexe dran." ["We must call the Witch to our help after all!" (Goethe, *Faust*, Part I.)]–the Witch Metapsychology. Without metapsychological speculation and theorizing–I had almost said "phantasying"–we shall not get another step forward. Unfortunately, here as elsewhere, what our Witch reveals is neither very clear nor very detailed. We have only a single clue to start from–though it is a clue of the highest value– namely, the antithesis between the primary and secondary processes. (p. 225)

Here, as elsewhere, he comes round again to the discovery that he saw as his first and major one: "the most valuable of all the discoveries it has been my good fortune to make" (Freud, 1932, from the preface to the third [revised] English edition of "The Interpretation of Dreams").

The duality of the primary and secondary processes of thought has been considered by many psychoanalytic scholars as Freud's most original and fundamental idea, and as central to a psychoanalytic account of the mental apparatus (Jones, 1953; McLaughlin, 1978). A psychological theory that fails to account for this fundamental dichotomy cannot be applicable to psychoanalytic concepts; the major developmental theories of Piaget and Bruner have failed in this respect, as Noy (1979) has pointed out:

Almost all of the contemporary theories of cognitive development approach cognition as a one-track system, and its development as a linear process proceeding along a single developmental line. The fact is that although psychoanalysis has repeatedly attempted to assimilate part or several of these theories . . . it has never been able to adopt any of them *in toto*. The dual concept of primary and secondary processes is so deeply rooted in psychoanalytic conceptualization, that any developmental theory which does not view cognition as being composed of two systems, forms, modes, levels–or, at least, as a continuum stretched between two organizal centers–can never be integrated into psychoanalytic metapsychology. (p. 170)

While the distinction between the primary and secondary processes is central to a psychoanalytic model, the theoretical ground remains far from solid here. Freud's formulation of the primary and secondary processes was rooted in energic concepts (1895a, 1900) and thus retains all the difficulties of this theoretical base. The primary process, as characterized by shifting or unbound cathexis, provides the mental basis for immediate drive discharge in the service of the pleasure principle.

The binding and neutralizing of energy enable the delayed discharge and reality focus of the secondary process. On a formal or structural rather than dynamic or economic level, Freud described the primary process as operating by mechanisms such as condensation, displacement, imagery and symbolism, while the secondary process operates by the mechanisms of verbal, logical thought.

In the topographic model, the primary process is associated with the system Ucs. and the secondary process with the Pcs.–Cs. In the structural theory, the primary process was seen as the operating mode of the id and the secondary process as the mode of the ego. The structural theory defines the concepts of primary and secondary processes in terms of varying degrees of mobility of cathexis, without linkage to the qualities of mind. Here, fantasies, daydreams, and dreams are all described in terms of selective and variable ego and superego regression, and mutual interaction among forces of the id, ego, and superego. In contrast to the topographic model, fantasy activity is viewed as continuous throughout mental life, intruding into conscious experience as well as underlying dreams (Arlow, 1969). While the regulation of cathectic discharge is seen as an ego function, the correspondence is confounded, in that patterns of rapid discharge of cathexes may presumably mark the operation of id, ego, and superego (Arlow & Brenner, 1964). Freud's (1940) attempt at reconciliation leaves the organization of the system further confounded; it is not surprising that many theorists, including Arlow and Brenner (1964), question the sense in which Freud may have intended his final comments.

Gill (1967) has pointed to an "ambiguity" in which the primary process is characterized on the one hand as the original mode of mental functioning guided by the pleasure principle and on the other as "motivated" by defense, resulting from the impact of repression on verbal thought. This relates to the distinction noted by Fenichel (1945) between "archaic symbolism as a part of prelogical thinking" and the traditional psychoanalytic notion of symbolism as a "distortion by means of representing a repressed idea through a conscious symbol" (p. 48).

Loewald (1978) has argued that the ambiguity noted by Gill may be resolved by introducing the concept of regression: "The primary process is 'primary' because it is the first and more primitive. Defense—repression—leads to a regression to this old mode of mental functioning; it does not *create* primary process" (p. 243, emphasis in original). Primary process mentation is "unitary, nondifferentiating, nondiscriminating," conveying a "uniform density" (p. 258). Differentiation of this "unitary, global, unstructured oneness" occurs through linking of thing-presentation and corresponding word-presentation, which he terms "an act of *con-scire*" (p. 261). The representational field is undifferentiated prior to the linking of

thing and word presentations: "Thinking in terms of elements or components of an experience or act already bespeaks secondary process thinking" (p. 258).

The notion of regression in the service of the ego (Kris, 1936)
presupposes a similar view of nonverbal representation, which is also
rooted in—or trapped within—the economic concepts of the metapsychology. Thus, nonverbal, primary process mentation entails a "primi-
tivization of ego functions" based on "mobile energy discharge" (p.
312). In some cases, the ego is able to regulate the regression and make
use of it rather than being overwhelmed by it. Thus, imagery may
account for extraordinary achievements in mathematics and science as
well as in art. However, the advanced forms of thought still somehow
remain within the purview of the inherently regressive primary process,
as contrasted with the forms of verbal reasoning associated with secondary process thought.

The ambiguities inherent in the psychoanalytic model emerge in
all these formulations. While clearly acknowledging the role of imagery
in mental life, Kris and Loewald also retain the metapsychological view
concerning the regressed and primitive nature of nonverbal thought.
On a general level, we may question whether advanced and creative
achievements in science and art may be appropriately characterized as
regression. On a very specific level, in applying Loewald's formulation,
we may ask how a single "thing-representation" may be initially separated out of the global undifferentiated "oneness" to be linked to a
word-presentation if the linking to words is itself the means by which
the differentiation is postulated to occur. In the simplest formulation
of this problem, if word-presentations are to be linked to corresponding
thing-presentations, then the thing-presentations must somehow first be
formed. In other words, there must be a process that moves the mental
organization from global oneness to a field in which there are discrete
things, *prior* to the application of the word, in order for the word to
have an entity to which to apply. The point that Loewald and many
others overlook is that the initial differentiation of the representational
field must depend on a nonlinguistic or prelinguistic organizational
process. Once distinctions and categories are developed on a nonverbal
level, language may then provide further organization of these forms.

The explanation of phenomena such as unconscious fantasies and
daydreams has been a problem for the metapsychology throughout its
history. As early as 1915, Freud raised a basic question with respect to
the status and role of unconscious fantasies:

> Among the derivatives of the *Ucs* instinctual impulses . . . there are some
> which unite in themselves characters of an opposite kind. On the one

hand, they are highly organized, free from self-contradiction, have made use of every acquisition of the system *Cs.* and would hardly be distinguished in our judgement from the formations of that system. On the other hand, they are unconscious and are incapable of becoming conscious. Thus *qualitatively* they belong to the system *Pcs.*, but *factually* to the *Ucs.* (pp. 190–191, emphasis in original)

As Arlow (1969) points out, consideration of such inconsistencies initially contributed to Freud's questioning of accessibility to consciousness as a basis for differentiation of psychic systems and thus represented a foreshadowing of the structural hypothesis. However, the ambiguities concerning the status of organized fantasies and the difficulty of conceptualizing unconscious fantasies, dreams, and other phenomena of primary process mentation remains within the structural model as well.

According to Beres (1962), fantasies are organized mental representations "derived from instinctual drives and cathected by the energies of these drives" (p. 318). They may be conscious or unconscious, depending on the strength of the countercathexes supplied by the ego defenses. However, as he points out:

Unanswered questions remain. It is easy to postulate unconscious mental processes which are recognized by their derivatives. On the other hand, it is difficult to conceptualize unconscious mental content. Does the unconscious fantasy exist in verbal form? Or as imagery? We do not know. However as stated earlier, I consider all imagery as conscious and that it is necessary to assume some other state for unconscious mental content. Similarly, I would say that the unconscious fantasy is without verbal content and that verbalization is part of the process of making the fantasy conscious, though not an essential one. (p. 322)

In the terms of the metapsychology, the representation of mental contents in organized form, reflecting delay of discharge, is the province of secondary process thought. It is contradictory to claim that unconscious fantasy may be represented in such form. Arlow (1969), consistent with Freud (1915), has argued that in addition to being consistent and organized, unconscious fantasies may also include elements with fixed verbal concepts. In examining these and related problems, Arlow says:

Thus it would appear that unconscious fantasies embarrass our methodology. The evidence is clear that such fantasies exist but precisely where is one to place them in our conceptual frame of reference? What is their nature and in what form do they exist? (1969, p. 4)

ALTERNATE VIEWS OF THE PRIMARY
AND SECONDARY PROCESSES

Several writers have attempted to retain the concepts of the primary and secondary processes, while separating these concepts from the inconsistencies of the metapsychology and defining them in new ways. Noy (1969, 1973) has claimed that the primary process should not be conceptualized as representing a lower developmental level than the secondary process: "Both groups of processes are to be regarded as equally developed, structured, refined, and efficient" (Noy, 1979, p. 172). According to Noy, the primary and secondary processes differ only in their organizational modes, reflecting the differences in the functions carried out by each process. The secondary process handles perception, action, and communication with the external world, and is characterized as reality oriented; the primary process handles functions related to the regulation and integration of the self, and is characterized as self-centered. Noy also argues that the characterization of the primary and secondary processes as separate but equally well-developed organizational modes is supported by recent research on cerebral lateralization.

McLaughlin (1978), like Noy, rejects the view of the primary process as primitive, archaic, and irrational. According to McLaughlin, the primary process undergoes "a developmental progression that is pre-existent to, then coexistent and thereafter commingled with secondary process and its development" (p. 238). The development of both modes of thought continue throughout life, reflected in a wide range of rich and complex nonverbal functions. McLaughlin has suggested that primary process thought is largely localized in the recessive hemisphere, usually the right hemisphere for right-handed adults, and he associates the primary process with the creative, nonverbal functions of music and art, and skilled motor behavior of all types, as in sports and the dance. He has also suggested an association of peripheral vision with primary process and central vision with secondary process. He argues that research on subliminal perception by Shevrin (1974) and Kepecs and Wolman (1972), showing a relationship between perception outside of awareness and the primary process mode, provides some evidence for this hypothesis. A related position, assigning the primary and secondary processes to the right and left hemispheres, is also taken by Hoppe (1977).

In an attempt to systematize the concept of the primary process and render it coherent, Holt (1967b) has rejected the energic formulation and has characterized the primary process in terms of the goal of wish fulfillment and the formal properties of thought. The primary process does not involve an undifferentiated form of cognition; instead, it should be understood "as a special system of processing information," "a type or system of thinking, with autistic or magical as well as wishful properties" (p. 267). The organization of such thought presupposes the operation of stable structures and "must be the product of a considerable development":

> When Freud proposed the radical conception that dreams, neurotic and psychotic symptoms, and other such primitive and seemingly incomprehensible forms of thought and behavior could be interpreted, he pitted his new theory of the primary process against the prevailing view that such phenomena were essentially random, stochastic, and intrinsically meaningless. Freud's view was not only that determinism must be assumed to apply to all corners of psychology, but that the functioning of the unconscious or the id was something like an ancient, secret language. Its grammar was strange and perverse, yet it did follow rules that he could formulate, and with the aid of a symbolic dictionary to its vocabulary he taught us to translate so that sense could be made out of what others had considered inherently senseless. (pp. 278–279)

Holt had developed a system for empirical examination of the motivational and structural aspects of the primary process, using Rorschach responses as manifestations of this mode of thought. The psychoanalytic theory postulates a relationship between contents associated with repressed wishes and structural characteristics of primary process thought, such as condensation and displacement. In Holt's work, an association between wishful contents and structural properties was confirmed in a large sample of Rorschach responses. In further examination of these findings, however, using the techniques of factor analysis, the category of wishful contents was found to include not only the more primitive, raw, and blatant forms of unconscious wishes, which one would ordinarily expect to be repressed, but also more socialized forms, which might be better categorized in secondary process terms. Gill (1967) also noted that aspects of displacement and condensation may occur with secondary process as well as primary process contents.

The association postulated by psychoanalytic theory between wishes and particular formal features of thought has not been supported in Holt's results. In his research, he has found forms of thought that do not fall into the categories of either the primary or secondary processes, that is, where primitive wishful contents do not coincide with the structural characteristics of primary process thought, and mixed forms have also been found. As Holt suggests, a new typology appears to be required. As he also points out, the problem is not resolved by considering the dimension of the primary versus secondary processes as a continuum rather than a dichotomy; the problems remain of systematically defining the continuum (or continua) and the poles.

Following his research efforts, Holt (1976b) was finally drawn to a negative conclusion concerning the viability of the construct of primary process mentation:

> In its present state, the theory of the primary process is in sad disarray. Its empirical referents are only generally specified, too imprecisely to give firm guidance to concrete attempts at measurement. Taken either as a low-level clinical theory, or in its higher-level metapsychological guise, it is fundamentally lacking. (p. 301)

Thus, we are left with a fundamental and distressing problem. On the one hand, the concepts of the primary and secondary processes are widely seen as central to the psychoanalytic model; on the other hand, these concepts are also seen as ambiguous and incoherent—"deeply flawed," "fundamentally lacking," "in sad disarray."

CHAPTER 2

The Metapsychology, the Clinical Theory, and the Psychoanalytic Method

Several decades ago, Rapaport (1960), Holt (1962), Klein (1976), and others were engaged in an attempt to systematize the metapsychology, to master the Freudian text so that its "elusive meaning would then become clear" (Holt, 1962, p. 72), and to formulate coherent propositions that could be tested empirically, in effect, taking seriously Freud's scientific claims. The failure of this attempt has been well documented elsewhere (Gill, 1976; Eagle, 1984; Holt, 1985; Thomae & Kaechele, 1987). The general conclusion that was reached, after years of such effort, was that neither the structural organization nor the dynamic principles of the metapsychology survived this attempt at scientific cure: "The operation was successful though the patient died" (Holt, 1985, p. 342).

On the basis of these investigations, Rapaport (1960) argued in favor of separating a clinical psychoanalytic theory of neurosis and treatment from a general or metapsychological one. According to Klein (1970, 1973, 1976) and Gill (1976), the abstract explanatory level of the metapsychology should be abandoned, and the clinical theory, focused on questions of meaning and intent, should be developed into a self-sufficient and systematic framework. Gill (1976) argued that psychoanalysis should be categorized not as a natural science, but as having a different framework, as a "science of meaning." However, Holt held that the clinical theory and the metapsychology were "much more closely intertwined than

Rapaport had suggested, and that there was no simple or obvious way to produce a set of excerpts from Freud's writings that would give the clinical theory definitive exposition" (1985, p. 327).

Among practicing analysts today, the most common position seems to be one of ambivalence: a general view of the metapsychology as irrelevant to their work, coupled with implicit acceptance of concepts that have meaning only in that theoretical context. As Holt (1985) has pointed out:

> At present, I think it is fair to say that metapsychology is virtually dead. Fewer voices defend it explicitly, and more join the chorus of those who find it wanting. To be sure, most practicing analysts have not paid much attention to the demise, never having put much stock in "that abstract stuff" anyway. What they do not realize is that they are far more committed to it than they know. For everyday terms like ego, id, instinct, and psychodynamics are integral parts of metapsychology rather than the clinical theory. They share with more outlandish terms like anti-cathexis and defusion the fatal property of not referring to anything even indirectly observable and of contributing nothing to discourse beyond the nonrational gratification many of us get from speaking a recognizably psychoanalytic jargon. . . .
>
> I recognize the harshness of the above indictment, but do not make it lightly or with any pleasure. It is anything but a comforting reflection to realize that most of one's career has been devoted to as worthless a theory as metapsychology proved to be. (pp. 326–327)

Psychoanalytic theory today is in a period of explosive and diverse reformulation. Virtually all of the classical positions, including the universality of the Oedipus complex and the fundamental drive–conflict model, are being questioned and are undergoing change. We are no longer committed to Freud's clinical theories concerning the sources and nature of conflict and of pathology for females or for males. A new psychoanalytic perspective on the psychology of women is emerging that moves away from the classic conception of penis envy and postulates distinct female developmental lines. As Wallerstein has noted, we have seen a transition of psychoanalysis from a unified theoretical structure "into the present-day worldwide theoretical diversity in which we have existing now side by side the American ego psychological (and by now post-ego psychological) school, the Kleinian, the Bionian, the (British) object-relational sometimes narrowed down to the Winnicottian, the Lacanian . . . Kohut's self-psychology," and many other alternative theoretical perspectives (1988, p. 7). Many of the new theoretical approaches that have been developed, including object relations and self psychological perspectives, share an increased concern with earlier (preoedipal) sources of psychopathology; a range of subclassifications may be identified within each of these approaches. Brenner, who has been a major proponent and interpreter of the structural theory (Arlow & Brenner, 1964), has recently disavowed the concepts of the agencies of mind, while nevertheless retaining the energic framework and the concepts of drives in conflict (Brenner, 1992).

With all this manifest change and diversity, however, the clinical theories retain their underlying metapsychological roots in some explicit and some implicit ways. It is clear that the variants of the classical position, including the ego psychology and Brenner's purportedly radical reformulation, retain the basic metapsychological concepts of libidinal and aggressive drives. Rather than moving away from energic concepts, Brenner has in fact extended them, so that conflicts resulting from drive derivatives and the quest for instinctual gratification are now seen as ubiquitous in all the experiences and actions of life; in these terms, every perception, thought, word, and action is a compromise formation.

Object relations theories differ explicitly as to whether Freud's dual drive theory is retained and combined with the object relations approach, as in the work of Klein (1948), Mahler (1968), Mahler, Pine, and Bergman (1975), or Jacobson (1964), or object relations are seen to replace drives as the motivational system for human behavior, as proposed by Fairbairn (1954) and Sullivan (1953). A wide range of intermediate positions on this issue may also be distinguished. Thus, for example, Winnicott (1971) and Sandler (1987) retain the drive theory but see the infant–mother relationship as crucial in determining the development of drives. Kernberg also retains Freud's dual drive theory but considers "drives as supraordinate motivational systems, with affects as their constituent components" (1995, p. 451). Object relations theorists also differ as to the development of aggression and its role, as well as the degree to which unconscious fantasies versus reality experience contribute to determining the internalized object relational world.

The influence of energic concepts remains, even among theorists who have explicitly rejected them. For example, in Fairbairn's fundamental concept of ego splitting, an internalized bad object is split into an "exciting object" and a "rejecting object," and these are repressed by the central ego. Parts of the ego structure, which remain attached to these objects, are also repressed; these include a libidinal ego attached to the exciting object and an antilibidinal ego attached to the rejecting object. The change that is introduced by Fairbairn is not so much in the fundamental elements and relationships of the metapsychology as in the particular organization and modes of operation of these components. Thus, Fairbairn's concept of libido is now defined as a function of the ego and, therefore, as fundamentally object seeking and reality oriented.

The erotogenic zones are viewed not as the origin of libidinal energy but as channels for expression of libidinal needs related to objects.

The self psychology of Kohut also moves away from the traditional Freudian position: "From the beginning the drive experience is subordinated to the child's experience of the relation between the self and self-objects" (1977, p. 80). Nevertheless, in Kohut's terms, the formation of internal structures occurs through withdrawal of "narcissistic cathexis" from self-object images. Here again, cathexis and its withdrawal are energic concepts, although with different objects and different contents than in the classical drive models.

It seems apparent that writers such as Kohut and Fairbairn assign different meanings to the concepts of libido and cathexis, and even to the concept of drive itself, from those assigned by the metapsychology and also from one another. Unfortunately, it is impossible to know to what extent the concepts differ, since these concepts have never been clearly defined in Freud's system or in any other. With the failure of the energy model, libido and cathexis, and related notions remain concepts in search of a definition, without consistent meaning in theoretical or empirical terms. The clinicians and theorists who have offered new and important insights, still stated in the old energic terms, have not provided such a new, general theory, nor, apparently, have they seen the need for one.

It is not possible to avoid this problem by keeping words such as drive, drive derivative, libido, and cathexis out of our professional vocabularies; the problem is too pervasive for that, as Holt has pointed out. The central concepts of the psychoanalytic theory; the notion of unconscious mentation; the processes of repression, defense, conflict, structural change; the primary and secondary processes of thought; and the concept of mental dynamics itself are all defined—explicitly or implicitly—within the energic framework of the metapsychology, or else undefined and without meaning. In the absence of an alternative explanatory context, the structures of the energy theory will inevitably be drawn in to provide some coherent system of meaning for the central notions upon which clinicians must rely.

Wallerstein (1988) has argued that the clinical theory and clinical practice constitute the shared common ground of psychoanalysis, holding the profession together in the face of the growing diversity and pluralism: "My thesis is that what unites us is our shared focus on the clinical interactions in our consulting rooms, the phenomena encompassed by the 'present unconscious' (the Sandlers) or the 'clinical theory' (George Klein)" (p. 19). However, to the extent that the concepts of the clinical theory are defined differently in the various diverse theoretical formulations or are not systematically defined, such unity as may appear is necessarily limited or spurious. A general theoretical framework is required to compare the different approaches and to define the areas of convergence or disagreement among them in a systematic way.

THE PSYCHOANALYTIC METHOD

Freud saw the psychoanalytic method that he developed as necessary and sufficient for the scientific verification of psychoanalytic propositions and for the development of the metapsychology, and as essentially equivalent to the physicist's use of experimentation to test propositions concerning the physical world. He continued to voice unqualified confidence in the scientific power of his method to the end of his career:

> We make our observations through the medium of the . . . perceptual apparatus, precisely with the help of the breaks in the sequence of "psychical" events: we fill in what is omitted by making plausible inferences and translating it into conscious material. In this way we construct, as it were, a sequence of conscious events complementary to the unconscious psychical processes. The relative certainty of our psychical science is based on the binding force of these inferences. Anyone who enters deeply into our work will find that our technique holds its ground against any criticism. (1940, p. 159)

Whereas consciousness constitutes the starting point for the investigation of the psychical apparatus, these conscious processes do not form unbroken sequences; there are gaps in them. We assume that there are ongoing physical or somatic processes that are concomitant with the conscious ones but that also are more complete than those, ongoing even during the gaps in the conscious processes. "If so, it of course becomes plausible to lay the stress in psychology on these somatic processes, to see in *them* the true essence of what is psychical . . . " (Freud, 1940, p. 157). The basis for the psychoanalytic method lies precisely here: From the gaps in immediate conscious experience, we infer to the psychical experience that is not conscious.

In the treatment, the patient follows the fundamental rule and provides the material of his free associations. The analyst offers interpretations that address gaps emerging in this flow of material, gaps of which the patient is generally not aware. The interpretations may be viewed as propositions or hypotheses concerning the "unknowable" contents of the patient's unconscious; they are guided by the psychoanalytic theory and the application of this to the individual case, and are verified by the effects on the patient, and his response.

Freud was aware of criticisms of the psychoanalytic method as a scientific verification procedure, in particular that the patient's response is likely to be influenced by the power of the relationship, which is so central to the therapy, as well as by the interpretation itself. However, he believed his method incorporated verification procedures that were proof against such critiques.

One approach to verification was based on the efficacy of an interpretation in relieving symptoms: "After all, his conflicts will only be successfully solved and his resistances overcome if the anticipatory ideas he is given tally with what is real in him" (Freud, 1916–1917, p. 452). Another source of evidence was based on the patient's direct verbal response. While there are obvious problems with making inferences from the patient's utterances, Freud (1937b) claimed that the safeguards built into his method were proof against these:

> The direct utterances of the patient after he has been offered a construction afford very little evidence upon the question whether we have been right or wrong. It is of all the greater interest that there are indirect forms of confirmation which are in every respect trustworthy. One of these is a form of words that is used (as though by general agreement) with very little variation by the most different people: "I didn't ever think" (or "I shouldn't ever have thought") "that" (or "of that"). This can be translated without any hesitation into: "Yes, you're right this time—about my *unconscious*." . . . An equally valuable confirmation is implied (expressed this time positively) when the patient answers with an association which contains something similar or analogous to the content of the construction. (p. 263, emphasis in original)

Some psychoanalytic writers today, such as Brenner (1980), who accept Freud's formulation of the metapsychology as an adequate working model, also view the psychoanalytic method as a necessary and sufficient means of empirical validation. According to Brenner, the theoretical concepts of psychoanalysis are testable by the psychoanalytic method invented by Freud and have been continuously developed and refined by this means. Brenner views his own recent repudiation of the structural model as providing an example of such scientific development (1992). The critiques of the metapsychology, by Gill, Holt, Klein, and others, and their questioning the status of psychoanalysis as a natural science, reflect misunderstanding of the nature of Freud's theory and his scientific method:

> Psychoanalytic theories depend for their support on observational data that derive from the application of the psychoanalytic method. Those data are not accessible in any way other than by applying that method.

They were essentially unknown before Freud developed the analytic method and would still be so today without it. . . .

It is particularly significant, therefore, to observe the almost complete lack of reference to the psychoanalytic method in the works we have reviewed. In view of this omission I wish to emphasize that however different are the data of psychoanalysis from the data of other natural sciences, its method is the same: observation and accumulation of data by the best available method(s) that is (are) suited to the purpose. . . .

In discussing psychoanalytic theories one must keep in mind that it is the psychoanalytic method that has made them possible, that offers the data to support them, and that seems most likely at present to supply new data that will result in their revision and development. (Brenner, 1980, pp. 206–207)

CRITIQUES OF THE PSYCHOANALYTIC METHOD

The validity of the psychoanalytic method as Freud formulated it is accepted implicitly or explicitly by many, perhaps most clinicians. The responses of their patients, including verbal responses and behavioral and symptomatic change, provide the necessary and sufficient evidence for the validity of their view of a case and their therapeutic work. However, there are many criticisms of the psychoanalytic method from many sources that are not as readily discounted as Brenner's claims would suggest, and the method has proven to be as problematic as the metapsychology itself.

The "Tally Argument" and Its Flaws

Grünbaum (1984) has referred to Freud's (1916–1917) claim of verification of an interpretation based on its efficacy in reducing symptoms as the "Tally Argument." Grünbaum restates Freud's claim as a conjunction of the following two causally necessary conditions, including an explicit mediating function of insight, which is implied in Freud's formulation:

1. An accurate interpretation is necessary to provide the patient with insight into the unconscious basis of his neurosis.
2. Such insight is necessary to bring about symptomatic change.

Given these conditions, the occurrence of symptomatic change is sufficient to demonstrate that an interpretation is accurate. The problem, however, is that the claims of Freud's "Tally Argument" in fact assume the very conclusions that they purport to test, and these claims have been effectively refuted in empirical research, as Grünbaum and others have demonstrated (Bucci, 1989). Many factors in the treatment, other than accurate interpretations leading to insight, may contribute to change; such factors include suggestion, support, and the general effects of the relationship. Other types of therapy, as well as experiences outside of treatment, may also have mutative effects. The impact of nonspecific factors in bringing about change has been demonstrated in a wide range of studies (Bergin & Strupp, 1972; Strupp & Binder, 1984).

As Freud also recognized, the meaning of symptomatic change in psychoanalysis cannot be understood outside the context of the transference, and the actuality of change cannot be assessed until the transference is worked through. However, he did not confront, in this context, the issue of the transference persisting well after termination, even throughout life, or the question of whether conflicts may ever be fully or finally resolved and resistances overcome, which he addressed in later, more sober times (Freud, 1937a). In this later view, the definition of symptom alleviation, or cure, becomes inherently unclear; one can never be certain of the extent to which apparent cure is to be attributed to the persisting power of the relationship—the power of suggestion to which the critics of psychoanalysis referred in Freud's time, and to which they continue to refer today.

Even more basically, in a domain whose subject matter is meaning—private representations in the patient's mind rather than external, observable events—the significance of apparent symptomatic change or reduction of resistance must itself be questioned. Psychoanalysis is inherently concerned with the meaning of these symptoms and behaviors to the patient, rather than their outward manifestation. Apparent improvement, even decreased symptoms or expressions of positive feelings, may reflect dependence, compliance, or an unconscious wish to please or reassure the analyst; apparent regression in such indicators and temporary exacerbation of complaints may indicate undoing of repression, weakening of defenses, arousal of previously inaccessible feelings, or intensification of the transference, all of which may have positive, mutative significance. The issue of changing meanings versus overt symptomatic effects becomes even more crucial in the context of the long-term characterological issues that are addressed in psychoanalysis today, in contrast to the acute and specific symptoms that were more generally the focus of treatment in Freud's time (Bucci, 1989).

The Shifting of Reality in Freud's "Psychical Apparatus"

As Grünbaum also points out, the reference to insight as a mediating factor does not mitigate the problem, since insight is a private, internal event that cannot be observed. This leads us to the pivotal criticism of Freud's verification procedure, which relies on the patient's verbal response, as well as to symptomatic or behavioral change, as evidence that an interpretation has "hit the mark." The individual case reports that constitute the source of evidence for psychoanalytic propositions are inherently flawed as a scientific database (Grünbaum, 1984; Reiser, 1985). The case report method relies on a single observer whose reliability is not assessed, and who is a deeply involved participant in the situation that is being observed. All of this operates in addition to the impact of the analyst's theoretical assumptions, which constitute the foundation for his work.

As Spence (1982) argues, the very process of verbalization in the free association is likely to reorganize and distort the representations of experience that are being expressed. The analyst's processing of this material then further compounds the problem, both through his attempt to impose structure on what he hears and his tendency, which is pervasive, but which he may fail to recognize, to impose his own personal context in interpreting the patient's words. All of this applies on a basic communicative level in any discourse context but is unavoidably exacerbated by the special problems of suggestion and influence that are inherent in the psychoanalytic relationship.

The fundamental problem of the psychoanalytic method, underlying the problems that have been outlined earlier, derives directly from the flaws in Freud's formulation of the psychical apparatus itself and its statement of the ontological and epistemological status of mental representation: *what we know,* and *how we know it.* The psychoanalytic method was proposed as a way of making inference from conscious experience to the unconscious, filling in the gaps in what is immediately accessible by inference to what is unconscious. The problem that Freud inexplicably appears to overlook is that the only conscious experience to which one has immediate access is one's own; the analyst does not have access to the patient's *consciousness* but only to his behavior and speech. The mental processes of another person are, inherently, theoretical entities that must be inferred from indirect indicators, as for any other theoretical event. The need for inference is the same for the conscious processes of others as for their unconscious ones. The analyst listens to what the patient says, watches his actions, and infers what is in his conscious as well as unconscious mind. The significance of the patient's observable response as an indicator of his internal state cannot be assumed but requires verification as well. Before we can infer in a "trustworthy" manner from a patient's language and behavior to his private mental representations, conscious or unconscious, the systematic relationships—or in modern terms, the correspondence rules—between the observable words and behaviors and the theoretical mental representations must be independently developed.

On the other side of the psychical apparatus, the unconscious is defined both as "the true essence of what is psychical" (Freud, 1940, p. 157) and as equivalent to the ongoing underlying somatic or biological processes. In the first formulation, Freud creates the psychic space whose "working-out is a scientific novelty" (p. 145), and whose neurological localization "would give us no help towards understanding" (p. 145) the processes of consciousness; in the second formulation, he disregards this. As Gill (1976) and others have argued, he was always ambivalent concerning the psychological versus neurological status of the psychical apparatus; this ambivalence is reflected directly here.

Thus, the postulated method of predicting from the stream of what is conscious to what is unconscious is inherently problematic. On the one hand, we lack access to the postulated independent variable—the conscious experience *of another person*—and must infer this. On the other hand, we lack a coherent formulation of the postulated dependent variable, the unconscious experience, to which we wish to predict.

The conclusion of this discussion is that the claim of psychoanalysis to scientific status cannot be left to rest on the observational data of the psychoanalytic method, as introduced and developed by Freud and as applied by some analysts, such as Brenner, today. The method is inherently flawed in assuming immediate access to the mental processes of a particular patient. The problem is further confounded if an attempt is made to predict from observation in the clinical setting to theoretical formulations of the case, or to more general theoretical propositions concerning principles of operation of the psychical apparatus.

Problems of Verification: Two Case Examples

The problems of evaluating theory process and outcome, and the related issues of verification of interpretations have been raised by thoughtful practitioners of psychoanalysis, as well as by researchers and critics. The occurrence of multiple treatments provides a controlled naturalistic design in which the issue of verification of interpretations in the treatment may be examined and the problems may be seen. Grossman and Stewart (1976) discussed two cases in which interpretations accepted with conviction by patients in their first analyses were viewed as spurious and as supporting avoidance of underlying material by the analysts in their second. Both patients were young women who expressed envy of men and an inability to accept femininity; in both cases, the first analysts felt that the patients' penis envy was the central issue, and interpretations of the unconscious wish for a penis were given and accepted.

The first patient, a young woman of 21 at the time of beginning treatment, accepted the interpretation to such a degree that she considered traveling to Denmark for a penis transplant. At the same time, she showed apparent symptomatic improvement, according to the treating analyst. For the first time in her life, she established a relationship with a man whom her parents found acceptable and decided to marry him. At this point, the analyst, "with some satisfaction with the apparent improvement . . . decided to terminate the analysis—a decision the patient accepted" (p. 292).

During the succeeding years, "the patient adopted the role of the upper middle-class 'devoted wife and mother with healthy outside interests' " (p. 292); she also became progressively more depressed and dissatisfied. After a period of about 10 years, she reached the point of wishing to separate from her husband and to reenter analysis. Her previous analyst, unavailable at the time, referred her to one of the authors.

In her second analysis, the issues centered around narcissistic issues of worthlessness, damage, and deprivation. These were expressed in terms of the disadvantages of being a woman; however, "the issue of wanting a penis never came up in that form" (p. 294). It was not so much that the patient's issues had changed, and that new contents had come to the forefront following the work of the first analysis and through the life events of the intervening years. Rather, Grossman and Stewart say:

> It became apparent that she had taken the interpretation of her "penis envy" in the first analysis simply as the "proof" of her worthlessness. She had not seen it as an interpretation, but rather as an accusation and a confirmation of her worst fear that she was in fact hopeless and worthless. . . .
>
> The focus of her complaints about being a woman dealt more with the fear of humiliation and ridicule than with the sense of castration— that is, anal and masochistic features were the most prominent. Since admiration always led to rivalry and envy, and sexual interest to aggression, the only permanent tie to the object was of a sadomasochistic nature. She chose the masochistic role and the defense of a mild paranoid attitude. Indeed, the "helpless acceptance" of the penis envy interpretation in the first analysis seemed masochistically gratifying. (p. 293)

The second patient, 28 years old at the beginning of treatment, described herself as homosexual and alcoholic. Her first analyst, a woman, felt that the patient identified with men and was pretending to be a man, and, as in the previous case, focused on interpretations of penis envy. The patient accepted the interpretation, agreed that this was her central issue and the reason for her coming into treatment. She then saw no point in continuing the treatment, since her wish to have a penis and be a man could not be fulfilled. She experienced the analyst as treating her like a criminal; consequently, she refused to listen to what the analyst said or to tell anything meaningful about herself.

In the face of this "sadomasochistic impasse," the patient was referred to one of the authors. In her second analysis, it emerged that she had been severely neglected as a baby and lived in a perpetual state of panic with delusional contents; her alcoholism and homosexuality were ways of diminishing the panic. It also became apparent that she experienced all interpretations, including that of penis envy, as accusations. According to Grossman and Stewart (1976): "The interpretation of the penis envy exploited a metaphor, which seemed to represent both her fears and her defense against them. It created a type of delusional formation that brought order into her thoughts" (p. 297).

In both of these cases, the classical psychoanalytic formulation of penis envy was given by the first analysts and accepted with apparent conviction by the patients. In the first case, the analyst judged the treatment as successful and the patient's apparent symptom reduction and life course seemed to verify this, until feelings of depression and dissatisfaction became dominant. In the second case, the treatment became stalemated. In both cases, Grossman and Stewart (1976) have offered theoretical formulations that differ from the first analyst's position and from the classical theory. In both cases, they argue that the interpretation of penis envy enabled each of these women to continue her avoidance of her own specific underlying issues and worked as an impediment to change:

> The patients clearly did not respond to the interpretation of their "penis envy" in a way that was useful to them. They heard it as a final immutable truth. Although they readily agreed to the interpretation, it was with a feeling of despair—for it confirmed their worst fears of being worthless. (p. 301)

We are left here with a situation in which two analysts see previous treatments as having been based on false premises and theories that did not accurately apply to these cases, and as having destructive effects on patients' lives. Such occurrences are presumably not unfamiliar to analysts working with patients in their second (or later) treatments. Psychoanalysis is a treatment of enormous power for good or ill. In discounting the possibility that an inaccurate interpretation may harm a patient, because it will not connect to his inner experience, Freud (1937b) appeared to deny the great power of the treatment, and in particular of the relationship, which he fully acknowledged in other contexts.

Freud (1916–1917, 1937b) recognized that the patient's direct acquiescence is of no more value than his denial in validating the truth of an interpretation, so that indirect means of verification are required. What he did not acknowledge is the extent to which patients may be capable of bringing in apparent evidence to support an analyst's formulation and coming to believe in this: in some cases, in the interest of compliance and mutual gratification; in some cases, in grateful acceptance of the inaccurate interpretation as providing new protection against the actual representations that are feared and warded off, and in the direct service of maintaining pathology.

In both of the cases described by Grossman and Stewart, the second analyses were seen as successful; this is implicitly interpreted as evidence for the new formulations on which these analyses were based. However, we may note that the first analyst in the first case also reported the treatment as a success in his terms. In the absence of a coherent theory of what is meant by change in psychoanalytic terms and procedures for defining evidence for change, it is not possible to demonstrate reliably that the claims of the latter were valid, while the former were not. The scientific problem remains, although the reader of the case material presented by Grossman and Stewart may feel fully convinced.

The differences in interpretation from the first to the second analyses in these two cases seem to reflect, in part, changing styles in psychoanalytic theory. However, the suggestion that interpretations are determined by fashion, rather than by the specific emotion structures of each patient's life, does not explain away the problem but in itself attests to the need for procedures to monitor the work of the consulting room.

CHAPTER 3

The Role of Empirical Research

The problems that have been identified in Freud's scientific method do not negate his claims concerning the potential parallels of procedures in the physical and psychological sciences, and concerning the scientific role of an abstract psychical apparatus as necessary to enable inference from observable to private mental events. We can perhaps have even more confidence in that approach today than Freud could in his time. It was Freud's creative insight to recognize the need for a theoretical apparatus from which to make inferences to unconscious processes. We need to recognize that such inference is also required for the *conscious processes of other people,* for all inner representations that cannot be jointly observed; we need to continue the enterprise that Freud began.

In recent work, attempts to test psychoanalytic propositions that go beyond the psychoanalytic method have been carried out from two perspectives: (1) experimental research focused primarily on the concepts of the metapsychology and (2) psychotherapy research focused primarily on the clinical theory.

TESTING PSYCHOANALYTIC PROPOSITIONS WITH EXPERIMENTAL RESEARCH

Freud treated the use of experimental methods with some disdain. Thus, he devalued the work of experimentalist Saul Rosenzweig in a cavalier manner in his letter of 1934:

> I have examined your experimental studies for the verification of the psychoanalytic assertions with interest. I cannot put much value on these confirmations because the wealth of reliable observations on which these assertions rest make them independent of experimental verification. Still, it can do no harm. (quoted in Grünbaum, 1984, p. 101)

Freud viewed the psychoanalytic method as both necessary and sufficient for validation of the psychoanalytic theory. Those analysts who continue to rely on the "psychoanalytic method" in the face of accumulating evidence regarding its failure also tend to devalue experimental findings and other empirical research outside of the "method." On the other hand, some experimental researchers have continued to work toward validation of the concepts of the metapsychology and are, ironically, more accepting of these concepts than many clinicians today.

The innovative research of Erdelyi (1985) is just such an attempt to validate the metapsychology in its own terms. His approach has been to select certain psychoanalytic concepts and propositions, in some cases redefine them, then subject them to empirical test. He does not view the inconsistencies in Freud's model or its reliance on energy constructs as vitiating this project. Like Brenner, he sees the rejection of the metapsychology by many psychoanalytic researchers as reflecting misunderstanding of Freud's scientific methods and of scientific method in general:

> A major contemporary school of psychoanalytic thinking, for example, has gone as far as to reject the formal psychological theory of psychoanalysis (often termed *metapsychology*) because its mechanistic (cause–effect) formulations conceptually channel the field into out-moded physicalist notions such as "force," "energy," "etiology," and "hydraulics," which derail it from its true cognitive-psychological domain, semantics and intentions (see especially Gill and Holzman, 1976; Holt, 1965, 1976a; G. S. Klein, 1973, 1976; Schafer, 1976). . . . [This] criticism . . . fails to take into account Freud's use of multiple metaphor premises . . . and the likelihood that each, including the mechanistic framework, may complement the other. (pp. 54–55, emphasis in original)

Thus, Erdelyi argues, the mechanistic constructs that Freud employs are equivalent to the type of analog premises drawn from other domains, which are used as the basis of theory construction in all sciences today. Such models or metaphors are formulated and reformulated to map "reality" and to allow testable propositions to be generated. The inconsistencies in Freud's theory, which have troubled psychoanalytic researchers, in fact reflect his flexibility in attempting to map reality more accurately and constitute a strength rather than a weakness of his approach:

What then *is* the metaphor premise of psychoanalysis? The answer seems to be that psychoanalysis is unique; unlike major "schools" or "movements" in academic psychology, it adheres to no single analogic medium. Psychoanalysis is a mixed-metaphor system. Freud, unlike major academic theoreticians, was not willing to be fettered by any single metaphor premise. When one analogic medium failed to elucidate some facet of psychological reality, he was willing to try out new analogic tools rather than simply to ignore, as traditional academic psychology has typically done, the recalcitrant reality. In this respect psychoanalysis, despite its experimental provincialism, is much closer to the spirit of twentieth-century physics than contemporary academic psychology. (p. 111)

Erdelyi has focused particularly on the concepts of the unconscious, repression, and the defenses, and the effect of free association as a means of recovering previously inaccessible material. In one of his basic experimental studies, Erdelyi's goal was to investigate the psychoanalytic hypothesis that free association facilitates retrieval of previously inaccessible material. Subjects were shown a complex picture stimulus in a tachistoscopic presentation and were immediately asked to draw and label everything in the picture. The experimental subjects in the free-association condition were then asked to talk freely for 40 minutes, while the control subjects used the same time period for an unrelated, nonverbal task (throwing darts). Following this, a second test of recall was made. All experimental subjects recalled more stimulus items in the second test than in the first, while controls did not, indicating a positive effect of free association on retrieval of the contents of the picture stimulus and thus supporting the psychoanalytic hypothesis.

However, questions were then raised as to whether the increased recall following free association may have reflected a relaxed criterion for *reporting* remembered material, rather than the actual increase in *capacity to access* such material that was claimed, and also whether different types of subject matter may have different effects. In subsequent studies, a forced recall paradigm was used to differentiate the effects of criteria for reporting what is remembered from actual capacity to access material, and different types of subject matter were also compared. From this series of studies, Erdelyi concludes that there is not evidence for an effect of free association on the *recovery* of previously inaccessible memories. Rather than enabling subjects to remember more stimulus items, what free association does is enable them to be freer as to what they are *willing to report*. Erdelyi also found that the effects of free association applied only to picture stimuli and did not hold for memories of word lists. Erdelyi interprets these findings as providing evidence for an effect of free association on reporting of material that is suppressed but accessible, rather than retrieval of material that had previously been inaccessible or "repressed." Furthermore, this is not a general effect but operates only for memory images and not for linguistic memories.

Many other experimental studies focusing on questions of repression and the unconscious have been carried out, summarized in Kline (1981). Some of the findings of these studies, like those of Erdelyi, are of considerable interest in themselves, independent of what they have to say concerning clinical psychoanalysis or psychoanalytic theory. As Erdelyi has pointed out, the experimental approach has demonstrated attempts to avoid painful stimuli, the occurrence of mentation outside of awareness, and selective rejection of information from awareness.

What remains to be clarified, as Erdelyi also points out, is the specific theoretical relationship of such facts to psychoanalytic clinical concepts. In this context, the issue of Erdelyi's (1985) own redefinition of psychoanalytic concepts also needs to be addressed. Thus, for example, he separates the concept of the unconscious from the concept of repression:

> It is possible to believe in the existence of the unconscious, even of an active, intrusive and therefore "dynamic" unconscious, without necessarily espousing the proposition that repression accounts for all or even some of the unconscious. (p. 64)

He uses inaccessibility as the criterion of "unconsciousness proper" (i.e., the dynamic unconscious) and treats repression (and the defenses) as a separate issue. He also assumes no distinction between conscious and unconscious repression, arguing that Freud, as well, treated these concepts interchangeably:

> If the question of unconsciousness should be at issue in a particular clinical or experimental context one need only qualify the defenses under consideration as conscious or unconscious—conscious vs. unconscious repression, conscious vs. unconscious displacement, and so forth. (p. 221)

Erdelyi's concept of the unconscious also eliminates any systemic implications. He states that "the problematical systemic Unconscious is abolished by Freud in 1923, becoming the id" (pp. 64–65); thus, he argues, it is a mistake to assume that unconscious processes follow different rules than conscious ones.

While Erdelyi has made the claim that his project has been to test Freud's model, this needs to be qualified; Erdelyi's project was to test Freud's model as defined in Erdelyi's terms. Since he has explicitly redefined the concepts of repression, defenses, and the unconscious, the relevance of Erdelyi's findings to the operation of repression as an unconscious defense, the operation of free association as it occurs in the treatment situation, or its effect on memories that have been defended against or warded off, remain unclear.

Erdelyi's contention that his approach is somehow justified by Freud having "abolished" the systemic Unconscious is similarly problematic. As we have seen, Freud struggled continuously with the implications of the mental qualities and, in fact, retained their systemic implications to the end. He never abandoned the position that unconscious processes follow different rules than conscious ones; the difference in the nature of these processes remains the essential core of the psychoanalytic approach throughout his work. As he says: "We have found that processes in the unconscious or in the id obey different laws from those in the preconscious ego" (1940, p. 164).

We may also note that Erdelyi appears to overstate the case a bit or to be perhaps a bit sanguine concerning the relationship of the multiple-metaphor premises of psychoanalysis to those of the physical sciences. While physics may have multiple models and multiple mathematical systems for different domains, the concepts and the relationships between them are specifically defined for each model and each domain. It is not the multiplicity of psychoanalytic models of the mental apparatus but the *lack of any coherent one,* in any domain, that constitutes the problem for our field. Freud himself was seeking such a coherent theory, even while struggling with his mixed and multiple metaphors. In his final summary formulation, Freud (1940) not only implicitly realigned the two topographies, but also explicitly expressed his general dissatisfaction with the inconsistencies of his disparate formulations and actively sought the underlying reality that would provide the basis for their reconciliation.

On a more general level, the objection may be raised here, as in all experimental designs, as to whether processes that are inherently relational may usefully be tested outside of a naturalistic interpersonal context. The issues concerning testing propositions with interpersonal contents in the experimental laboratory have been raised from a number of different vantage points, by Neisser (1976), Thomae and Kaechele (1987), Yuille (1986), and many others.

Shevrin's Subliminal Paradigm

The work of Shevrin (1995) and his colleagues, using the subliminal laboratory method, links psychoanalytic, cognitive, and neurological concepts in an experimental paradigm. Shevrin's design addresses some of the general objections that the experimental paradigm is inapplicable to actual clinical concepts by incorporating in-depth evaluation of patients by experienced psychoanalysts, who provide a psychodynamic formulation of each case. The cognitive component of Shevrin's design consists of tachistoscopic presentation of words at both subliminal and supraliminal rates. The words that are presented include both unconscious conflict and conscious symptom words, selected specifically for each patient on the basis of the clinical evaluation. The subliminal presentation operationally determines the status of the stimulus as *descriptively* unconscious. For each word presented, either subliminally or supraliminally, a brain response is electrically recorded; this constitutes the neurological component of the design. Shevrin found that the time-frequency patterns for brain responses to the unconscious conflict words were the inverse of those for conscious symptom words, and the patterns were reversed for subliminal versus supraliminal presentation. He argues that these findings support the validity of a causative psychological unconscious by demonstrating differences in the temporal organization of neural processes as a function of level of consciousness and the specific contents of unconscious conflict for each individual.

This innovative paradigm and its findings are clearly of considerable interest in bridging the gap between cognitive and psychoanalytic concepts and methods. He develops operational definitions of concepts derived from both cognitive and psychoanalytic domains and uses neurophysiological indicators as an independent source of evidence.

Here, as in Erdelyi's work, however, the question arises as to the relationship between the construct of the causative psychological unconscious, as defined and tested in Shevrin's paradigm, and the concept as defined in the psychoanalytic model of the psychical apparatus in either the topographic or structural formulation. Shevrin's approach is based on accessibility to awareness as the major determinant of mode of cognitive processing, as in the topographic model. However, in relying entirely on verbal stimuli, he assumes linguistic organization in the unconscious, which is obviously at variance with the topographic formulation. If there is indeed a linguistic component within the causative unconscious, as Shevrin's work would indicate, the systemic implications of this within the psychoanalytic theory need to be traced.

From either the psychoanalytic or experimental perspectives, it seems crucial that we agree on what the model is that we are testing before we can understand the meaning of the results that are obtained. The work of Shevrin and Erdelyi yields results that seem of considerable interest to the psychoanalytic approach and that raise important questions concerning the structure of the psychical apparatus. However, the lack of a coherent model of the psychical apparatus limits the degree to which we can trace the implications of their research in psychoanalytic terms.

The Metapsychology and Computer Simulation

Wegman (1985), working within the domain of artificial intelligence rather than in the experimental laboratory, has also attempted to demonstrate the compatibility of psychoanalysis and cognitive psychology and to show that psychoanalytic propositions are capable of empirical validation outside of the therapeutic context. Wegman's project has been to show that a particular aspect of Freud's theory—the trauma theory of hysteria—can be examined through a computer formulation. He outlines a computational sketch of the case history of Miss Lucy R. (Freud, 1895b) based on the format of script programs introduced by Schank and Abelson (1977). Scripts are models of expected sequences of behaviors as these are manifest in repeated events. Using the script sequence as a model, gaps or unexpected elements can then be objectively identified, and their dynamic or emotional meanings can be explored. While Wegman does not carry out this simulation, he outlines it sufficiently to demonstrate its plausibility. The basic notion that aspects of Freud's model can be the subject matter of scientific investigation is supported by Wegman's attempts, as by Erdelyi's and Shevrin's work. Given Freud's attitude toward experimental research, however, even when carried out with human subjects from a clinical perspective, it is interesting to imagine a letter from Freud to Wegman about the computer simulation of the case of Miss Lucy R.

The position of this book is in agreement with the core assumption of the empirical researchers whose work has been sampled here, which is also the core assumption of the field of cognitive science: Complex mental representations and processes can be the subject matter of empirical, scientific research. However, we must always question the extent to which the concepts that are tested in the empirical studies outside the therapeutic context are equivalent to the clinical psychoanalytic concepts, or are in fact different constructs with different features, identified by the same terms. On the one hand, all types of evidence may potentially be relevant, given a coherent theory and a coherent statement of the relationship of the evidence to the theory. On the other hand, no observations within the analytic context or in the experimental laboratory, or anywhere else, can be assessed in relation to the theory unless the propositions and constructs are well defined in conceptual and in operational terms.

THE FAILURE OF THEORY AND PSYCHOTHERAPY RESEARCH

The field of psychodynamic psychotherapy research may be seen as a rigorous and focused attempt to apply the methods of empirical science to the propositions of clinical theory, while abandoning the metapsy-chological framework. From another perspective, the field of psychother-apy research might also be seen in certain respects as a modern version of the psychoanalytic method. Essentially, the research looks at the effects of particular treatments or particular interventions on measures of proc-ess and outcome, as Freud (1916–1917, 1937b) claimed to do, while attempting to correct the shortcomings of the psychoanalytic method, as outlined earlier. The researcher assesses process and outcome effects using objective procedures that meet acceptable standards of reliability and validity, rather than relying on his own individual and possibly biased observations, as in the standard case reports. The tools of process analysis transform a record of the session, usually a verbatim transcript, into a form that may constitute scientific data in the usual sense.

Psychotherapy researchers do not see their studies as testing the propositions of the metapsychology itself, as the psychoanalytic method was originally understood to do; this goal has been laid aside. The terms "metapsychology" or "energy" are not indexed in the handbook of *Psychodynamic Process Research* (Miller, Luborsky, Barber, & Docherty, 1993). Nevertheless, the field of psychotherapy research is increasingly concerned with theory in some form, rather than simply demonstrating differential treatment or "dosage" effects. As Dahl (1988) has pointed out, psychodynamic psychotherapy researchers have moved in the past several decades from a focus on demonstrating treatment outcome to fundamen-tal questions about the nature of psychopathology, the ways in which psychotherapy addresses pathology, and how treatment brings about change; all of these issues may be seen as intrinsic aspects of the psychoanalytic clinical theory. To accomplish these aims, psychotherapy researchers have attempted to develop operational measures of conflict and the processes of change. A wide array of such measures of clinical content have emerged in recent years. These include Luborsky's (1988) measure of the "core conflictual relationship theme" (CCRT); Hoffman and Gill's (1988) coding of the "patient's experience of the relationship with the therapist" (PERT); the "configurational analysis" of Horowitz et al. (1984), a systematic method of case formulation; the "cyclical maladap-tive patterns" of Strupp and his colleagues (Schacht, Binder, & Strupp 1984); the "frame structures" of Teller and Dahl (1986), which are recurrent sequential-event structures extracted from a patient's discrete narratives; and Weiss, Sampson, and the Mount Zion Psychotherapy Research Group's (1986) concept of the patient's "unconscious plan."

Entities such as conflictual relationship themes, the patient's experi-ence of the relationship, and unconscious plans are all internal subjective events, accessible directly only to their experiencer, the patient, and often inaccessible even to him. In modern scientific terms, the possibility of doing empirical research that involves such private, subjective events entails a particular epistemological stance, although this question is not directly addressed in the psychotherapy research field. Thus the researcher is, at least implicitly, taking some version of the following positions concerning clinical concepts such as transference, conflict, or structural change, and how we know them:

1. These entities may be viewed as having the status of hypothetical constructs, inferred through their effects on observable events such as language and behavior, and well defined in these terms. However, this position requires a coherent theoretical framework, which has been lacking in the field.

2. In the absence of a coherent theoretical framework, the alternative is to adopt some version of a behaviorist position:

a. The most straightforward behaviorist position is that we are not concerned with hypothetical constructs or intervening variables but simply with observable measures and groups of these. This is an unwieldy approach, which has been rejected in its own field of learning theory. In the field of psychoanalysis, which is concerned with meaning and inner experience, we cannot do without constructs and concepts in some form, as I have discussed in detail elsewhere (Bucci, 1989).

b. The researcher may recognize the need for theoretical constructs but may attempt to work without a general theoretical framework, building up each concept from the empirical side through the development of consistent operational measures. This is similar to the approach used by some psychometric researchers to define elusive concepts such as intelligence, that is, taking the position that the measure *is* the concept. Thus, intelligence is no more or less than what intelligence tests measure; similarly, we have and require no theoretical formulation of concepts such as transference and psychical structure beyond the operational indicators of these.

c. Alternatively, the researcher may hold a bootstrap variation of the pragmatic "as-if" position accepted widely in the psychoanalytic clinical domains. Thus, the psychoanalytic researcher proceeds as if concepts such as transference, psychic structure, and structural change were sufficiently well defined that we know what we are measuring; the operational definitions developed in the research then may help to clarify their meaning. This seems to be the more common, if implicit, epistemological position in the field.

The problems associated with proceeding without a theoretical framework, in most cases implicitly relying on alternative 2c above, may be seen in comparing several of the most widely used measures of content, all of which have been interpreted as measures of the transference, without transference itself being systematically defined. The CCRT was initially designed by Luborsky as a measure of the patient's "general relationship pattern" (Luborsky & Crits-Christoph, 1988, p. 100) and is now widely accepted as a measure of transference. The CCRT is identified by examining narratives of interactions between the patient and other people. These are identified in "relationship episodes" (REs), which are stories of past and current interactions, and also include episodes in the relationship with the therapist. The structure of the CCRT includes three major components: the patient's wishes, needs, or intentions toward the other who figures in the story; the responses of the other; and the responses of the self. The CCRT was initially proposed by Luborsky as a measure of central relationship themes. "It was only later that experiences with the CCRT led him to realize that he had hit upon an operational definition of the transference," Luborsky says, referring to himself (1988, p. 100).

Hoffman and Gill's PERT and Dahl's (1988) "fundamental repetitive and maladaptive emotion structures" (FRAMES) are now also characterized as transference-related measures, and the correspondence of these procedures with one another and with the CCRT has been examined (Luborsky, 1988). The PERT was explicitly designed as a measure of transference, analyzed by clinical judgment. In contrast, the concept of FRAMES is related to the notion of stereotyped knowledge structures, as defined by Minsky (1975) within the artificial intelligence field. FRAMES are characterized as "structured sequences of memories of emotions," which meet a number of additional specific criteria, and which "provide the framework for a theory of change independent of any particular theory of technique" (Dahl, 1988, p. 61).

The concepts of the patient's experience of the relationship with the therapist (PERT), repetitive and maladaptive emotion structures (FRAMES), and general relationship themes (CCRT) presumably intersect. However, it is also the case that they have different origins and different definitions, and their theoretical relationship needs to be clarified before their empirical relationship can be understood. The concepts of 'emotion structure" and 'core relationship pattern" have the status of psychological constructs. They differ as to explanatory level from the notion of the patient's phenomenological experience, which lies at the core of the Gill and Hoffman measure. From a concrete or substantive perspective, it might certainly be argued that the patient's experience of the relationship may arise from reality considerations concerning the person and behavior of the analyst, rather than reflecting only, or primarily, the patient's own emotion structures or relationship patterns projected onto a neutral screen. Different predictions concerning the empirical correspondence of the measures might be made on this basis.

The point that emerges from these comparisons, and that has not been addressed by psychotherapy researchers, is that convergence of operational measures is validation for them *if and only if* they are supposed to be measuring the same thing; it is not validation and may in fact be seen as invalidating them, if they are supposed to be measuring different things. The significance of convergence or divergence of observations as a basis for development of construct validity depends on the definition of the constructs within a nomological net. Without a general theory, within which theoretical constructs may be consistently defined, we cannot postulate the expected relationship between measures, nor the implications of their divergence or convergence; we are on constantly shifting ground. The fundamental notion of construct validity, as dependent on a theoretical framework, is built on this premise.

Problem of Demonstrating Treatment Effects

While the field of psychotherapy research has increasingly, and appropriately, been concerned with understanding the process of treatment, the necessity to demonstrate treatment effects also remains central. Whether we talk of treatment process or outcome, we are basically interested in how to bring about changes in internal representations or meanings—how we feel, how we perceive things, what we believe, rather than changes in behaviors or symptoms alone.

Beyond this, it is necessary to distinguish positive improvements that are fragile and spurious from others that are likely to persist. As a related question, it is important to distinguish to what extent the apparent improvements reflect the direct impact of the transference or other factors in contrast to the effect of an interpretation in facilitating insight. The question is made still more complex by the possibility of transference continuing in internalized form after termination. Such internalization may in fact be deeper and more long lasting in successful treatments.

If we can determine by our measures that structural change has occurred, we can then address the question of how this change has taken place. In so doing, we need to distinguish among such factors as insight based on valid interpretations, the continuing effect of the relationship, and other means of change. The issues that have been raised here speak directly to the need for theory-based empirical research. The use of transcripts and systematic research methods can potentially provide the observable indicators of inner experience; the scaffolding of a theoretical model is necessary to permit consistent interpretation of the measures that have been developed. The theory redefines subjective events as psychological constructs and connects the events observed by the researcher (or the clinician) to these.

We may also note that such a general formulation is needed to address a central—but not sufficiently heeded—problem of the psychotherapy research field: To what extent do treatments in which an observer—the researcher—is implicitly present resemble treatments in which the intimacy of the dialogue is undisturbed? The observations may occur with varying degrees of intrusiveness, from the minimal presence of an audiotape recorder to the more intensive imposition of video recording, ongoing physiological measurements, and additional sessions with research staff. Only in the context of a general model of pathology and process can we hope to know to what extent the concepts that are being studied in the different types of research treatments correspond to the concepts in clinical use. These issues will be discussed further in Chapter 18.

The failure of theory, and the lack of acknowledgment of this failure, present dangers in practice for all participants in the psychoanalytic enterprise. Analysts and researchers alike continue to function, as they must, with an implicit "as-if" position—as if they know to what the concepts of the theory refer, and as if the absence of a general theory does not affect the work. Thus, analysts who explicitly reject the energy theory, and recognize the ill-defined nature of concepts such as cathexis and libido, nevertheless continue to use terms such as "id," "drive," "repression," and the "primary and secondary processes," as if they do understand what these words mean.

Thomae and Kaechele (1987) have emphasized the pervasive effect of the crisis of theory on the practicing clinician:

> The striking, graphic language of Freud's theory suggests similarities between physical and psychic processes which in fact do not exist. If the suggestive power of metaphors leads the analyst to apply them in areas where the comparison is no longer valid, his therapeutic action will also be inappropriate. The crisis of theory cuts deep into psychoanalytic practice. (p. 30)

Here they refer to the highly evocative concepts of the drive discharge model as rooted, in an unacknowledged manner, in the processes of male sexuality, and as deriving much of their meaning, metaphorically, from this source. Many other dangers of interpretation also stem from the implicit effects of the metapsychology. The "witch," as Freud (1937a) characterized the metapsychology, continues, unacknowledged or not, to cast her spell.

While the epistemological issues have not been directly addressed, the problems of mapping psychoanalytic concepts onto empirical indicators, which we have illustrated here, are not unrecognized by thoughtful psychotherapy researchers. At the close of his comparison of the three measures mentioned earlier, among which he found considerable empirical correspondence, Luborsky has presented his own version of this philosophical issue:

> Each of these systems embodies some reasonable approximation between the concept of transference and their particular measure of it. But there might be some differences of opinion about how closely they approximate the concept. Apropos of that, I was amused by an experience I once had. I heard two men telling riddles to each other. One riddle seemed very appropriate to our difficulty of matching the transference concept with each operational measure of it. The first man, Sam, said: I have a riddle for you. What is it that is green, hangs on a wall and whistles? The second man, Joe, sitting next to him, thought a while and said: I don't know, what? Sam: A herring. Joe: A herring isn't green. Sam: So you paint it green. Joe: But it doesn't hang on a wall. Sam: So you hang it on the wall. Joe: But it doesn't whistle. Sam: So who cares if it whistles? (1988, p. 114)

In an alternate version of this parable, from another source, Sam's final comment is different: "You wouldn't expect me to make it too easy." The problem for psychotherapy researchers, as represented here, is similar to the problem we have encountered in the discussion of experimental research on clinical concepts and is not at all an easy one. To what extent do the concepts of transference or conflict or structural change, as measured by the PERT, CCRT, or FRAMES, correspond to one another, or to the concepts that clinicians understand and use? To what extent must psychotherapy researchers paint the clinical concepts green, hang them on walls, and deny their failure to whistle, as we have suggested that experimental researchers such as Erdelyi have also done? In the absence of a general theory, within which the clinical concepts may be systematically defined, the questions remain.

CHAPTER 4

Networks of the Mind
TOWARD A PSYCHOLOGICAL MODEL FOR PSYCHOANALYSIS

In order to talk about the nature of the universe and to
discuss questions such as whether it has a beginning or an
end, you have to be clear about what a scientific theory is. I
shall take the simple-minded view that a theory is just a
model of the universe, or a restricted part of it, and a set of
rules that relate quantities in the model to observations that
we make. It exists only in our minds and does not have any
other reality (whatever that might mean).
                              —STEPHEN W. HAWKING (1988, p. 9)

A new explanatory theory is required for psychoanalysis to fill the gap
left by the failure of the metapsychology. The need for theory can be seen
in clinical work, as in the attempts of researchers to study treatment
effects. The question then arises as to what kind of theory it should be,
the specific nature or level of the psychoanalytic theoretical domain, and
the level of explanation that we require. The universe of psychoanalysis
is emotion and mind—the representation of private emotional experience,
its communication to another person, and its transformation in treatment.
While a psychoanalytic theory must be about private emotional meanings,
the sine qua non of science is that events be jointly observable. This has
been seen as the central dilemma for the field, which Freud and others
since have attempted to resolve in a variety of ways. In tracing Freud's
position and that of other psychoanalytic writers since his time, my goal

57

is not to establish some historical truth, but to examine and resolve several issues that continue to confuse the field today.

Freud's position was complex and variable in characterizing the level of explanation represented in the metapsychology. In his earlier work, Freud attempted "to furnish a psychology that is a natural science; that is, to represent psychic processes as quantitatively determinate states of specifiable material particles" (Freud, 1895a, p. 355). In the same period, in a letter to Fliess dated March 10, 1898, which has been widely quoted and discussed, he writes:

> It seems to me as if the wish-fulfilment theory gives only the psychological and not the biological, or rather metapsychological explanation. (Incidentally, I am going to ask you seriously whether I should use the term "metapsychology" for my psychology which leads beyond consciousness.) (1954, p. 246)

Here Freud appears to equate the metapsychological with the biological level of explanation and distinguishes these from the psychological level represented by the wish-fulfillment theory. Nevertheless, he refers to the metapsychology as a "psychology," the one that "leads beyond consciousness"; and in his writings from 1900 on, Freud generally disavows the biological account. For example, in 1900 he writes:

> I shall entirely disregard the fact that the mental apparatus with which we are here concerned is also known to us in the form of an anatomical preparation, and I shall carefully avoid the temptation to determine psychical locality in any anatomical fashion. I shall remain on psychological ground. . . . (p. 536)

In the "Introductory Lectures" (1916–1917), he makes a similar point:

> No philosophical auxiliary science exists which could be made of service for your medical purposes. Neither speculative philosophy, nor descriptive psychology, nor what is called experimental psychology (which is closely allied to the physiology of the sense-organs), as they are taught in the Universities, are in a position to tell you anything serviceable of the relation between body and mind or to provide you with the key to an understanding of possible disturbances of the mental functions. . . .
>
> This is the gap which psycho-analysis seeks to fill. It tries to give psychiatry its missing psychological foundation. It hopes to discover the common ground on the basis of which the convergence of physical and mental disorder will become intelligible. With this aim in view, psychoanalysis must keep itself free from any hypothesis that is alien to it, whether of an anatomical, chemical or physiological kind, and must

operate entirely with purely psychological auxiliary ideas.... (pp. 20–21)

STATUS OF METAPSYCHOLOGY: RECENT VIEWS

Throughout his subsequent writings, up to and including his final summary formulation, Freud (1940) continued to refer to the psychical apparatus as an abstract theoretical model and to disclaim interest in anatomical localization. Nevertheless, Gill (1976) has argued that Freud remained ambivalent as to the status of the metapsychology, and that it is inherently a theory about the nervous system, despite Freud's explicit claim of "psychological ground." According to Gill, the metapsychology represents a reduction of psychological concepts to their biological substrate, such as Freud attempted at the time of the Project, rather than the abstract psychological theory that he claimed from 1900 on. The problem with Freud's formulation is its failure to recognize the fundamental nature of a psychological stimulus:

> A stimulus cannot be psychologically characterized by its external dimension, whether that stimulus arises inside or outside the skin. A stimulus is psychologically definable only in terms of its psychological significance in the psychological universe of meaning, or intentionality, or whatever other term is chosen to indicate the psychological perspective. (p. 96)

A "pure" psychology is required, which deals with intentionality and meaning, and which is based on data such as those of the psychoanalytic situation. Such a psychology "can be a science that is valid in its own right" (p. 103).

In opposition to the views of Gill, Klein (1973, 1976), and others, Rubinstein argued that a psychological model cannot provide an acceptable level of explanation for a psychoanalytic theory. According to Rubinstein (1965), there are two ways in which psychoanalysis might be said to be a psychological rather than neurophysiological theory. According to one approach, the theoretical terms of the psychoanalytic theory, for example, "id," "ego," and "superego," would be interpreted as referring to "*actual* divisions of an *actual* mental apparatus," which exists on some level or in some form separate and distinct from its physical substrate, and "would not be translatable into neurophysiological terms" (p. 45, emphasis in original). Such an interpretation, Rubinstein says, assumes a dualist view of the mind–body relationship, that is, a "fundamental mental substance," distinct from physical reality, in the philosophical terms of Descartes, and would not be seriously advanced by scientists or philosophers of science today. It is unlikely that "psychoanalysts who speak as if they used the high-level theoretical terms in this manner are willing to accept the dualistic implication of their usage" (p. 45).

An alternative formulation of a psychological model involves speaking in a dualist language but with metaphoric intent. Rubinstein characterizes this as a "metaphorical interpretation," an "as-if dualism or *pseudodualism*":

> This interpretation, as is readily seen, successfully avoids the mind–body problem; but in doing so it reduces itself at best to a low-level theory. The theoretical terms, having no actual referents, are definable more or less exclusively in terms of the inferred relationships between observed and/or inferred psychological (i.e., phenomenal and behavioral) events. . . . In its core meaning the pseudodualistic interpretation is thus describable as a modified . . . form of behaviorism or of operationism. Obviously, psychoanalytic theory can be said to be a "purely psychological" theory according to this interpretation as well. (1965, p. 46)

Rejecting either "actual" or "pseudo"-dualism, and seeing no other alternative, Rubinstein (1965) concludes that the only acceptable empiricist interpretation of psychoanalytic theoretical terms is as referring to neurophysiological entities: "By this interpretation the terms would, in other words, be completely translatable to neurophysiological terms—i.e., they would be protoneurophysiological" (p. 47). The empiricist neurophysiological interpretation may then be combined with the "pseudodualistic" position, so that "theoretical terms would be definable both neurophysiologically *and* in terms of psychological relationships" (p. 47). Rubinstein's approach does not require every concept of the psychoanalytic theory to have been translated into neurophysiological terms, or even to be translatable at the current stage of our knowledge, but does require that neurophysiological criteria be used in development and evaluation of these psychoanalytic concepts.

According to the empiricist criterion, as Rubinstein formulates this, many of the high-level concepts of the psychoanalytic theory, such as the id–ego–superego classification, or the concept of psychic energy itself, are unacceptable as elements of a systematic scientific theory. Such concepts are not translatable into physiological terms, and there is no indication that neurophysiology is moving in a direction to make this translation possible. Rubinstein concludes that to meet the criteria of the empiricist interpretation, the obsolete, high-level concepts of the psychoanalytic theory must be eliminated and replaced with terms referring to mental events, such as unconscious wishes or fantasies, for which a physiological substrate is more likely to be identifiable.

Grubby Facts and the Unruly Body:
Holt's Critique

Holt (1967a) has agreed with Rubinstein in rejecting a "pure psychology" and calling for a model with a physiological basis, although he develops his argument on somewhat different grounds. As Holt argues, a psychoanalytic theory must account for the interaction between mental and somatic events; a psychological theory will necessarily fail in this respect, as Freud implicitly recognized:

> The usual account is that after recognizing the failure of the Project, Freud rejected the mechanistic doctrine of physicalistic physiology; turned resolutely to a pure psychology; and created an abstract psychic apparatus in place of the nervous system, in which the operative quantity was psychic, not physical energy.... But through his years of constructing theories, whenever it was necessary to consider somatic events such as conversion symptoms, Freud unhesitatingly spoke as if cathectic energy was *not* psychic but physical (neural). It is to his everlasting credit, and to the huge benefit of psychoanalysis, that whenever the facts demanded it—even grubby facts involving the connection of the abstract mind with a heavy, smelly, affect-shaken, unruly body—Freud reverted to a psychosomatic view of the organism as a whole. If he had been consistent, if he had insisted on a pure psychology in which there *could* have been a consistent concept of psychic energy, psychoanalysis would have lost its principal claim to scientific interest: that it alone really takes into account all the facts about human beings, their secret desires, their somatic aches and lusts, the pervasively psychosomatic nature of behavior and thought. (Holt, 1967a, pp. 153–154, emphasis in original)

Holt's statement seems to confound the abstract character of a theoretical model with the character of the domain that it models, as if the domain of a psychological theory must somehow be restricted to accounting for the processes of disembodied thought. Theoretical models are indeed abstract but may be about any type of psychological or physical events—including "grubby" ones—and their interactions. In Holt's statement, the issue of mind–brain relationships also is confounded with the issues of psychosomatic interaction. The theoretical relationship between the level of mind (psychological constructs) and the level of brain (the neural substrate) needs to be distinguished from the relationship between mind and body in a broader sense, that is, the relationship of mental to somatic events, which may include visceral, motoric, and sensory representations and processes.

We may note that psychological theories and psychological research have traditionally dealt with the types of bodily functions involved in sensation and perception, as well as sensorimotor coordination, and the interaction of these with concept formation and language. Models have not yet been developed that account for the interaction of cognitive functions with somatic, including visceral, events, but the epistemological framework is in place to develop such theories. The type of abstract model that Freud sought to develop for psychoanalysis, and that we now seek to develop in the context of the cognitive science of today, must be a model of emotional information processing, not information processing only, and must account for the relationships among motoric, perceptual, and visceral functions, and the interactions of these with language and abstract thought.

Holt assumes that a formulation based on neurophysiological functions will account for the interaction of mental with somatic and emotional functions in a way that a psychological model cannot. This is a spurious assumption. Explanations for the interaction of cognitive and somatic processes can be and need to be developed on both psychological and neurophysiological levels, that is, on the level of mind and on the level of brain. Thus, in the former case, for example, we might pose our question in terms of the effect of depression on susceptibility to physical illness; in the latter, we might wish to investigate the relationship of changes in specific neurotransmitter levels to immune system effects.

We may also point out that just as we construct theories of the universe of mind, so we also require theoretical networks to model the universe of brain. Neurophysiological processes and relationships, which figure in theories of brain function, themselves have the status of constructs and must be inferred from observation in the context of a theoretical frame. We do not directly observe the working of the intact brain; we infer to it from observable indicators that are functions of these operations. The observable indicators may include behaviors or, very often, readings on dials, printouts, or other electrical signals. The pen markings that reflect the evoked potential are not themselves the evoked potential; we infer from the pen markings to the brain function. Studies using positron emission tomography (PET; Petersen, Fox, Posner, Mintun, & Raichle, 1988) now permit immediate imaging of areas of cerebral blood flow while the subject is engaged in particular tasks. Even with such techniques, however, we remain several inferences away from the firing of the neuron itself, and areas of uncertainty in this inference remain. The PET method does not have a clearly known threshold, so that lack of activation does not rule out activity at a given site (Posner & Rothbart, 1989). The images from PET scans are averaged from multiple readings rather than representing a single scan, so that actual information at any point in time is not retained. We should also note that the subject of the magnetic resonance imaging technique must lie in a metal cylinder, so that the relationship of the processes that go on in such circumstances to processes as they occur naturally in the interpersonal world must be seen as problematic.

Beyond this, we take many inferential steps on a different level in connecting indicators of evoked potential or variation in cerebral blood flow to specific mental contents—the representations of images and words, the experiences, conscious or unconscious, that may be associated with these. The meaning of an experience cannot be associated directly to a particular reading of the evoked potential, or the blood flow in the brain, but must be inferred.

Once we understand that the concepts of neurophysiological models (like concepts of all physical systems, and like those of psychological models) have their existence within formal theoretical networks, with their own systematic, defining rules and operational links, then the tools and rules of the modern science game are in place, and the traditional mind–body problems, which so concerned Rubinstein, take a new and constrained form. As Mandler (1984) has argued:

> Much of the difficulty that has been generated by the mind–body distinction stems from the failure to consider the relation between well-developed mental and physical theories. Typically, mind and body are discussed in terms of ordinary-language definitions of one or the other. Because these descriptions are far from being well-developed theoretical systems, it is doubtful whether the problems of mind and body as developed by the philosophers are directly relevant to the scientific distinction between mental and physical systems.
>
> Once it is agreed that the scientific mind–body problem concerns the relation between two sets of theories, the enterprise becomes theoretical and empirical, not metaphysical. If, however, we restrict our discussion of the mind–body problem to the often vague and frequently contradictory speculations of ordinary language, then, as centuries of philosophical literature have shown, the morass is unavoidable and bottomless. (p. 29)

For Holt (1967a), it appears somehow that a psychological model can only work to account for the reality of psychosomatic interaction by drifting into theoretical inconsistency. The approach of cognitive science permits a different, more optimistic view. I would suggest that it is precisely the inconsistency of Freud's model that has brought us to the philosophical morass in which we find ourselves today and has led to the abandonment of hope for a scientific theory of the psychoanalytic process by many who have devoted their careers to this goal. We need to move toward theoretical coherence at the same time as we accept clinical reality, or we will not be able to achieve either.

THE NATURE OF A PSYCHOLOGICAL MODEL

Gill was fundamentally correct in arguing that physiological concepts cannot provide an adequate level of explanation for psychological events. However, in viewing psychological significance as equivalent to intentionality or phenomenological experience, Gill, like Klein (1973, 1976), seems—inexplicably—to restrict a psychological model to the level of conscious events. Rubinstein was seeking a level of explanation that was not restricted to conscious experience, but to develop such an explanatory theory, he found it necessary to go beyond the mental or psychological and into the physiological domain.

The positions of Rubinstein and Holt, from one vantage point, and those of Gill and Klein, from another, may be understood as a reflection of the limitations of scientific psychology prior to the advent of the cognitive revolution of the past quarter century. While important as a response to the formulations based on phenomenology and intentionality, which were put forth by Klein and Gill at the time, the objections to a psychological model that were raised by Rubinstein and Holt appear anachronistic in the scientific context of today. The construction of a psychological theory to account for nonconscious as well as conscious mental representations and processes is the day-to-day work of the cognitive science field (Baars, 1986; Mandler, 1984). The theory that we ultimately seek is a network that, as Hawking formulates this, relates concepts and quantities in the model—mental representations and processes—to one another and to observations that we make. The field of cognitive science, and its related disciplines, using the approach of all modern science, has introduced the means by which such a theory may be developed.

In cognitive science, mental representations and processes—whether conscious or unconscious—are treated as hypothetical constructs defined in terms of other concepts and inferred from observable events in the context of a general theoretical framework. Psychological entities, defined in this way, have the same theoretical status as particles and quarks, dark matter, the big bang, and life in the Bronze Age. All are theoretical entities that are not directly observable but are defined at varying levels of directness through connection to one another and to observable events. Subjective meanings have a role in a scientific enterprise when considered as such theoretical entities; they cannot be studied scientifically without such a framework. It is the power of the theoretical framework that enables a science of subjective meaning, such as psychoanalysis, to be constructed.

If we accept a characterization of such theoretical networks as metaphoric, pseudodualistic, or low-level theories, as Rubinstein suggests, we must also recognize that all of psychology, and on a broader level, all of modern science, operates in this way. The existence of "black holes" or extra matter is inferred from readings of the speed or trajectory of planets, using computational formulas derived from a theoretical model. Similarly, the mass and behavior of particles are inferred from indicators of their effects. Such inference to unobservable events is also the way in which archaeologists construct knowledge of times long past.

In such a network, there may be different levels of theoretical entities, reflecting different degrees of inference from observable events (Feigl, 1956; Margenau, 1950). Thus, a psychoanalytic theory might include intervening variables, which are lower level, experience-near concepts—for example, desiring, feeling sad, feeling angry—inferred relatively directly from observables, such as facial expression, speech, and action; and may in principle include hypothetical constructs that are more abstract, such as id, ego, superego, the systems conscious and unconscious, and the primary and secondary processes of thought. The second and higher order constructs may represent interactions among the lower level, experience-near variables, or composites of these. The difference in levels of abstraction of the constructs is reflected in the number of inferential steps. In contrast to Rubinstein's position, a consistent psychological theory can potentially incorporate higher order concepts, but can only do so to the extent that they are systematically defined.

In constructing a theoretical framework or "nomological network" of this sort, the scientific challenge arises in the development of reliable and valid observable indicators and inferential rules that determine how mental events are defined. A mature science is characterized by a high ratio of observable indicators in proportion to the hypothetical constructs and intervening variables, and by multiple defining connections within the theoretical net (Margenau, 1950). Psychological theories (and theories in the social sciences generally) differ from theories in the natural sciences, not in their level of explanation, as dependent on hypothetical constructs, but in their relatively minimal development of observable measures and defining links. In these terms, the basic scientific problem of the metapsychology is not so much that the propositions of the theory have been disconfirmed, but that the actual scientific work of constructing and testing the systematic networks of definitions and developing their linkage to observables has really never been carried out.

The danger of a psychological model is not that it is "dualistic," or an "as-if dualism," or even a "metaphoric position," in the terms used by

Rubinstein. A scientific theory must be built on a framework of hypothetical constructs; there is no other way. The real danger is the kind of wild reification that has proliferated in the psychoanalytic theory, with endless multiplication of empty theoretical terms. Psychoanalytic theory has indeed been particularly burdened with a multitude of highly abstract theoretical terms, which are not linked systematically to one another, or to observables. This, rather than the use of conceptual terms per se, is the self-defeating legacy of the metapsychology.

While Rubinstein has advocated elimination of higher order theoretical constructs in favor of constructs that are more directly observable, we suggest this is not a necessary or even a desirable step. Our goal must be to provide multiple defining links for the conceptual nodes of the model and multiple connections to observables, rather than to attempt to do without hypothetical constructs because they are subject to reification when improperly used. In this attempt, those higher order terms that can be systematically defined in the theoretical network will be retained; concepts that are not linked consistently to other nodes of the network, or to observables, will ultimately be dropped.

Paradoxically, in a psychoanalytic model, it may be easier to accept the higher order concepts as having the status of hypothetical constructs in the scientific sense than lower level concepts—terror, love, rage, fear of abandonment, and expectations of attack, loss and annihilation—which are so experience-near. The characterization of experiential states as hypothetical constructs may be more understandable if we consider the anxiety, love, and interpersonal expectations of other persons rather than our own. Like any other hypothetical entities, the inner states of other persons must be inferred from observable events. This need for inference applies to the conscious as well as nonconscious mentation of other people. Thus, rage or anxiety as it exists in another person is inferred from a range of operational indicators that may include facial expressions, verbal and motoric behaviors, and biological measures. The category of observables may also include one individual's conscious experience as an indicator of the experience of another, as in the use of countertransference reactions or judges' ratings of various types. We all work with implicit theories concerning the emotions of others in our daily interactions with them, and we all use systems of operational indicators derived from our implicit theories. The approach of cognitive science as applied in this book is obviously not to deny or to "cognitivize" emotions, but to find a way of incorporating the emotions, conscious and unconscious, into a systematic scientific model, which has the potential to expand our understanding of our clinical work. What the scientific theory attempts to do is to systematize and integrate the kind of inferences that we work with into a general model, which may be investigated in systematic ways.

It should be clear that the approach used here does indeed characterize a stimulus in terms of its psychological significance, in Gill's terms, but without restricting the domain of psychological significance to conscious thought. We should also stress that the restriction of experiential terms—love, hate, sadness, rage—to their systematic definitions within a theoretical net does not imply disinterest in the subjective meaning of everyday experience but is necessary to enable scientific study of such experience on both conscious and unconscious levels. The identification of conscious or unconscious rage, or anxiety, in another person can only proceed on the basis of a theory of how such feelings are defined and manifested; this in no way denies the existence or the meaning of the subjective experience. We may note that the identification of unconscious processes in oneself requires inference in the same sense.

FREUD'S THEORETICAL MODEL: THE ENERGY THEORY

Freud's attempt to build an abstract theoretical model of the psychical apparatus predates the approach of model building in cognitive psychology today. Brenner and Erdelyi understand Freud's approach in this way, each from his own very different perspective. Hartmann (1950) made similar claims in asserting that the structural theory was constructed in terms of groupings of psychological functions, ultimately definable in operational terms.

Like many abstract psychological models, the metapsychology was based on structures and processes derived from physical domains; in the case of Freud's energy theory, it was based on principles of Newtonian mechanics. This approach to model building works to the extent that the structure of the explanatory domain provides a good fit for the domains of emotion and mind. What is crucial but sometimes tends to be forgotten in carrying out this approach is that the propositions that are generated from a model need to be tested in their own terms. It is not sufficient, and in fact not relevant, to test the basic premises of the model in their original domain, as discussed in Chapter 1.

The energy theory has been tested to some degree and found wanting in the physical and biological domains. It is also the case, however, that the findings in the biological domain do not disconfirm the propositions of the metapsychology as a psychological model, although they may lead us to question the applicablility of the model. Conversely, perhaps even more difficult to accept, the evidence of Pribram and Gill (1976), purportedly supporting aspects of Freud's energy theory on a biological level, does not provide validation for the psychological theory.

The particular model of the psychical apparatus, developed by Freud based on the processes of Newtonian mechanics, has not yielded the systematic and coherent explanatory account that we require; this in no way implies that we should turn away from model building as a strategy. The failure of the metapsychology was at least in part because the fit of the energy model to the functions of mind has not been good; the human organism cannot usefully be construed as the kind of closed system in which the principles of energy distribution, as postulated in the metapsychology, might apply (von Bertalanffy, 1950). Cognitive science has begun to address the challenge of building theoretical nets for mental processes based on domains of information processing that seem to have a better fit. The classical approach to cognitive science has been based on the architecture and function of information processing in the von Neumann computer, as we shall see in detail in Chapter 5. This has been a productive source of hypotheses concerning human mental functions, although its limits are now being recognized to an increasing degree. New psychological models based on neural networks are now being developed in cognitive psychology that account for aspects of mental function that classical symbolic models cannot. These include aspects of processing or "computation" associated with the primary process and the dynamic unconscious, as these are understood psychoanalytically. Studies of parallel preattentive processes and automaticity, among others, have provided operational methods for exploring processes that are outside of awareness. As Posner and Rothbart (1989) point out, cognitive psychologists are now "coming to understand that much of our mental life is structured outside of consciousness and that our intentional control of mental events represents only one, perhaps small, part of the mind" (p. 451). Thus, in the development of a systematic psychological theory for psychoanalysis, we are not restricted to the domain of phenomenology or intentionality, as Klein and Gill appear to have assumed, but can systematically address unconscious processes as well.

ESCAPE FROM THE MIND–BODY MORASS

The modern approach to doing psychological science that has been advocated here now frees us to identify, and distinguish, a bundle of different "mind–body" questions or ways in which mental and physiological events and the relationships between them may be defined, in place of the monolithic "mind–body problem" with which Rubinstein was concerned. In developing a theoretical framework, we need to distinguish three levels of theoretical relationships involving constructs of emotion and mind:

1. Relationships between mental and emotional constructs and observable events. These include relationships of *reference, inference, explanation,* and *prediction.*

2. Relationships between mental and emotional constructs, and neurological constructs (mind and brain). These include relationships of *translatability,* which do appropriately apply, and relationships of *reducibility,* which do not.

3. Relationships between mental and emotional constructs and somatic constructs (mind and body proper). These include relationships of *interaction* and *representation.*

Relationships between Mental and Emotional Constructs and Observable Events

1. The theoretical terms of psychoanalysis *refer* to or signify mental or emotional representations or processes, which are hypothetical constructs defined within a theoretical framework or nomological network.

2. Variation in these constructs and the relationships between them are *inferred* as a function of variation in specified observables; the functions are based on the relationships specified in the nomological network. For a psychological theory of mind, the observables may include language and behavior; they may also include neurological and biological observations; they may include judgments by observers as well.

3. Theories *explain* or account for data; theories do not explain other theories, and data do not explain theories. The theoretical constructs and relationships between them are successful to the extent that they account for observations.

4. In the terms of these relationships, we make *predictions* from theories to variations in observable events. Models are validated or disconfirmed in terms of their ability to account for or predict observable data, not their correspondence to other models.

The kinds of conceptual relationships we have just discussed—*reference* or *signification, inference, explanation,* and *prediction*—concern the relationships between hypothetical constructs and observable events within the theoretical framework of a model of mind. These relationships need to be distinguished from the relationship between psychological and neurological levels, that is, between the sets of hypothetical constructs that constitute the separate theoretical networks of "mind" and "brain."

Relationships between Mental and Emotional Constructs and Neurological Constructs

In modern psychology, as in neurology, it is assumed that the brain is the organ of mental activity and that the different levels of mind and brain must in principle be *translatable* to one another, although the translation might be too cumbersome to carry out in practice. The level of Newtonian mechanics is in principle translatable to the level of particle physics; particles make up all matter. However, the assumption of translatability needs to be differentiated from the fallacious position of viewing mental constructs as *reducible* to physiological ones. The engineer would rely on the principles of Newtonian mechanics, not of quantum mechanics or particle physics, to design a rocket or a bridge. The computer scientist works on the level of the program, not the individual binary switches that constitute the hardware of the system. The tennis instructor works on the level of coordination of sensory and motoric behavior, not in terms of the cells that make up the muscles or the neurons that feed the sensory systems. In all these contexts, the nomological networks of one theoretical level chunk the domain of observation differently from the other; they are not reducible to one another. The analyst works on the level of cognitive, linguistic, somatic, and emotional systems in an interpersonal context. Although each of these systems is assumed to have neural substrates, the analyst could not frame his psychological models in terms of neurons, any more than the engineer could make his computations in terms of particles.

We may note that the theoretical frameworks of the psychical apparatus and the neural substrate may account for some of the same observable data, while formulating the underlying theoretical structure in quite different ways. Failure of correspondence in the predictions and inferences of such theories would raise questions for each of them; the finding of correspondence would strengthen theoretical positions, as I will illustrate in the specific models of mental function to be presented in Sections Two and Three.

We may also note that the relationship between constructs of mind and brain may include the use of neurological data as indicators of variation in mental constructs. Just as behavioral observations may provide evidence concerning psychological theories, so neurological observations may provide evidence of their own sort. For example, in research by Shevrin and his colleagues (as discussed in Chapter 3), electrically recorded brain responses are used as indicators of unconscious and conscious mental events. Similarly, hippocampal activation provides evidence concerning differences in memory functions in different types of task situations, as we shall see in Chapter 6.

Widlocher (1990) has addressed the issue of the relationship between neurobiology and psychoanalysis, in current terms, and has
incorporated some of the distinctions that have been made earlier. He
states the necessary condition of translatability as follows: "The guiding
principle is to make compatible the notional system of psychoanalysis
with that of neurobiology. . . . That which expresses itself in one area
must be able to exist in the other" (p. 341).[1] At the same time, he also
recognizes that the establishment of such correspondence requires a
psychological model:

> Our conclusion will be that one cannot establish a direct compatibility
> between psychoanalysis and neurobiology and that we need an interme-
> diate operator, a kind of transformer, in order to pass from one domain
> to another. As did Kandel, although with other arguments, we suggest
> that the so-called "cognitive" psychology allows the building of such an
> operator. (p. 341)[2]

The position of this book is in agreement with Widlocher concerning
the need for a psychological model. However, rather than conceptualizing
the psychological model as a mediating operator between psychoanalysis
and neurobiology, I argue that a psychological model potentially functions
as a unifying theoretical framework that encompasses the clinical concepts of psychoanalysis on a continuum with other functions. The overall
study of cognition may be understood as comprising several separate
domains of study, including perception in various sensory modalities,
memory, language, and reasoning, and also as comprising a psychoanalytic sector. Just as the study of perception incorporates the interaction
of mental representations and functions with the activity of the sensory
apparatus, the psychoanalytic sector of the cognitive domain would focus
on emotional experience and unconscious, including warded-off mentation, its interaction with somatic events, and the effects of verbalization
on these processes.

Reiser (1985) recognizes the status of the metapsychology as a
psychological theory, but also argues for an explanatory level based on
neurophysiology. As Reiser argues, it was Freud

---

[1]Le principe qui nous guide est de rendre compatible le système notionnel de la
psychanalyse avec celui de la neurobiologie. . . . Ce qui s'exprime dans un domaine
doit pouvoir l'être dans l'autre (trans.: J. Maskit).

[2]Notre conclusion sera que l'on ne peut établir de compatibilité directe entre
psychanalyse et neurobiologie et qu'il nous faut un opérateur intermédiaire, une
manière de transformateur, pour passer d'un domaine à l'autre. Comme Kandel, mais
avec d'autres arguments, nous poserons que la psychologie dite "cognitive" permet de
construire cet opérateur (trans.: J. Maskit).

who took the lead in abandoning nineteenth century physiology, but he did so without giving up hope and "belief" that brain science would ultimately provide relevant and useful explanatory information. I, for one, cannot imagine that he would dismiss or turn away from the neurobiologic information now available, some hundred years later. (p. 16)

I would agree with Reiser's position, except for the claim of brain science as providing explanatory information. On the basis of the distinctions that have been made here, we can see that it cannot be the case that neurobiological data will *explain* psychoanalytic concepts. As we have seen, theories account for or explain data; information (data) does not explain theoretical concepts. Reiser's point is well taken, provided neurobiological observations are seen as providing *evidence* rather than *explanation* for a psychological model. Thus, inferences may be made from neurophysiological data as well as from behavioral and linguistic data, to psychological constructs and psychological theories, and such data may contribute to the construction and testing of psychological theories, as in the work of Shevrin and his colleagues discussed earlier. We would also hope that psychoanalytic theory would contribute to an explanation of the neurological observations.

Relationships between Mental and Emotional Constructs and Somatic Constructs

In addition to the relationship between the conceptual levels of "mind" and "brain," there is another type of relationship that needs to be studied, and that has a somewhat different epistemological status. This concerns the *interactions* among mental and somatic functions: the extent to which mental functions direct or regulate somatic ones, and the extent to which somatic events are represented in the mind. Here we are concerned with accounting for the effects of wishes, beliefs, fears, anger on physiological systems; the interaction by which emotion may cause headaches, ulcers, hysterical paralysis, and even suppress the operation of the immune system in a more general sense; and also with the question of how our physical state may affect mental functions.

As we have already noted, the issue of psychosomatic interaction would need to be considered whether we talk about mental events on the level of psychological or neurological models. Psychological models, as noted earlier, have customarily accounted for activation of the sensory and motoric apparatuses. All that we are adding here is that it is necessary to expand psychological models to include interaction with somatic and visceral systems as well; this is particularly important for an emotional information-processing model.

Another type of relationship between mind and body, which is related to, but distinguished from, their interaction, is the fact that somatic experience, including visceral, kinesthetic, and motoric, as well as sensory experience, may be *represented* in the mind. Like sensory representations, these representations—temperature, respiratory changes, gut feelings of all sorts—may be conscious or unconscious. The features of somatic representation require definition within a psychological model, exactly as do the forms and contents of the various sensory modalities. In psychological models, the factors affecting perception have been elaborated extensively for the visual and to a somewhat lesser extent for the auditory modalities. Psychophysiological and other forms of perception research in these modalities are traditional domains of research in experimental psychology. There is now also beginning to be a psychology of the olfactory sense, as will be discussed in Chapter 7. The psychology of somatic or visceral experience may be developed in precisely this way.

CONCLUSIONS: WHAT KIND OF THEORY DO WE NEED?

A new theory is required that is able to account for the processes of mind and emotion, and for the interaction of mind and body, with which psychoanalysis is fundamentally concerned. The concept of "mind," including conscious and unconscious events, has been formulated in terms of hypothetical constructs defined by relationship to observables and to other constructs within the theoretical framework of a nomological net. "Mind" may be said to have moved (graduated) from the philosophical to the scientific realm of discourse by this means. Two types of mind–body interface have also been distinguished: the relationship between mind and brain, the neural substrate; and the relationship between mind and the entire range of somatic events. Subtypes of relationships have been distinguished within each of these categories.

The position of this book is that Freud's general concept of an abstract psychical apparatus remains sound, although the metapsychology has failed. It is not necessary to reject Freud's goal of developing an explanatory theory of the mental apparatus because the first attempt did not succeed. A clinical theory is not adequate as a general explanatory model; an overarching theoretical framework is required to provide definitions for clinical concepts. The variety of alternate clinical hypotheses that are being proposed today can only be formulated in coherent and potentially testable form, and distinguished systematically from one another within a consistent theoretical framework. While the psychological theory that is needed must be potentially translatable into neurophysiological terms, it cannot be reducible to that level, but must develop its own concepts and its own definitions on the psychological level.

No theory has yet been developed within cognitive psychology that provides the account we require for psychoanalysis—an account of the human organism as a multicode emotional information processor, with substantial but limited integration of systems. In the following chapters, I will develop such a theory based on current work in cognitive psychology, emotion theory, and theories of cognitive and emotional development. I will then show how this multiple code theory can provide a framework for developing consistent definitions of the basic concepts and processes of psychoanalysis and a foundation for empirical research. I also expect that some of the ideas in this model, which are directed by insights of psychoanalysis, and which are potentially testable in the psychoanalytic situation, may feed back to inform the cognitive psychology field.

As cognitive scientists recognize today, the challenge to the field does not lie in determining the ontological status of mental (or emotional) events. The ontological questions, the status of the domains of emotion and mind, have now been resolved, in pragmatic terms, in the mainstream fields of psychology as in the physical sciences. Psychologists have shifted their focus from the metaphysics of ontology to the pragmatics of epistemology—the question of *how we know* these domains—and have achieved a resolution that allows us to do our scientific work. We can now afford a more sanguine view concerning the possibility of constructing a coherent psychological model to account for the "powerful emotions and drives of real life" than Holt, Rubinstein, Klein, or Gill could take in the limiting context of the behaviorist psychologies of their time.

SECTION TWO

COMPONENTS OF THE MULTIPLE CODE THEORY: CURRENT RESEARCH

As we have seen, Freud's theory emphasized the operation of two distinct modes of thought: the primary process, which is the mode of operation of the unconscious or the id and is associated with nonverbal functions; and the secondary process, the mode of conscious thought or of the ego, associated with verbal forms. Freud's theory also emphasized the role of verbalization in psychical organization and psychical change. The crucial discovery that talking can cure emotional and even bodily ills is now widely recognized, even beyond psychoanalysis. However, Freud's metapsychology, which is rooted in energic concepts, does not help us to understand these interactive effects in psychological terms.

The dual code model (Bucci, 1985) was a first attempt to apply concepts of modern cognitive science to develop a general psychological theory of the psychoanalytic process. The field of cognitive science has expanded exponentially since that paper was written. The view that the human information-processing system is characterized by multiple, disparate representations and processes is far more widely accepted today than it was a decade ago. The controversies that are central now primarily concern the characterization of the disparate modes of representation, the bases for their differentiation, and the level at which the differentiation occurs. The new research has also begun to address the issue of the integration of emotion in the human information-processing system and has examined the roots of these processes in cognitive and emotional development, and the effects of the interpersonal world. We are now in a position to formulate a more comprehensive and elaborate model of mind and emotion, as this applies to the general development of adaptive processing modes, to their breakdown in pathology, and to the modes of repair in the psychoanalytic process, than was possible a decade ago.

In this section, I outline the basic research that has contributed to our formulation of the multiple code theory. I begin with a discussion of models of the architectures of mind, the enduring, hypothetical structures that are postulated as accounting for human information processing and human memory. I turn then to issues of the multiple functions that information processing and memory must serve, including functions that are specific to particular sensory modalities, then to the relation of emotion and cognition, as this develops in children and continues in adult life. I will also cover neurophysiological evidence that is relevant to our new psychological model.

In essence, what I will do in this section is initiate the basic construction of the nomological network within which the underlying representations and processes—the hypothetical constructs—that make up the multiple code theory may be defined. This section develops the constructs that will be used in the multiple code theory. In the next section, I can then go to a formulation of the multiple code theory and to a multiple code account of pathology and its repair in treatment.

CHAPTER 5

The Architecture of Cognition
SYMBOLIC AND
SUBSYMBOLIC PROCESSING

The "architecture" of cognition refers to the general structures underlying human information processing. The symbolic architecture has, until recently, been generally accepted as the dominant, if not only possible approach in artificial intelligence and in cognitive science. More recently, models based on contrasting types of architecture have been postulated, which have been variously termed subsymbolic, connectionist, or parallel distributed processing (PDP) models.

THE SYMBOLIC ARCHITECTURE

According to the classical symbolic approach, intelligent beings are symbol systems operating on representations that have the format of symbolic codes. The two main classes of intelligent beings are human beings and computers. The concept of the symbol and the process of symbolizing are defined here in their general information-processing sense (Fodor & Pylyshyn, 1988). Symbols are entities that refer to other entities and have the capacity to be combined in rule-governed ways, so that an infinite array of meaningful units can be generated from a finite set of elements. Symbols may be images or words; symbols in the psychoanalytic sense constitute a subset of these.

The classical symbolic architecture follows the general design of the von Neumann computer. This includes some version of the following types of processing units:

1. Buffer memories, which are extremely brief, modality-specific memories connected to the sensory organs.
2. Short-term memory, with rapid access and limited capacity, which operates within attentional focus and serves as the gateway to the long-term memory store.
3. Long-term memory, with longer access time, not within attentional focus, and with virtually unlimited capacity.
4. Control structures overseeing the operation and integration of these processing units.

The buffer memories, which are composed of modality-specific elements connected to different sensory organs, are necessarily multiple in format. There is also general agreement within cognitive science as to the operation of multiple processing channels within short-term memory, as well as specific mechanisms for processing language and imagery. The controversy concerning coding format, among the various types of single code theories, including verbal or perceptual dominance, dual or multiple code theories, and common code models, concerns the long-term-memory component of the symbolic architecture.

Verbal Dominance Theory: Then and Now

Verbal dominance or verbal mediation theories view thought as encoded in verbal form; in some instances, this is a heuristic permitting empirical research; in others, it is a substantive theoretical position. Verbal learning and verbal behavior models have been dominant in the study of human cognition from the time of Watson (1913) until the cognitive revolution of the 1960s. In several forms of this paradigm, language was viewed as determining, mediating, or even constituting thought. The cultural relativism of Whorf (1950, 1964) and, in a different way, the verbal mediation position of Vygotsky (1934) reflect this point of view. Implicitly, the verbal mediation position has been deeply influential in psychology and philosophy, as well as in psychoanalytic theory, as examined in the first section of this book and as discussed elsewhere (Bucci, 1985).

The theory of Chomsky (1957, 1965), with its formulation of deep and abstract syntactic structures, may be characterized as a current, more sophisticated version of verbal dominance theory. According to Chomsky, the capacity to acquire and use language is species specific and innate, with its own developmental line, which is distinct from other aspects of cognitive development. While the specifics of language learning are necessarily environmentally driven, in that children learn the particular native language of the country into which they are born, Chomsky argues that there are universals of language syntax that are shared by all languages and reflect the innate structure of the human brain.

Most cognitive scientists today accept the view of language as a specifically human function that emerged relatively late both phylogenetically and ontogenetically and is learned by virtually all humans, regardless of intellectual level, and by no other species. While nonhuman primates show considerable capacity for problem solving and some sign-using behaviors, there are enormous differences in the level of such behaviors that can be acquired by humans and apes, and enormous differences in the necessary acquisition contexts. Primates other than humans require long and intensive repetition to acquire a level of sign-using ability that is far below that acquired without focused training by retarded human adults. The intensive attempts to teach aspects of language to nonhuman primates (Gardner & Gardner, 1969; Premack & Premack, 1983) have, in fact, had the converse effect of supporting the species-specific nature of language (Pinker, 1989).

On the other hand, there is less general support for Chomsky's strong position concerning the modularity of language, the operation of innate linguistic universals, and also less support for the role of linguistic forms in determining or mediating thought. Many cognitive scientists today, representing a wide range of approaches, argue that communicative language arises from application of general cognitive capacities to the function of communication over vocal and auditory channels (Simon & Kaplan, 1989; Anderson, 1983; Minsky, 1975). The emphasis on linguistic mediation is also diminished by the general recognition of complex, nonlinguistic forms of thought in normal adults, as will be discussed, and by the existence of complex thought processes in prelinguistic infants and nonhuman animals, as well as in deaf persons who lack any form of language. Based on various lines of investigation, there is little support today within cognitive science for linguistic forms as providing the underlying structure in which knowledge is stored.

Imagery Theories: Prototypic Organization in the Perceptual System

The basic controversy concerning imagistic versus linguistic forms as underlying the representation of knowledge in the mind is as old as experimental psychology. The study of imagery was central in introspectionism and associationism (Titchener, 1910; Wundt, 1912), although systematic methods for its operational definition and empirical study had not yet been developed. With the advent of behaviorism (Watson, 1913) and neobehaviorism (Hull, 1943), imagery was excluded as not amenable to scientific investigation and having no role in a scientific theory. The study of imagery remained out of scientific favor until the work of Paivio and others in the early 1960s. In the current cognitive approach, "imagery" is defined in general terms as transient mental representations that are generated on the basis of information stored in memory rather than through direct, ongoing perceptual experience, but that are essentially equivalent to perceptual activity in any given modality (Paivio, 1986; Kosslyn, 1987).

The modern position of perceptual dominance is represented most closely by recent work demonstrating categorical organization based on properties of the perceptual system itself, without mediation by language. In several studies, building on the work of Berlin and Kay (1969), Rosch (1975) has shown that color categories are processed in terms of such prototype organization, reflecting the internal structure of the color domain. Prototypic organization has also been found in studies in which the shapes of objects were compared. The prototypic level was the most inclusive level at which an averaged shape of an object, formed by drawing outlines of normalized, superimposed shapes, could be recognized. Rosch has also proposed that the general concept of internal perceptual structure, which had previously been specified only for natural perceptual domains such as color and form, was applicable as well to objects whose categorization does not have an apparent perceptual basis. In one experiment, Rosch found prototypic objects to be the most general classes to have patterns of motor sequences in common.

Based on her findings, Rosch has argued that basic objects might be the most inclusive categories for which it is possible to form a mental image isomorphic to the appearance of members of the class as a whole. The more prototypic an object is of its class, the more features of this type are shared. Functions, motor movements, perceptual features, and visual images all lead to the same basic level of categorization. As would be expected, these are also the first categories of concrete objects named by children. Thus, children identify "dog" or "cow" before "animal," "table" before "furniture," "apple" before "fruit." The basic conceptual categories are most likely to be represented by "best examples" (rather than some kind of statistical averaging). An alternative way to represent general categories as images would be a grouping of instances, for example, a grouping of different kinds of fruit in a bowl.

The general conclusions reached by Rosch on the basis of her research is that the material objects of the world are classified in categories based on co-occurrence of attributes of function or form. Rosch has also suggested that her analysis in terms of prototypes and basic categories applies to the organization of the flow of experience in terms of events as well as to identification of basic categories of objects. When subjects are asked to describe prototypic events, there is considerable agreement as to the kind of unit into which the event is segmented, and these tend to involve interactions at the basic object level. Furthermore, event boundaries tend to be marked by factors such as "changes of the actors participating with ego, changes in the objects ego interacts with, changes in place, and changes in the type or rate of activity with an object, and by notable gaps in time between two reported events" (Rosch, 1978, p. 44). This corresponds to the finding of Dodd and Bucci (1987) that narrative units are marked by statements of time, place, and person that set the scene and introduce a character in relation to oneself. This also corresponds to the formulation, to be presented in Chapter 12, that emotion structures are organized as prototypic episodes stored in memory, based on the repeated events of one's life—events whose contents and sequential organization are isomorphic in function and form.

Dual and Multiple Code Models

Rosch's research demonstrating independent organization in the nonverbal system prior to and independent of language has been characterized as supporting a perceptual dominance theory. However, this view is also compatible with a dual code theory (Paivio, 1971, 1986; Bucci, 1985), as well as with the new multiple code theory that is presented in this book. Thus, forms of perceptual processing, and of verbal processing, may be considered as components of a model incorporating several different types of codes, rather than there being a single or dominant underlying form in which all information is necessarily represented. Dual coding postulates separate channels of verbal and nonverbal processing rather than dominance of one code. The dual code theory, as formulated by Paivio, focused primarily on visual imagery within the nonverbal system. The new multiple code theory that is the focus of this book and will be presented in detail in Section Three, incorporates representations and processes in all sensory modalities, as well as motoric and visceral information, as contributing to the human information-processing system. These diverse representational forms operate at the level of long-term or semantic memory at which meaning is assigned, not only in short-term or buffer memory. The psychological meaning of an external event, a verbal or perceptual stimulus, is defined by the total set of modality-specific verbal and nonverbal reactions that it typically evokes; these may include word associations, images of objects, nonverbal motor reactions, and affective reactions. Bucci (1985) reviewed a large body of evidence in support of dual coding; additional experimental evidence concerning multiple coding will be presented throughout this section of the book.

Common Code Theories

In the ongoing controversy concerning encoding formats within the cognitive science field, the major opposition to a dual or multiple code theory comes from the common code paradigm rather than from single code perceptual dominance or verbal dominance theories. The classical symbolic paradigm is most closely associated with the abstract common code or propositional approach. According to common code theories, there is a single abstract underlying code, which is common to all information processing, within all sensory modalities, and which underlies verbal as well as nonverbal processing. While short-term or buffer memory may contain specialized systems for language and imagery, the common code approach postulates a single common set of mechanisms used for all forms of thinking—one unified system of semantics shared by all subsystems that deal with meanings. The same system accounts for assignment of meaning to expressions of ordinary language, formal logic, and the number system, and also accounts for nonverbal functions such as imagery. This common code is essential for translation between propositional and image-like informational input.

Several different types of abstract code theories have been proposed. According to one dominant approach, knowledge is encoded by a system of symbolic codes that are structured much like a language (as in the logical calculi); thus, information would be represented in the form of propositions or networks of propositions (Pylyshyn, 1973; Simon & Kaplan, 1989; Fodor & Pylyshyn, 1988). Propositions may also be stored in memory in a variety of formats, for example, as strings similar to natural language sentences, in the notation of the predicate calculus, or as components of networks.

There are also common code theories built on nonlinguistic underlying formats. These include models in which information processing is viewed as a process of heuristic search for problem solutions, using representations that may be image-like and that model the problem domain in certain respects. Images may be stored in memory in pictorial or diagrammatic form, as arrays of points, or as node-link structures incorporated in networks (Simon & Kaplan, 1989).

According to Johnson-Laird's (1989) version of a common code approach, reasoning is based on mental models that are equivalent to internal symbols and represent the *reference* of verbal discourse; they are internal representations of the situation that the discourse describes. Thus, while Johnson-Laird accepts the fundamental common code approach, he has extended this to a formulation of mental models that integrate information from the senses with general knowledge, providing representations that are isomorphic with or correspond to the structure of the situation being represented, rather than an abstract description of it. In these terms, the specific nature of the content will determine the relationships that are expressed and the reasoning that is carried out; not formal rules of inference alone. Johnson-Laird's model may be viewed as a kind of hybrid common code theory (or perhaps a virtual multiple code model), which includes concrete, content-sensitive as well as abstract, structure-determined components.

Evidence for Dual or Multiple versus Common Code Theories

The operation of distinct pictorial and linguistic formats is now generally recognized at the processing stages of stimulus input and short-term memory, even by common code theorists. As Simon and Kaplan (1989) point out, human beings have or acquire the ability to discriminate among phonemes in their native language, to recognize word boundaries, and to parse syntax in their native language. They also have or must acquire the ability to "discriminate among the features of visually presented stimuli, to recognize familiar kinds of objects, and to detect and recognize the relations among objects in a visual scene" (p. 16). Other species, without language, nevertheless give evidence of knowledge of objects and their relationships, and function in a world that requires such knowledge. "It seems parsimonious, even apart from the empirical evidence of brain localization, to postulate that there are specialized mechanisms for processing linguistic messages, on the one hand, and visual stimuli, on the other" (p. 16).

The major controversy, as we have said, concerns the existence of separate representational systems at the level of long-term memory at which knowledge is stored and meaning is derived. A wide range of evidence has also been developed supporting such multiple rather than common code representation at the long-term memory level. One line of evidence, developed by Paivio and his colleagues, is based on the dual code postulate that the nonverbal imagery system, which is linked to perceptual experience, is more likely to be activated by concrete objects and events; the verbal system dominates in abstract and formal tasks. A corollary of this is that the referential connections, in either direction, between words and referent objects are more active and direct for concrete words and the entities to which they refer and less direct for abstract concepts and things. Therefore, reaction times for imagery arousal are expected to be faster for concrete than for abstract words. This hypothesis has been supported in many studies. In addition, concrete words have been shown to facilitate learning and memory in a wide range of tasks (Paivio, 1966).

Another major premise of dual or multiple code formulations is that imagery is functionally and structurally similar to perception in each modality and uses at least some parts of the same processing systems. A wide range of studies of visual imagery has demonstrated equivalent effects of perceptual and imaginal conditions in facilitating learning and recall. Learning of concrete words is facilitated in a highly similar way by showing pictures of objects designated by the words, and by instructions to create visual images of these objects (Denis, 1975). Similar results were found for memory for phrases describing actions (Engelkamp, 1986) and for positions of letters in a matrix (Peterson, 1975).

In a study by Kosslyn, Ball, and Reiser (1978), subjects were instructed to study a map of a fictional island and then asked to estimate distances between particular locations from memory. The reaction time was longer for pairs of locations that were actually farther apart on the map, indicating that the mental map functions as does the real perceived one, and that subjects were mentally scanning from one object to the other.

In a series of studies comparing visual functions in perception and imagery, Shepard and his colleagues have also shown that images may be processed by mechanisms similar to those that apply to percepts and with similar results. Shepard and Metzler (1971) presented drawings of pairs of three-dimensional objects in different orientations and asked subjects to determine whether two shapes in a pair represented objects that were the same or different. For identical objects, the time to make the decision was proportional to their angular disparity; the same results have been replicated in many studies with a wide range of stimuli. According to Shepard and his associates (Shepard, 1975; Shepard & Cooper, 1982), the results indicate that subjects carry out a mental rotation process to bring the two images into alignment; larger angles of rotation require proportionally more processing time.

In contrast to the large body of evidence that has been developed in support of dual coding, the empirical research supporting common code theories is rather weak. Several studies have found that subjects are unable to remember whether they saw a particular sentence or a simple drawing expressing the same meaning, and bilingual subjects are frequently unable to remember whether a sentence they saw was in French or English (Bransford & Franks, 1971; Rosenberg & Simon 1977). However, the results in this research paradigm have been found to vary with the nature of the material and the means of testing (Roediger & Blaxton, 1987). Subjects will remember either the general or the surface form, depending on how the testing is carried out. Thus, the question of the format of encoding in long-term memory is confounded with the method of retrieval; this objection applies to many of the experimental results that have previously been interpreted as supporting common code theories.

The arguments put forth for common code theories are framed largely on conceptual grounds and as theoretical or methodological critiques of the dual code research, rather than derived from empirical findings. Some common code theorists (Pylyshyn, 1973; Anderson, 1978) have argued that results supporting imagery or dual coding theories may be accounted for by subjects' tacit knowledge of the experimenter's expectations and the characteristics of perceptual stimuli. In response to these critiques, investigators have carried out a number of studies that ruled out the effects of tacit knowledge or compliance with experimenter expectations, and that continued to support previous findings in favor of dual or multiple coding at the underlying level of meaning. Thus, for example, investigators have shown that the activation of perceptual pathways by imagery extends to certain effects of this activation of the type that subjects would not be able to infer, including differential afterimage (Finke & Schmidt, 1978) and image-resolution effects (Kosslyn, 1975, 1983; Finke & Kosslyn, 1980). Also in response to these methodological critiques, investigators have shown that differential reaction times in imaginal tasks are determined by factors similar to those determining reaction times in the corresponding perceptual tasks (Podgorny & Shepard, 1978). Selective, modality-specific interference of function has been found for imaging as well as perceiving; imaging and perceiving in the same modality are likely to interfere with each other more than imaging in one modality and perceiving in another (Segal, 1972; Segal & Fusella, 1970; Baddeley, 1986; Brooks, 1970). Subjects are unlikely to have knowledge—tacit or explicit—concerning such technical features of visual perception as the particular pattern and hues of color aftereffects, size, and other features of the field of focal resolution, or complex interference and facilitation processes. Unless one could account for acquisition of such knowledge, the results must be interpreted as dependent on use of similar visual-processing mechanisms for imagining an object, as for perceiving it directly, and thus, as demonstrating modality-specific rather than abstract, propositional encoding underlying imagistic representations.

Neurophysiological Evidence

Studies using techniques such as measures of regional cerebral blood flow measured by PET scans, electroencephalography (EEG), and event-related potentials (ERPs) with samples of normal subjects have provided additional compelling evidence showing that imagery occupies the same channels as are occupied by perception that cannot be explained by subject knowledge or compliance effects. Roland and Friberg (1985) found different patterns of cerebral blood flow in visual imagery tasks compared to mental arithmetic and auditory imagery tasks. Goldenberg, Podreka, Steiner, and Willmes (1987) found greater visual-area activation for questions requiring visual imagery (e.g., "Is the green of pine trees darker than the green of grass?") in comparison to abstract questions (e.g., "Is the categorical imperative an ancient grammatical form?"). Using EEG techniques, Davidson and Schwartz (1977) found the site of maximum alpha suppression, associated with increased brain activity, over the visual (occipital) area of the brain in a visual imagery task (imagining a flashing light) and over the tactile (parietal) areas in a tactile imagery condition (imagining one's forearm being tapped). From the perspective of multiple coding, this is a very important study in showing effects for imaging parallel to perceiving in the tactile as well as visual modalities. In several studies Farah (1988) and her colleagues have found highly localized increases in positivity of ERPs at the occipital electrodes in visual imagery conditions.

Studies of brain-damaged patients have revealed specific deficits in imagery ability that parallel their perceptual impairments. Patients with acquired cerebral color blindness are unable to state the colors of common objects from memory, although their general imagery function appears to remain unimpaired (Sacks & Wasserman, 1987; Riddoch & Humphreys, 1987). Patients with bilateral parieto-occipital disease are unable to localize visually presented objects and to indicate their positions either verbally or by pointing, although they retain their ability to identify objects and to orient to tactile and auditory stimuli. Conversely, patients with temporo-occipital disease, characterized as agnosic, have generally adequate visual and spatial capabilities but are unable to recognize and identify visually presented objects; their impairment is also modality specific and does not extend to identification of objects by touch or sound. For both these types of impairments, Farah (1988) and her associates have found corresponding dissociations in the patients' imagery systems.

The phenomenon of "visual neglect," in which patients with right parietal lobe damage may fail to detect stimuli presented in the left half of the visual field, provides dramatic evidence for imagery effects. Bisiach and Luzzatti (1978) asked two patients with such damage to imagine viewing a familiar square, the Piazza del Duomo in Milan, from a particular vantage point; both patients omitted from their descriptions the landmarks that would have fallen on the left side of the scene. When these patients were asked to imagine the same square from the opposite vantage point, the converse results were obtained; the patients now reported the landmarks that had previously been omitted and omitted those that currently fell on the left side of the image. We may conclude that the bulk of empirical evidence supports dual or multiple formats of representation and processing, not only at the sensory or short-term memory level, but also at the level of long-term-memory at which meaning is assigned. The experimental and neurophysiological research have fully addressed the critiques based on subject knowledge or compliance with anticipated results.

We may also say a word about the conceptual arguments that have been put forth by common code theorists. These include arguments based on internal theoretical criteria, such as simplicity, and claims that the nature of a propositional theory is such that it is inherently not susceptible of disconfirmation, that is, that any format is in principle restatable in propositional terms (Anderson, 1978).

It is not clear that Occam's razor is on the common code side. At the very least, it seems to cut both ways. As we have seen, Simon and Kaplan (1989) argue that it seems parsimonious to postulate specialized mechanisms for linguistic messages and visual stimuli; they would presumably include mechanisms for processing stimuli in other sensory modalities as well. If this is so, then at the very least, there must be processes for translation from the various different input formats to the common semantic representation in which they are encoded, as well as from the common code to words. Rather than simplifying the system, the necessity for a two-step process—images to common code to words (or the reverse)—seems to add a step over and above a direct translation between imagery and words. In general, while there may be many sources of complexity in any of the translation processes that have been postulated, it appears difficult to assess relative simplicity of processes that are not at all well understood. On the most basic level, in any case, it is questionable to what extent simplicity is a useful guide for a system such as human information processing that presumably developed in complex multidetermined ways rather than through application of a unified design.

The variation in input format, which is recognized even within common code theories, has other implications that seem to raise difficulties for that approach. It seems likely that the postulated translations from the various input formats will vary as to their immediacy, directness, accuracy, and completeness, depending on the nature of the particular format. Input formats that are more like the underlying code are likely to be translated more quickly and completely than those whose formats are quite different. Along these lines, it seems obvious to many people, including analysts and analytic patients, creative scientists, painters, musicians, poets, and lovers—but is apparently not obvious to cognitive scientists—that there are many important ideas that cannot be fully represented in verbal form. If some types of input information are translated far more adequately than others, and some in fact cannot be translated at all, then we end up with a system that seems tantamount to a multiple code theory. This line of evidence for dual or multiple coding, which psychoanalysis is in a position to augment materially, will be discussed further in Chapter 11.

We may also comment briefly on Anderson's argument that any format is in principle statable in propositional terms, so that a propositional theory is by its very nature not susceptible of disconfirmation. First and most obviously, such an argument taken at face value strips the propositional model of any scientific interest. On the other hand, if we accept the position that any code could be stated in propositional form, this still leaves open the interesting question of whether there is *one or more than one* underlying type of propositional form at the level at which meaning is assigned. The general claim of multiple coding is that there needs to be more than one type of code; this could in principle be satisfied by a system incorporating several types of propositional codes. However, we can now see that the controversy goes beyond this as well. The argument that all types of input information are representable by some form of propositional symbolic code has also been questioned from a new perspective, within the connectionist or PDP approach.

Subsymbolic Processing: The PDP Paradigm

Both common code and dual code theories assume the basic symbolic architecture. On a different level, another controversy has arisen concerning the format of processing that goes beyond the distinction between language and imagery, and the question of whether or not these two modes of representation may be derived from a single underlying code. There is now increasing recognition within cognitive science of a wide range of systematic human information processing for which symbolic processing models—whether common code or dual or multiple code theories—do not provide an adequate account. These include representations and processes in which the elements are not discrete, organization is not categorical, processing occurs simultaneously in multiple parallel channels, higher level units are not generated from discrete elements, and explicit processing rules cannot be identified. As some researchers have argued, complex nonsymbolic computation of this nature underlies creative problem solving, fluent linguistic behavior, practically all skilled performance in animals as well as humans, and many other types of intuitive and implicit processing.

We each draw upon an essentially infinite array of rapid and complex computations, often carried on outside of awareness, often without explicit metrics, dimensions, or units, in most of the common acts of everyday life—in entering a line of traffic, taking down a heavy book from a high shelf, or picking up a piece of paper that has fallen behind the desk:

> Hundreds of times each day we reach for things. We nearly never think about these acts of reaching. And yet, each time, a large number of different considerations appear to jointly determine exactly how we will reach for the object. The position of the object, our posture at the time, what else we may also be holding, the size, shape, and anticipated weight of the object, any obstacles that may be in the way—all of these factors jointly determine the exact method we will use for reaching and grasping. (McClelland, Rumelhart, & Hinton, 1989, p. 4)

The cat uses computations of this nature to select a landing place on a table filled with objects; the football player to throw a ball to where he expects a teammate will be; the tennis player to hit a ball to where he hopes his opponent will not be. The analyst uses computations of this nature to infer the patient's emotional state from all the manifold indicators that are presented to him, including the feelings that are activated in response to the patient, and to decide when and how to intervene.

In such information-processing domains, meanings are expressed in formats that go beyond words or even discrete images. The abstract painter does not set his plans for a project verbally and often does not wish to—indeed, cannot—explain his vision in words. His plan is set by patterns that are not necessarily representational and that are generated within his visual system itself. It is difficult for dancers to break down the sequence of body movements and expressive actions into separate units, and even more difficult to translate them into words. Dancers' modes of representation are motoric; their mode of communication is primarily to demonstrate and to guide with movement. The master chef must illustrate, not verbalize, the feel of dough that has been kneaded sufficiently, the look and feel of egg yolks that have thickened enough but not too much. The same applies, in different ways, for other nonverbal processes and skills. Apprenticeships rather than textbooks are generally required for acquiring such abilities. All of these constitute forms of information processing, but we must broaden our notions of information and our theories of information processing to account for them.

The type of rapid and complex intuitive processing illustrated here calls for simultaneous consideration of many pieces of information (or "constraints"), which may occur at many levels of awareness, and which may be poorly defined, unclear, and occur too quickly to process completely. Such processing requires the capacity to compute accurately with degraded and partial information input and to tolerate considerable amounts of noise (in an informational sense). We recognize the people we know well from any angle, in any posture, and under virtually any conditions—seen at dusk, at a distance, or through a window, and under many transformations—as they gain or lose weight, grow older, become pregnant, change hairstyles or hair color, wear bikinis or heavy winter coats. We recognize a painter's style from a quick glance; we recognize a piece of music from the first two notes; we identify a patient's emotional state from a minor change in vocal tone or a slight difference in the bodily position on the couch. We carry out such recognition immediately, often with certainty, and usually without being able to identify the specific factors or features to which we respond. Obviously the stimulus can be degraded or noise increased to a point where such recognition is blocked, as in the mistaken-identity farces of Shakespeare or Gilbert and Sullivan. However, the unusual nature of such recognition failure is reflected in the fantasy quality of entertainments of this nature.

The paradigm of PDP, also referred to as subsymbolic or connectionist models, directly recognizes the massively parallel, implicit, and noncategorical nature of such processing, and focuses on this in the model development. According to PDP theorists, people are smarter than computers—at least those in use today—because the brain employs a basic computational architecture with different features. Some of the important characteristics of neuronal functioning, which have "inspired" or constrained connectionist models, and which are not reflected in the classical symbolic models, include the following, as discussed by Rumelhart, McClelland, and the PDP Research Group (1986):

1. Neurons are much slower than computer components. Basic operations in modern serial computers are measured in nanoseconds (one-billionth of a second), while neurons operate at speeds measured in milliseconds (one-thousandth of a second) or longer. Humans are able to carry out very sophisticated processing—as in the activities mentioned earlier—in a few hundred milliseconds. If processing were serial, this would permit only about 100 steps, whereas computer programs for even simple tasks require many thousands of operations.

2. There is a very large, but not unlimited, number of neurons in the brain—generally estimated on the order of ten to the tenth or eleventh powers. This permits massive parallelism but also sets limits for the most complex models.

3. Each neuron receives input from many other neurons. It is estimated that a single cortical neuron may have from 1,000 to 100,000 synapses on its dendrites. Activation of any given neuron requires building up of a sufficient number of action potentials; this suggests that human computation depends on statistical processes rather than on the all-or-none categorization of logic circuits.

4. Related to this is the processing feature that Rumelhart et al. have termed "graceful degradation." There is no single neuron whose functioning is essential for any particular cognitive operation, and no single critical point at which processing breaks down. While loss of an entire region of the brain may have a measurable and specific effect, performance within regions deteriorates gradually and proportionally as more neural units are destroyed. This gradual deterioration cannot be modeled by the usual serial, symbolic processing models, which imply all-or-none function rather than partial loss. The failure of a single step in a huge program in the standard symbolic models will usually degrade the entire program.

5. The control of brain function is distributed rather than central; there is no executive system overseeing the overall flow and coordination of processing, no part of the cortex on whose operation all the other parts depend. Instead, the organization emerges through all parts working together, influencing one another, with each region contributing certain functions, constraints, and sources of information.

Formal Description of the PDP Paradigm

The structure of PDP models is compatible with the basic characteristics of the brain that have been outlined earlier. While specific PDP models can only be understood fully in terms of the mathematical systems and programming languages in which they have been developed, the defining concepts of the theory can be outlined to provide a flavor of this approach.

A PDP system is a network with a finite set of nodes, each connected to every other, each in a different state of arousal. The state of the system is the state of each of the nodes at a given time, that is, its level of arousal. The level of arousal of any node at any given time is dependent on the arousal levels of all nodes at the previous time. The values are calculated from the state of arousal for each node and a matrix of weights; the individual's learning and experience determines the nature of the weights. The network and matrix of weights may be described as a dynamical system, which can be iterated. Given the input of a particular state of arousal for each neuron, the system assigns a new state of arousal for each, which can then be used as new input for the system. The systems continue this iterative process, testing the match with the desired schema and evaluating the error, the difference between the actual and desired position, until the error is small enough to proceed. The dimensions and metrics used by the system for the evaluation of error are specific to each problem; the system is characterized as content sensitive in that sense. One may observe this process in the many decisions of daily life. A young child trying to climb down from a table reaches down a bit at a time with his leg while evaluating the distance visually between his foot and the floor; he does not let go until the visual distance matches the schema of safe-jump distance that he has constructed and stored. In picking up a teakettle whose weight will vary widely depending on the amount of water it contains, without the difference being visible, we do a series of rapid, implicit estimations by applying different amounts of force, which are not great enough to lift the kettle, so as to determine the amount of force that is required.

The PDP approach does not incorporate the classical symbolic distinctions among buffer, short-term-memory, and long-term-memory zones. Schemas are understood in terms of activation or process, continually reforming, rather than as fixed structures, as the long-term memory component has been construed. Each time the child attempts his move toward the floor, the computation is different; the schema of the safe jump changes with his increasing skill and strength, and with where he is. In this sense, PDP models are not representational. Storage in PDP models takes place primarily in connections among units and the distribution of weights. This means that knowledge is implicit in the structure of the device that carries out the task, rather than explicit in the contents of the units. The strengths of the connections and the levels of arousal of the nodes continue to change simultaneously as new equilibria are attained.

It also follows that the PDP networks are not conceptualized as having a certain fixed capacity. Instead, there is simply more interference and blending as the system gets overloaded. Because many units participate in the storage of all patterns, the information value can be retained over degradation of the stimulus or loss of a few components. These features of the parallel distributed processing environment account for ability to function with a relatively high noise to signal ratio, and with degraded and partial stimuli, and also accounts for partial, continuous, or gradual learning, as stored patterns or schemas are built up.

Applications of the PDP Paradigm

The PDP models have been developed primarily at the level of relationships between individual neurons. The fundamental processing unit may be understood as an abstraction of a neuron. The core application of the PDP models, as currently understood, is to the microlevel of processing, the massively parallel and distributed organization of processing at the unit or neuronal level. The positive results in modeling human information processing within the connectionist paradigm have been achieved at the level of very specific, definable tasks such as finger movements by a skilled typist in typing a single word (Rumelhart & Norman, 1982, reaching for an object without losing one's balance while standing (Hinton, 1984), and particular examples of stereoscopic depth perception, for example, in random dot stereograms (Marr & Poggio, 1976). Other models have been developed accounting for the perception of occluded letters in visually presented words, and for the phonemic restoration effect, in which listeners hear sounds that had been cut out of words as if they had been actually present.

PDP Systems as Models of Mind

The PDP heuristic may be characterized as replacing the computer architecture that has dominated cognitive science with a brain architecture, to provide a better fit to the processes of mind. While PDP models are "neurally inspired" and strongly neurally constrained, the PDP or connectionist paradigm remains within the cognitive science and, in particular, the artificial-intelligence research domain. PDP models are psychological models, not neurological ones. They do not focus on "neural modeling" or detailed analysis of particular circuitry and organs of the brain. Rather, brain function is used as a basis for modeling particular types of information processing, within the PDP paradigm, in the same sense as principles derived from the domain of Newtonian mechanics served as a basis for Freud's model of the psychical apparatus, and principles derived from the structure and function of the von Neumann computer served as a basis for modeling information processing in the classical symbolic paradigm.

As in other psychological models, the PDP concepts have the status of hypothetical constructs, defined within the nomological net of the connectionist approach. PDP models are not *reducible* to neurological models, but, like any mental models, must ultimately be translatable to them, when and if the constructs in each are sufficiently well defined. Computers are used to simulate systems in the PDP as in the symbolic paradigm, and the models are defined using mathematical and programming terminology. The distinction between the PDP and symbolic models in this regard is that the former make use of hypothetical constructs drawn from the neurological rather than computational domain, and they also place greater emphasis on neurological constraints than the symbolic models have done.

It may take a particular leap of imagination to recognize that the brain, which is, of course, the physiological seat of mentation, is used here as the basis for building a model of mind, rather than on its physiological level. The peculiarity of this approach is in fact shared with Freud's approach to modeling the psychical apparatus. As discussed earlier, when we talk of energy as "unbound" in the unconscious or the id, we are referring to theoretical relations among hypothetical constructs, not to something that is measurable on a physical metric in ergs or amps. Neural nets as these figure in PDP models are abstract and hypothetical constructs, in the same sense.

The Relationship between Symbolic and PDP Systems: One Architecture or Two?

While PDP models have thus far been successfully applied only at the level of specific low-level tasks, some cognitive scientists also view these models as having potential application to higher level functions, including the type of complex, intentional, goal-directed processing that is central to the symbolic paradigm. Conversely, some researchers within the symbolic approach argue that their models can potentially be adapted to account for the intuitive processing—involving fine distinctions made on continuous gradients, without explicit dimensions or metrics, and without discrete units—that is associated with the subsymbolic domain.

The controversies concerning PDP and symbolic systems somewhat parallel the earlier controversies within the symbolic approach, among perceptual dominance, verbal dominance, common code and dual code approaches, as discussed by Bucci (1985). A variety of positions have been proposed concerning the relationship between PDP and symbolic systems; these include single-format systems as well as several proposals for integrating the symbolic and PDP models.

On the one hand, some advocates of symbolic models take what might be characterized as a "symbolic dominance" approach. For example, according to Fodor and Pylyshyn (1988), symbolic processing can in principle be carried out in implicit formats outside the focus of attention, and even in multichannel, concurrent modes:

> It seems extremely likely that many Classical symbolic processes are going on in parallel in cognition, and that these processes interact with one another (e.g., they may be involved in some sort of symbolic constraint propagation). Operating on symbols can even involve "massively parallel" organizations; that might indeed imply new architectures, but they all share the Classical conception of computation as symbol-processing. (pp. 55–56)

Along these lines, several specific proposals for parallel symbolic processing networks have been proposed (e.g., Hewett, 1977; Hillis, 1985), but
the application of the symbolic paradigm to the intuitive processing and
skilled performance that is the domain of PDP models has not been
developed.

At the other extreme is the position that only PDP accounts of mental
functions are scientifically valid; accounts at levels higher than those of
connectionist nodes and links, including symbolic models, would have no
scientific standing. This might be characterized as a "subsymbolic dominance" position. According to connectionist researchers holding this
position, subsymbolic models may ultimately be developed in which
"sequential behavior is captured in the successive settlings of a parallel
network or set of networks" (Rumelhart et al., 1986, Vol. 2, p. 548), so
that models of high-level processing might ultimately be developed based
on emergent properties of individual connectionist nets:

> We see no reason to suppose that the mechanisms that control cognitive
> processing are not themselves constructed of the same underlying
> parallel hardware as the other aspects of the cognitive systems, and . . . we
> prefer to view the system not so much in terms of controlled and
> controlling modules, but in terms of more distributed forms of control.
> (Vol. 2, p. 549)

Thus, these researchers argue that PDP models may eventually be developed that will account for human information processing at all levels,
from the specific, low-level tasks and intuitive functions that have been
modeled by PDP systems, to the higher levels that have traditionally been
accounted for within the symbolic domain.

However, no connectionist theorist or researcher has yet provided a
clear formulation of how the same processes that occur locally (at the unit
level) also occur globally—at the macrolevel of the schema or prototype.
The basic concepts of dynamical systems theory on which the models are
based apply at the level of the individual unit and relationships between
these, and must be reformulated if they are to apply recursively to units
composed of units, or to nets with embedded nets.

The question of how the highly specialized PDP models may be
integrated with one another is inherently problematic, as Dyer (1988)
points out:

> Since PDP models form their own patterns of activity through learning,
> the activity pattern learned by one network will generally be indecipher-
> able to another. As a result, it is very difficult to port knowledge from
> one area of memory to another. Most current PDP models are designed

> to perform a single task; the same network cannot be used for multiple
> tasks. (p. 32)

It follow that the PDP paradigm is not sufficient to account for all
information processing:

> The PDP system is fine for perception and motor control, fine for
> categorization. It is possibly exactly the sort of system required for all
> of our automatic, subconscious reasoning. But I think that more is
> required—either more levels of PDP structures or other kinds of system—
> to handle the problems of conscious, deliberate thought, planning, and
> problem solving. (Norman, 1986, p. 541)

From the viewpoint of this book, the PDP or connectionist design is
of potential importance in providing a systematic account, based on cognitive structure rather than content, for the type of intuitive and analogic
processing that escapes standard symbolic models and that analysts associate
with the primary process. On the other hand, this approach does not
account for organization of mental function, and no PDP applications have
been developed to account for higher order processing.

People can do multiple activities at the same time, some of them
related to one another and to shared goals; others are quite unrelated. As
Norman argues, PDP applications to the entire human information-processing system will require multiple units, perhaps many thousands of
independent PDP-like systems or networks, each settling into a particular
state at a given time. Given this inherent multiplicity of independently
operating PDP systems, there has to be a mechanism that enables
connections among them; there also has to be a mechanism that monitors
complex behavior to see if things are proceeding well, that decides what
the desired output should be, that evaluates performance and output, and
is satisfied or not. Norman argues that this organization requires a
second, evaluative system, which overlooks behavior and compares expectations with outcomes. Thus, he proposes a dual-system model, incorporating a second type of system that has features of symbolic processors,
along with the parallel processing modules:

> The point is that although the system is highly parallel and very fast
> when viewed at the level of computational operations, it is highly serial
> and relatively slow when viewed at the "higher level" of interpreting and
> analyzing the resulting state changes. This dual perspective is a strong
> virtue for the modeling of human cognition, for this duality reflects
> current understanding. . . . People do seem to have at least two modes
> of operation, one rapid, efficient, subconscious, the other slow, serial,
> and conscious. (Norman, 1986, p. 542)

Similarly, Schneider (1988) argues that symbol knowledge and pattern or connection knowledge may be quite different processes, implemented very differently in the architecture. Symbolic learning often occurs in a single trial, while connection learning typically requires thousands or millions of trials; human behavior appears qualitatively different in using these two kinds of knowledge. While forms of categorization that have manifestly symbolic features may be performed in connectionist architecture, hundreds of trials are required, and a specific control mechanism must be implemented that does not emerge directly from the associative input–output processing and thus is outside of the PDP design. In computer operations, the control-processing level moderates the interactions that occur when multiple messages need to be multiplexed serially to limit cross talk. In human information processing, this relates to the need for a processing level that deals with goal directedness and integration of systems. On the basis of his systems analysis, Schneider, like Norman, points to the need for "hybrid architectures that can better cover the space of human behavior" (p. 51):

> Connectionism is a major advance in the modeling of cognition and has already had a significant impact on psychology. . . . However, it must become a member of a team of concepts and tools for the study of cognition, rather than trying to produce a paradigm shift supplanting its predecessors. A wide range of architectures should be explored in trying to cover a space of human behaviors while using available physiological, behavioral, and computational constraints. Neurophysiologists tell a story that if you can think of five ways that the brain can do something, it does it in all five, plus five you haven't thought of yet. In the study of cognition we need to control our desire to have one answer, or one view, and work with multiple views. (1988, pp. 51–52)

The conclusion to be drawn from this survey is that an integrated, multiple architecture, incorporating both subsymbolic and symbolic architectures, each accounting for different functions, is required. This is the position that I take in this book. This conclusion is compatible with studies of the functions that human information processing must serve, as will be discussed in the next chapter.

CHAPTER 6

Multiplicity of Systems
EVIDENCE FROM THE FUNCTIONAL APPROACH

The theories and research I have discussed thus far have focused on different types of human information-processing architectures. These are conceptualized as enduring organizations or structures, and they are studied primarily in experimental designs or through computer modeling within the artificial-intelligence paradigm. From a different perspective, other scientists have approached the issue of organization of cognition by examining mental functions rather than structure and have also examined the evolutionary roots of these functions in species other than man. These theories have focused primarily on the organization of memory; many alternate classification systems have been proposed.

In contrast to the views in cognitive science a decade ago, the notion of multiple memory systems now seems to be widely accepted. The controversies concern the basis on which the functions of memory are distinguished and defined.

A growing number of investigators in cognitive psychology, neuropsychology, and neuroscience have argued for the existence of multiple memory systems. In most cases, dichotomous classifications of memory have been advanced, such as procedural versus declarative (Cohen, 1984; Squire, 1982), semantic versus episodic (Tulving, 1972, 1983), reference versus working (Honig, 1978; Olton, Becker, & Handelmann, 1979), semantic versus cognitive (Warrington & Weiskrantz, 1982), habit versus memory (Hirsch, 1974, 1980; Hirsch & Krajden, 1982; Mahut, 1985; Mishkin et al., 1984; Mishkin & Petri, 1984), dispositional versus representational (Thomas & Spafford, 1984), taxon versus locale (Jacobs & Nadel, 1985; O'Keefe & Nadel, 1978), and early versus late (Schacter & Moscovitch, 1984). However, distinctions among three and even more memory systems have also been put forward (e.g., Johnson, 1983; Oakley, 1983; Tulving, 1985). (Sherry & Schacter, 1987, p. 446)

From other perspectives, within the general framework of modularity of function, additional formulations concerning multiple memory systems have also been proposed by Minsky (1975), Fodor (1983), Gardner (1983), Gazzaniga (1983, 1985, 1988), Farah (1984, 1988, 1991), and Kosslyn (1987). The notion of modularity refers primarily to information-processing functions that are specific to particular tasks, viewed in some cases in psychological, and in some cases in neurophysiological terms. Researchers have also addressed the issue of modality-specific aspects of information processing and the implications of these distinctions for the overall information-processing organization.

In his distinction between the primary and secondary processes of thought, Freud also made particular assumptions as to the nature of the functional distinctions that were relevant for his model of the mental apparatus. A major reason for us to examine what is known about the functions of memory is to evaluate to what extent the systems as characterized by Freud retain validity in the light of this current work. We will briefly review the schemes for classification of human memory functions that have been most widely accepted and influential in recent years; then identify the basic functional distinctions that are most relevant to the formulation of a new theory.

DECLARATIVE VERSUS NONDECLARATIVE (OR PROCEDURAL) MEMORY

A distinction between declarative and procedural knowledge has been recognized by many memory researchers. Declarative knowledge denotes the store of knowledge whose contents one can bring to mind or "declare." Whereas declarative knowledge concerns *what* we know or *what* we learn, procedural information concerns habits and skills—learning or knowing *how*. This distinction initially emerged from an analysis of modes of representation in computer programs within an artificial intelligence context (Winograd, 1975). Here, the human information-processing system was viewed as analogous to a computer program that includes both a database (declarative memory) and a production system consisting of functions for manipulating this (procedural memory). Declarative memory has also been defined as concerning representation of the outcome of a processing operation that is available to conscious recall, procedural memory as involving acquisition of processing operations (Cohen, 1984; Squire, 1982).

Declarative memory was initially associated with processing that is verbal and conscious. However, as Squire (1992) has recently argued, the quality of being declarable or explicit does not necessarily apply only to verbal knowledge, although it will certainly include such ability. Thus declarative memory is now defined as including "memory for faces, spatial layouts, and other material that is declared by bringing a remembered image to mind," as well as verbal knowledge, and may also involve both general knowledge and memory for specific events (Squire, 1992, p. 205).

The term "procedural" was initially used to contrast with "declarative" and referred primarily to habit or skill learning. Squire now gives this category the more neutral designation of "nondeclarative," and defines it as including

> skillful behavior or habits (perceptuo-motor, perceptual, and cognitive skills), simple conditioning (including emotional learning), the phenomenon of priming, and other instances where experience changes the facility for operating in the world but without affording conscious access to specific past events. Whereas declarative memory concerns recollection, nondeclarative memory concerns behavioral change. (Squire, 1992, p. 210)

Thus, starting from a notion of the distinction between a database and production systems that operate on this within the artificial intelligence paradigm, declarative memory is now understood as including memory for specific events and general information, which is explicit, or can be made so, and is declarable in some sense but is not necessarily verbal or conscious. A representation of a past event that is recalled, or can be recalled as a specific memory, would be classified as declarative; a stored representation of a past event that is inaccessible to retrieval but that affects one's functioning would be considered part of procedural knowledge. Change in the procedural level could occur through input, retrieval, and reorganization in declarative knowledge, although the specific memories may not remain accessible. In this definition, procedural memory includes not only behavioral knowledge, but also certain types of registration of perceptual experience, which are not explicit and generally not accessible to retrieval. The type of functions associated with procedural memory would be modeled primarily in PDP formats, whereas the dominant features of declarative memory correspond to the formats of classical symbolic models.

SEMANTIC VERSUS EPISODIC MEMORY

Another influential approach to classification of multiple memory systems, and one of the earliest of these, was the distinction between semantic and episodic memory introduced by Tulving (1972). Here, episodic memory refers to the system that receives and stores information about specific, temporally dated events and relations among them, and also stores information about the relations of these events to the individual's personal identity as this is constructed in subjective time and space (Tulving, 1983; Claparède, 1911). Semantic memory, as initially defined by Tulving, denotes

> the memory necessary for the use of language. It is a mental thesaurus, organized knowledge a person possesses about words and other verbal symbols, their meaning and referents, about relations among them, and about rules, formulas, and algorithms for the manipulations of the symbols, concepts and relations. (1972, p. 386)

In Tulving's system, semantic and episodic memory are both forms of "what we know": on the one hand, general knowledge; on the other, memory for specific events. In terms of the previous dichotomy, both of Tulving's categories would appear to be within the declarative memory system. Tulving's dichotomy leaves out of account the process of behavioral change—"learning how"—which is encompassed in the nondeclarative domain. Both episodic and semantic memory have the features of symbolic systems. Tulving's dichotomy of function was also initially understood as reflecting a distinction between nonverbal (episodic) and verbal (semantic) knowledge. However, we can see that this leaves out of account both verbal knowledge of specific events and general, prototypic nonverbal information.

IMPLICIT VERSUS EXPLICIT MEMORY

Another functional classification, developed by Schacter (1987) and others (summarized by Schacter, 1989), contrasts explicit memory that denotes conscious recollection of specific recent experiences with implicit memory, in which evidence for the memory is found in behavioral indicators, although there may not be any conscious recollection of experiences in which the memory was laid down. Implicit memory has been seen as related to the psychoanalytic notion of the unconscious; however, implicit memory is more specifically defined and lacks psychodynamic implications. Implicit memory, as studied experimentally, is generally inferred from studies of changes in performance following particular experimental interventions characterized as priming, where there is no conscious awareness or recollection of the intervention. An example of priming would be subliminal exposure to a word, leading to increased accuracy or speed of identification of that word on subsequent exposure, although the subject does not recall having seen it before. Another example would be previous exposure to a set of words influencing contents or speed of word-fragment completion, without awareness of the effect. This dimension differs from both the procedural and declarative memory distinction, and the semantic versus episodic dichotomy in focusing on level of awareness rather than differentiation of contents or forms of knowledge.

Evidence for a basic, systemic distinction between implicit and explicit memory has been found in several neuropsychological and neurophysiological conditions. Some amnesic patients show a striking inability for explicit memory of recent experiences across even very brief (e.g., 5 minutes) retention intervals, while implicit memory is generally unimpaired, even for recent events (Milner, Corkin, & Teuber, 1968; Warrington & Weiskrantz, 1974; Squire & Cohen, 1984). For example, amnesic patients showed priming effects of studying a list of words on completion of word fragments a few minutes later, indicating implicit memory function, but were profoundly impaired, compared to controls, in explicit memory of the contents of the list (Warrington & Weiskrantz, 1968, 1974). Patients with blindsight (cortical damage producing blindness for a part of the visual field) are sometimes able to respond appropriately to stimuli presented in their visual fields without conscious experience of the stimulus, and with a phenomenological experience of producing the response by guessing (Weiskrantz, 1986); this provides evidence for implicit processing, while explicit processing is lost. Whereas patients with the deficit known as prosopagnosia are unable to recognize familiar faces explicitly, several studies have reported physiological and behavioral evidence for implicit facial recognition (Bauer, 1984; Tranel & Damasio, 1985).

There seems to be some correspondence between explicit memory and the type of functions characterized as declarative, and explicit memory, like declarative, might seem to be most adequately modeled by symbolic systems. Conversely, implicit memory has functions more closely associated with subsymbolic systems, although, as for all other correspondences that have been noted, the theoretical perspectives of these distinctions are different, and the correspondence is not complete.

INTENTIONAL VERSUS AUTOMATIC PROCESSES

The distinction between explicit and implicit memory is related in part to the distinction noted by Posner and Snyder (1975) between conscious and automatic processes. Bargh (1989) has characterized automatic processes as being "unintentional, involuntary, effortless (i.e., not consumptive of limited processing capacity), autonomous, and occurring outside of awareness" (p. 3). These contrast with conscious or controlled processes, defined as "those that are under the flexible, intentional control of the individual, that he or she is consciously aware of, and that are effortful and constrained by the amount of attentional resources available at the moment" (p. 4). However, other researchers have provided evidence that intentionality and control do not necessarily converge with level of attention and awareness; so that the construct validity of this dimension has been questioned (Zbrodoff & Logan, 1986).

SHERRY AND SCHACTER'S SYSTEM I VERSUS SYSTEM II

As Sherry and Schacter (1987) have argued, it is unlikely that each of the various dimensions of function now being studied refers to a distinct memory system. Given the multiplicity of dimensions that have been identified, a criterion is needed to select dimensions that identify distinct memory systems, and to differentiate these from distinctions that are of descriptive interest only. Sherry and Schacter have proposed an evolutionary basis for such differentiation of functional systems. They argue that certain adaptations that develop to serve particular functional needs cannot, because of their specialized nature, effectively serve others, and that such incompatibility of function then provides an independent basis for differentiation of memory systems (p. 439). They have distinguished two specialized memory systems that show incompatibility of function in this sense. The first system, which they refer to as System I, is devoted to gradual, incremental detection and registration of features that remain invariant across sets of events, without retaining the unique and idiosyncratic features of specific episodes. In contrast, System II is an episodic–representational system, whose major function is to preserve the contextual details that uniquely mark individual experiences—to preserve the differences between episodes rather than the invariance across them.

Examples of System I memory, as identified in many species, range from the learning of the songs of his subspecies by the male bird, learning of olfactory orientation cues by salmonoid fish, and learning of stellar orientation by migratory birds (Rozin & Schull, 1989; Sherry & Schacter,

1987; Shettleworth, 1983), to the human learning to type, ride a bicycle, play tennis, and ski, or differentiate shades of color or types of wine. The male songbird learns the songs of his species to defend his territory and to attract mates. The song types of the species are learned and retained across many types of contextual changes. They are retained from one breeding season to the next, are transmitted among all males of the species, and are recognized by them, regardless of the particular singer or location. This type of skill or performance learning, which involves acquisition of concepts and learning to discriminate members of a category from nonmembers, has also been demonstrated in experimental contexts such as discrimination and concept learning tasks. Such learning occurs gradually, reaching asymptotic levels after many trials.

An example of System II learning is a bird's acquisition of memory for food-cache sites. Such learning requires registration of a specific, unique spatial location that can be safely used only once. System II learning, which concerns memory for information specific to a single episode, in many cases based on a single exposure, is functionally incompatible with the type of memory processes that underlie song learning, where performance is repeated in many contexts, following the shared template of the species. Memories of particular incidents, people, and places, with their wealth of idiosyncratic features, involve System II. Such memory is also demonstrated experimentally in matching tasks in which lists of items are shown once, and subjects are later tested as to whether they can identify these and distinguish them from items not seen in that context before.

A distinction related to Sherry and Schacter's systems was identified more than 70 years ago by Smith and McDougall (1920). They found that performance on tasks that required gradual, incremental repetitive learning (such as learning to type) was uncorrelated with performance on tasks that tapped memory for unique episodes (e.g., recognition of pictures seen once).

Evidence for the System I–System II distinction has emerged in experimental studies of nonhuman primates and other animals, including rats and birds, and in studies of evolutionary patterns. In a developmental study, infant monkeys were able to learn visual discriminations as well as adult monkeys but were not equivalent on delayed matching tasks that required recognition of items seen only once (Bachevalier & Mishkin, 1984).

In certain amnesic patients, System II learning is affected, while System I learning appears relatively intact. These patients are characteristically impaired in their capacity to remember recent events and to learn many types of new information; they may fail to recall or recognize events after delays of a few seconds. Nevertheless, they are able to learn new perceptual and motor skills such as reading mirror-inverted scripts, responding to a repeated sequential pattern, puzzle solving, and mirror-tracing tasks, even without recollection of having performed the task (Cohen & Squire, 1980; Nissen & Bullemer, 1987; Brooks & Baddeley, 1976; Milner, 1962). Similar patterns of dissociation have been found in normal subjects injected with scopolamine; they showed normal rate of learning on a repeated-pattern task and substantial impairment on one-trial memory tasks (Nissen, Knopman, & Schacter, 1987).

INTERSECTION OF FUNCTIONAL CLASSIFICATION SCHEMES

Each of the memory systems that have been outlined here carve up the domain of memory or knowledge at somewhat different joints. Three fundamental functional categories may be identified in the several systems that have been reviewed:

1. Behavioral (habits and skills) versus representational knowledge reflected primarily in the declarative versus procedural or nondeclarative distinction.
2. General knowledge versus specific memories reflected in different ways in Sherry and Schacter's System I versus II, and in Tulving's episodic–semantic distinction.
3. Conscious versus unconscious knowledge underlying the distinction between explicit versus implicit and intentional versus automatic functions.

Several tripartite functional classifications have been identified that incorporate subsets of these basic dimensions. Tulving's initial dichotomy of episodic versus semantic memory reflected a distinction within the general domain of "what we know," leaving habit and skill acquisition out of account. Going beyond this dichotomy, Tulving (1985) later proposed a trichotomous classification incorporating, along with semantic and episodic memory, a system of "procedural memory," defined as underlying learned connections between stimuli and responses, including complex stimulus patterns and response chains.

Tripartite memory schemes similar to that suggested by Tulving have also been developed by other investigators. Ruggiero and Flagg (1976) proposed a model consisting of systems of stimulus–response, representational, and organized memory; and Oakley (1983) referred to associative, representational, and abstract memory systems. In both schemes, the first category is analogous to procedural memory and involves incremental learning and retention of skills. The second is similar to episodic memory in representing specific situations together with their spatiotemporal context. The third is analogous to semantic memory and enables storage of context-free facts abstracted from specific instances.

In general, as we can see, the relationships among the functional systems are unclear. We may also note that the distinction between verbal and nonverbal processing is essentially independent of any of these. For example, verbal and nonverbal processing have both been associated with declarative memory. Sherry and Schacter's System I–II distinction has been initially identified as applying to species other than man, thus intrinsically operating within the nonverbal mode. The other processing dimensions also cut across the verbal–nonverbal distinction. From the perspective of psychoanalytic theory, it is important to see that implicit processing has been shown with verbal as well as nonverbal processing, and also that intentionality and awareness do not necessarily converge.

What this research demonstrates unequivocally, regardless of how the intersection of functions is defined, is the existence of a wide range of systematic, organized, goal-directed mental functions that operate outside of the verbal or explicit or intentional functional domains, and that continue throughout normal, mature, waking life. The assumption of a unified process that is unconscious, nonverbal, associated with regressed or pathological forms, or with altered states, and characterized by contents of wish fulfillment, that is, with the features that Freud associated with the primary process, is essentially disconfirmed by these research findings. I will discuss the implications of these findings for our understanding of psychoanalytic concepts in more detail in Section Three.

NEUROLOGICAL CORRELATES OF FUNCTIONAL DISTINCTIONS

We may provide additional bases for multiplicity of systems, and perhaps some indications of how the lines may appropriately be drawn, by examining anatomical as well as functional constraints. While our goal is to develop a psychological model of mental and emotional processing, the neurological data provides an additional source of evidence for the psychological constructs. The functions defined as declarative memory have been shown to depend on the hippocampus and related structures in animals, as well as humans, in contrast to the more heterogeneous and vaguely defined collection of nondeclarative functions, which do not require the hippocampus. This conclusion is supported by selective memory impairments associated with hippocampal damage in amnesic patients and also in surgically treated animals, including rats and monkeys, as summarized by Squire (1992). The ability to remember that an event occurred and that it occurred in a particular context, which is associated with certain aspects of declarative memory, requires an interaction between the neocortex and the medial temporal lobe memory system to have been established at the time of learning. The hippocampus carries out such coordinating functions in perception and short-term memory, enabling integration of distributed sites of neocortical activity that represent multiple aspects of a particular event. While the neocortical activity itself is sufficient for perception and short-term memory, the possibility of long-term storage and explicit retrieval (in contrast to implicit memory recognized through its effect on performance) is dependent on this hippocampal coordination.

As would be expected, Sherry and Schacter find hippocampal involvement in System II functions, which require coordinating multiple features of a specific event, but not in System I. Lesions of the hippocampus and other limbic structures in monkeys impair performance on matching tasks but do not impair discrimination learning (Malamut, Saunders, & Mishkin, 1984). Similar patterns of dissociation have also been found in rats with hippocampal lesions (O'Keefe & Nadel, 1978). We can see here a convergence of data concerning the operation of the hippocampus as associated with a particular type of organizational function, as this occurs in the nonverbal as well as verbal systems, and including data on species other than man. As we will also suggest, the roots of the symbolizing function lie precisely here.

CHAPTER 7

Functional Distinctions in Specific Sensory Systems

We may gain an additional perspective on the multiplicity of human information-processing systems and some insight as to the distinctions that may be most fundamental by examining the distinction of functions as they occur in different sensory systems. I will examine processing in the two sensory systems whose functional operations are perhaps must distant and distinct; these are the visual and olfactory systems.

MULTIPLE FUNCTIONS IN THE VISUAL SYSTEM

According to Kosslyn (1987), the information-processing operations of the visual system may be understood through an analysis of the functions that the system is required to perform. Vision has two general purposes: (1) to recognize objects and parts of objects; (2) to navigate through space and to track movement. In carrying out these functions, the system needs to balance a number of opposing demands.

One such set of opposing demands concerns recognition of objects as the same over changes of position versus computation of the variations that occur. The same object will appear at many different positions in the visual field, and its image will fall on many different parts of the retina. Nevertheless, we can generally recognize a person we know, or a familiar object, regardless of its location in the visual field. On the other hand, we also know where an object is when we have seen it, and we remember this position. Thus, while we are able to store a representation of an object independent of its location, we are also able to store its position and changes in this.

A similar set of opposing demands applies for changes in shape. Many objects present wide, essentially infinite variations in shape, yet are recognized as the same. Animate objects are constantly changing in visual form; we recognize the people we know over virtually all such variations— standing up, lying down, standing on their heads, from the back, side, or front. Letters of the alphabet are recognized across manifestations in numerous fonts, sizes, and colors, as well as (most) individual handwritten forms. On the other hand, we are also able to recognize and distinguish variations in form and shape, to distinguish one person's handwriting from another, to tell when someone looks thinner, and to recognize subtle variations in facial expression.

Another type of opposing demands on the visual system concerns recognition of multipart objects as wholes versus recognition of individual parts. When an image of an object is stored in memory, it is organized and encoded as a whole and also as composed of its constituent parts. If a part of an object seen later matches a constituent previously encoded as such, recognition is easy; otherwise, it is not. Kosslyn uses the example of the Star of David: Triangles are readily recognized as constituents of that figure; the intersecting parallelograms are not. When parts are encoded and recognized separately, the shape-recognition function is independent of location, as is the case in the encoding of any unitary entity, whole or part. A triangle will be recognized as such regardless of its location or orientation. At the same time, the relative locations of parts is an important characteristic of whole objects. The encoding of the Star of David depends on the relative location of the triangles; the image of the American flag depends on the location of the stripes and stars; the encoding of a face or figure of a person depends on the relative location of its parts. To solve the problem of recognizing whole objects and their parts, there needs to be in place a system that encodes parts (stars, stripes; or eyes, nose, mouth, ears) independent of their location in a whole; a system that encodes relative locations (one eye on each side of the nose and slightly above, lips below, etc.); and a system that coordinates the "what" and "where."

Kosslyn argues that the types of functional opposition illustrated here call for two distinct operating systems, which he has characterized as *categorical* and *continuous*, within the visual modality itself.

The Categorical System: Prototypic Representation

There must be some kind of stable representation built up and stored in long-term visual memory to enable us to recognize a particular shape never seen before as a person, cat, tree, or mountain, or letter of the alphabet. Thus, one basic system identified by Kosslyn must register prototypic images of objects (the yellow house, Fido, mother, Mt. Rainier, a triangle, the American flag) stored in long-term memory, which may then be accessed by the ever-changing visual manifestations of that object, and which then permit all these manifestations to be recognized as such. These prototypic representations of objects and their constituent parts are stable over changes in location and changes in shape. They constitute the representations of the world of objects in the human—and primate—visual system. The range of visual variations that serve to access the prototypic image of a given object constitutes what Kosslyn terms a *functional equivalence class*. The categorical processor of the visual system ignores variation within such a class, responding to this range of manifestations as if they were the same.

In addition to representation of objects, the categorical system also has the capability of representing *relations,* particularly spatial relations that are prototypic, for example, a perceptual category of being on top, without specifying how far above; "connected to," "next to," or "between," without specifying how close or at what angle. Such relationships between objects, like objects themselves, are represented in memory in prototypic form. The class of visual manifestations of a particular relationship— things that are seen *on top of, inside, underneath, between* other things—constitutes functionally equivalent classes of spatial relationships that are themselves applicable across widely varying specific objects.

Continuous Processing Subsystems

The second type of functional visual system identified by Kosslyn is one that computes actual distances and angles, where a specific object is, and where one's self is in relation to that object. This is the type of visual processing that is necessary for purposes of navigation and search, for guiding motor actions, and for making fine discriminations. The basketball player uses such computations to shoot at a basket; the painter, to capture a particular expression of face or body; a cat, to guide his leap to the top of a wall. Here, the stable prototypic images that operate over variable manifestations are not what are needed; the processor must register variations on continuous dimensions to know the exact positions of objects, at a given time, in relation to one another and to oneself.

The implicit, continuous computations carried out within the visual system are not measurements in the usual mathematical sense but are systematic computations of a unique kind. Computation in the mathematical or arithmetical sense requires a metric system with explicit units and specified coordinates or base points. The visuospatial information-processing system lacks such an explicit metric. However, it does have available a system of computations of an intuitive and analogic nature, which serve quite accurately to guide motor action and permit anticipation of the movement of objects.

These opposing functions within the visual system correspond generally to certain of the functional distinctions outlined earlier. Continuous processing would be largely associated with procedural (or nondeclarative) knowledge, implicit memory, and Sherry and Schacter's System I. Categorical functions would be dominant in declarative and explicit memory, the System II, and in both episodic and semantic functions. The distinctions made by Kosslyn also correspond to the distinctions between subsymbolic and symbolic architectures. Kosslyn's continuous processing system would be modeled by subsymbolic or PDP architectures, whereas the categorical processing has features associated with symbolic systems.

Integration of Processing Systems

Kosslyn's formulation makes an additional crucial contribution in providing an understanding of how the disparate systems may be integrated with one another and also linked to language. According to Kosslyn, the general, implicit information in the continuous processing systems is chunked or funneled, through functionally equivalent classes of representation, to the prototypic images, including representations of objects and relationships.

The system of functionally equivalent classes leading to prototypic imagery thus plays a pivotal role both in the organization of the visual system itself and the connection of visual experience to language. Within the implicit, continuous computational system, there are no discrete units and no explicit coordinates to which labels can be assigned. We cannot verbalize the variations, on continuous dimensions, that underlie recognition of changes in position or that shape and guide motor action. Formation of functional equivalence classes must first take place in the nonverbal system, in order for prototypes to be formed and registered in memory, to which verbal labels may then be assigned. This progression provides the necessary foundation for the initial development of language and for the connecting of all manner of nonverbal experience to language.

Neurophysiological Evidence for Separate
Visual Subsystems

The functional dichotomy identified by Kosslyn within the visual system is supported by neuroanatomy and neurophysiology, as well as behavioral data (Desimone, Albright, Gross, & Bruce, 1984; Ungerleider & Mishkin, 1982; Van Essen, 1985). Ungerleider and Mishkin (1982) and Mishkin, Ungerleider, and Mack (1983) have identified two visual systems in the primate brain: a ventral system, running from primary visual cortex down to the inferior temporal lobe, which enables the visual identification of objects and also the association of visual objects with other events, such as emotions and motor acts; and a dorsal, parietal system that is involved in functions of orientation and spatial localization, such as the construction of spatial maps and the guidance of motor acts. Thus, the shapes of whole objects and their constituent parts would be encoded in the ventral temporal system without preserving location; the dorsal, parietal system represents location of objects in a scene, as well as spatial relations among parts of an object. As Mishkin et al. point out, a major question posed by these results is how these two sectors of information processing are integrated. Not surprisingly, they suggest that a potential site of such integration may be the frontal lobe and limbic system, in particular, the hippocampal formation. This suggestion is compatible with data outlined earlier, concerning the role of the hippocampus in establishing declarative memory as well as explicit memory for specific events, and also concerning Sherry and Schacter's finding of hippocampal involvement in System II. Again, we see a crucial role of the hippocampus in organizing nonverbal experience, and in organizing experience in species other than man.

The existence of separate subsystems carrying out encoding of objects and spatial relations is also supported by neurological findings by many investigators. Levine, Warach, and Farah (1985) found two patients with complementary imagery disorders: one could image shape but not locations, following damage to the parieto-occipital regions; the other could image locations and spatial relations but not shapes, following damage to the temporo-occipital regions.

Farah (1988, 1991) has also identified different systems for object recognition and spatial imagery within the visual system. The memory system that is needed for object recognition registers specific information concerning an object's literal appearance, including information about color, form, and perspective; another system shows the layout of objects in space with respect to the viewer and each other. Farah has also found evidence for multiplicity of representation within the object-recognition system itself, including a system that encodes information about function contrasting with one that registers specific visual features and characteristics, and a visual system that encodes specific parts of an object contrasting with one that encodes global patterns.

In a related finding, Schacter, Cooper, and their colleagues (Schacter, Cooper, & Delaney, 1990; Cooper, Schacter, Ballestros, & Moore, 1992) have identified a group of neurons in the visual representation system, which they have called a structural system, and which unconsciously or "implicitly" computes an object's global structure and its orientation with respect to a frame of reference; this type of representation is not affected by specific features, such as the object's size or color. A contrasting system, which they have called an episodic system, consciously or "explicitly" identifies the object's specific characteristics, enabling recognition of a particular object and differentiation from other objects.

Biederman and Cooper (1992) have also identified two distinct visual-system pathways originating in the same primary visual projection area. One processes an object's shape and geometric parts, and handles representation of an object separate from its environment or position in space; this pathway extends ventrally into the inferior temporal cortex. The other system, which mediates spatial memory, extends dorsally to the posterior parietal cortex. This system conveys information about location and orientation, and enables the attunement of action to an object's position, orientation, and size.

While the various analyses of distinct neurophysiological pathways represent somewhat different divisions of function and localization, they converge generally in differentiating a ventral system that supports identification of objects and association of these with other events, and a dorsal, parietal system that handles spatial functions. There is also general agreement that the site of integration of these systems is likely to be the hippocampal formation.

A CONTRASTING MODALITY: THE OLFACTORY SYSTEM

Different types of information processing may be identified in each sensory modality, as well as in visceral and motoric systems, in forms determined by the features of each modality. As Kosslyn has shown, the visual system incorporates both discrete categorical representations and continuous processing. The continuous processing would be modeled by subsymbolic systems and the categorical representations by symbolic processes. Within the visual system, however, even the processes of the continuous system, including processing of spatial relations, patterns, colors or shades, may be potentially capable of being mapped systematically on physical dimensions with specified metrics. Thus, the intuitive location of visual objects could be translated to identifiable spatial dimensions (e.g., right, left, up, down) and to metrics on these dimensions. Their color and shading features may also be specified on dimensions of tone, brightness, and saturation, with each dimension having a direct and systematic relationship to physical properties of the stimulus.

Olfaction contrasts with vision in most of these respects. The olfactory field is without discrete features or metrics, and without dimensions that are even potentially identifiable. It is generally assumed that the experience of smell results from the action of molecules emitted by an odorous substance on the olfactory epithelium. However, the precise mechanism underlying this effect is not well understood, and there is as yet no coherent basis for distinguishing among different types of odor on the basis of their physical or chemical properties. Each odor appears to be coded individually according to patterns of chemical activity in olfactory and other receptors, and no dimensions have been identified that would permit categorization of these effects. Attempts to develop a classification system for odor comparable to the system developed for color vision have failed. Henning (1916) proposed a model of an "olfactory prism," in which the vertices at the two ends were defined by six supposedly primary qualities (flowery, fruity, putrid, spicy, resinous, and burnt). All possible odors were then, in principle, definable by their position on the surface of the prism. However, attempts to demonstrate the validity of the prism by formal experiments and other means did not succeed (Engen, 1987). No systematic relationships have been found between Henning's prism, or any odor classification system, and the physical characteristics of either the stimulus or the olfactory receptors. There are no known physical or chemical correlates of odor similar to the well-established psychophysical correlates of the visual spectrum and no evidence of olfactory receptor neurons analogous to the rods and cones (Gesteland, 1986).

Olfaction and vision show significant differences in function that relate to the different organization of these modalities. Visual images are used as aids to thinking, learning, and memory. They provide knowledge of an object in its absence, in some cases enable identification of visual properties or features that may not have been attended to previously, and enable performance of mental simulations and computations. We may project an object's trajectory in imagination in order to determine where it will land; we may compute the number of windows in a house by viewing images of each room in turn and arrive at an answer never explicitly determined before.

In contrast, we do not ordinarily attempt to retrieve memories of smells to derive information from them. "The main function of the sense of smell, then, is not to recall odors for cognitive reasons, but to respond to odors actually encountered," as Engen points out (1987, p. 503). Olfaction appears to be primarily associated with motivational rather than cognitive functions—directing response to present objects rather than to images of absent ones, guiding avoidance and approach. Odors alert us to danger (fire, spoiled food), activate appetites for food and drink (smell of coffee brewing, the bouquet of wine), stimulate sexual desire, and arouse nurturance and love.

While odor representations are not amenable to retrieval or replaying of the type that is possible for visual imagery, there must nevertheless be memory for odors in some form to support the extensive recognition functions that have been documented. Humans, as well as animals, show clear evidence of olfactory representations stored in long-term memory, in complex, associative schemas. The trained dog registers the particular smell of a fugitive's clothes to guide the chase. For humans, memory for odor is long-lasting, and odors, like tastes, have the power to evoke memories of long-past events. As Proust says in *Remembrance of Things Past*:

> When from a long-distant past nothing subsists, after the people are dead, after the things are broken and scattered, still alone, more fragile, but with more vitality, more unsubstantial, more persistent, more faithful, the smell and taste of things . . . bear unfaltering, in the tiny and almost impalpable drop of their essence, the vast structure of recollection. (quoted in Engen, 1987, p. 497)

Nabokov has also stressed the power of odors to evoke memory, and has emphasized its unidirectional retrieval pattern. While odors bring visual imagery to mind, visual images do not operate to restore odors, as he says in his early novel *Mary*: "Memory can restore to life everything except smells, although nothing revives the past so completely as a smell that was once associated with it" (quoted in Engen, 1987, p. 497).

The mixed and asymmetric nature of odor memory has been demonstrated in research on odor learning and odor memory. The learning of odors and their registration in memory is characterized by a pattern of slow acquisition and long retention times, which is the converse of the learning pattern for vision and audition. In experiments on odor recognition with human subjects, odors are learned slowly and partially compared to visual learning, but once odors are learned, there is little forgetting over time, resulting in a characteristic flat forgetting curve. (Schab, 1991). In contrast, initial retention is essentially perfect for vision and audition, but considerable forgetting occurs over a period of 30 seconds (Campbell & Gregson, 1972).

The particular nature of odor processing is also reflected in the incompatibility that exists between the human capacities for odor discrimination versus odor identification. Contrary to some popular beliefs, the sense of smell itself is far from weak in humans. People show very sensitive abilities to detect the presence or absence of odors, and to discriminate odors presented side by side (Richardson & Zucco, 1989). The weakness in human olfactory perception arises not in detecting odors but in identifying them. On average, as many studies have found, subjects are able to identify less than half of common odors presented to them in single-trial, unaided, odor identification tasks (Sumner, 1962; Cain & Krause, 1979).

Subjects will often experience an odor as familiar but will be unable to retrieve its name. This phenomenon has been characterized as the "tip-of-the-nose" state (Lawless & Engen, 1977). In contrast to the well-known "tip-of-the-tongue" phenomenon (Brown & McNeill, 1966), subjects in a "tip-of-the-nose" state cannot provide any information about the name of the familiar odor, such as its first letter or the number of syllables; however, they are able to answer questions about its quality and context. Different subjects often generate widely varying names for the same odorants. Conversely, smells that are chemically different may activate the same name, even for a single individual (Engen, 1982).

Organization of Odor Representation in Long-Term Memory

In the capacity for fine discrimination on continuous dimensions, but without clear identification of these dimensions, and without identification of discrete features or metrics, odor processing appears to provides a model exemplar of the subsymbolic or PDP format. Yet, people are also able to categorize odors and have imagistic associations to them, indicating symbolic processing in some sense.

Engen (1987) explored the basis for odor identification and its relationship to the organization of odor memory using a recognition paradigm. Subjects were asked to identify common odors, which varied in familiarity and saturation. The usual results for odor recognition tasks were obtained, with a mean of less than 50% of subjects identifying each odorant accurately and considerable variation across odors (e.g., no correct responses for musk compared to 83% correct for licorice). Engen then analyzed the responses, including those scored as errors, to provide information about the nature of associations to odor as a basis for inference to the structure of odor memory. He found that 44% of responses were the correct identifying term or source (e.g., lemon, licorice); 3% of the responses were superordinate odor categories, (e.g., "fruity"); 1% were related sensation categories (e.g., bitter); 5% were not identified. The remainder of the responses, which constituted almost half (47%), referred to associated objects, including similar odors, aspects of the context in which the odors may be perceived (e.g., hard candy, cleaning products), and also including personal and idiosyncratic responses. The results showed that odor representations are likely to be identified by the contexts in which the odors are perceived, the objects they are associated with and sensory features of these objects in multiple modalities, and the episodes in which the odors occur, rather than by features or dimensions of the olfactory field.

Coding of Odor in an Episodic Context

The complex cross-modal and experiential registration of odor is illustrated in these lines from Baudelaire:

> There are odors fresh as the skin of an infant,
> Sweet as flutes, green as any grass,
> And others, corrupt, rich and triumphant.
> (Baudelaire, *Correspondences,* 1857; quoted in Stern, 1985, p. 155)

As Stern points out, in just these three lines, "Baudelaire asks us to relate smells to experiences in the domains of touch, sound, color, sensuality, finance and power" (1985, p. 155). Odor memory, as this occurs in real life, is based on "perceptually unitary episodes ... described in an idiosyncratic lexicon" as specific and distinct events (Engen, 1987, p. 501). The memory that is retrieved is not of an isolated odor, but of the odor embedded in an episode with particular people, places, and a particular emotional tone. As early as 1929, Achiles recognized that the first impression of an odor is

> not a pure sensation, as it can be and perhaps often is in vision and hearing, but a complex feeling state. It is the development of this state which takes time, for it entails interactions with other aspects of the situation. Although the odor perception is slow to come to mind, it may last long. (quoted in Engen, Kuisma, & Eimas, 1973, p. 225)

The nature of odor encoding in complex, cross-modal associative schemas accounts for many of its special processing features, including the very slow acquisition and the long, essentially ineradicable retention and evocative quality, as shown both in naturalistic observation and in experimental research.

Lawless (1978) provided an empirical demonstration of the relationship between the absence of identifiable features or dimensions in olfactory stimuli and the characteristic, slow acquisition and long retention times. He presented subjects with different types of stimuli, including odors, pictures of specific objects and visual free-form designs lacking specific, identifiable features, and tested recognition performance over a span of 4 months. The usual result of high initial memory but steep forgetting thereafter was obtained for pictures of specific objects, with slower, less complete development of immediate memory and little subsequent forgetting for odors, as in previous work. As predicted, the learning and forgetting functions for the visual free forms were found to be parallel to those for the odors, indicating similarities in the encoding processes. In other words, for stimuli for which identifiable features were absent, encoding was slow and retention long for the visual as well as olfactory stimuli.

Lyman and McDaniel (1986) proposed that the recognition of odors could be improved by providing an episode related to the odor or by a verbal label, in both cases elaborating the relatively featureless nature of the olfactory stimulus as experienced in the laboratory. Subjects were instructed to generate a name and a short definition for each odor, or to describe a specific episode in their lives when they had experienced each odor. Recognition of odors increased significantly under both conditions. The number of correct responses was directly proportional to the accuracy of the names generated in one case, and to the degree of specificity of the remembered experiences in the other.

Categorical and Continuous Processing in the Olfactory System

The findings that have been reviewed suggest that the distinction of function identified by Kosslyn within the visual system applies as well to olfaction, but in a manner determined by the particular requirements of that modality. The olfactory system operates directly to distinguish subtle differences in odor on continuous, implicit dimensions. However, ranges of smells are also chunked into discrete categories. There may be variation among the smells of different roses, but the fragrance of the rose can be distinguished from jasmine, lilac, and lilies. As in the visual field and other modalities, a continuous range of odors that serve to access a prototypic representation of an odor form a functionally equivalent class. Also, as in the visual system, such olfactory prototypes would have to be constructed before labels can be attached.

Whereas prototypic odor representations stored in memory are presumably sufficient to permit odor *discrimination,* and *judgments of familiarity,* odor identification—identification by a verbal label—generally requires that these representations be associated with objects or episodes with visual and other cross-modal features that incorporate discrete and specific elements that can be named. Discrete images and episodes constitute the organizers of the olfactory, as of the visual system, and also underlie the connection to language. However, in the olfactory system, the discrete images are generally drawn from other—usually multiply cross-modal—sensory domains.

Relationship of Odor Representation and Emotion

The olfactory modality is of particular interest for our project of developing a model for representation and expression of emotional experience, as this operates in the psychoanalytic process. Odor is closely related to emotion, both neurophysiologically and functionally. The neuroanatomy of human olfaction is characterized by relatively direct connections (few synapses) to brain structures implicated in memory and emotion, including the hippocampus, thalamus, and frontal cortex, and by relatively few connections to the neocortex and associated structures (Lynch & Baudry, 1988). The association of olfaction with limbic-system mechanisms is also reflected in the selective effects of brain damage on odor processing. Korsakoff patients have gross difficulty in all aspects of odor function, including detection, discrimination, and retention of odors. This dysfunction is also verified by direct recordings from electrodes implanted in the limbic region (Halgren, 1976). Other studies have found impairment of odor detection in patients with temporal lobe epilepsy, including patients who have undergone temporal lobectomy.

The relationship of odor representation to personal experience and emotion has been shown directly in several experimental studies. Kirk-Smith, Van Toller, and Dodd (1983) demonstrated that neutral odors may acquire affective values by being paired with emotionally significant events. Rubin, Groth, and Goldsmith (1984) found that odors evoke more emotional memories than do visual or verbal cues, and also evoke autobiographical memories that subjects had not previously retrieved.

Schab (1991) has suggested that identification of odors may be understood as a progression that begins with a judgment of pleasantness or familiarity judgments (e.g., "It smells good," "I'm sure I've smelled it before"), then moves on through a number of intervening steps to retrieval of the specific name ("It smells like a banana"). In agreement with the data reported by Engen (1987) and others, these intervening steps were most likely to include episodic and perceptual features of the odor and features of the events in which they occurred.

As Richardson and Zucco (1989) have suggested, "Olfactory traces, visual images and verbal representations might constitute three systems of cognitive processing that are functionally independent but at least partially interrelated" (p. 358). The interconnected processing sequence outlined earlier for odor is compatible in general terms with the process by which experience in all sensory modalities, and in somatic and motoric experience, is connected to symbolic imagery and to words. Such connections are central in the organization of emotion structures and their verbalization, as we shall see in Chapters 8 and 12. Before turning to current research on emotion and its verbal expression, I will look briefly at the operation of this processing sequence in the other sensory modalities, all of which figure in the emotion schemas in different ways.

THE SYMBOLIZING OF SENSORY EXPERIENCE

The accounts of imagery by Paivio, Kosslyn, and others focused almost entirely on the visual system. Kosslyn's formulation of a bipartite, visual operating system, including processing on continuous gradients and construction of prototypic images, provides a general model of the symbolizing process as this operates in the human perceptual system (and perhaps other species as well), with particular features and constraints imposed by each sensory modality. I have shown the application of this approach to the olfactory system, which differs significantly from vision, in its dominantly subsymbolic format and absence of discrete features or explicit metrics, and in its consequent reliance on prototypic images drawn from cross-modal domains. I suggest that a similar bipartite distinction can also be found in other sensory modalities, with varying formats specific to each modality. The nonverbal sensory organization operates prior to and independent of organization by language in all species, not humans only, but may also be affected in significant ways by language within the human information-processing system.

DISCRIMINATION AND IDENTIFICATION OF TASTES

The processes of taste appear to be essentially parallel to those of smell. People are able to make far finer and clearer distinctions between tastes than they are able to identify with words. When a taste, like a smell, cannot be specifically identified, people are also likely to refer to specific images or events, usually with cross-modal features.

The description of an entity by reference to other entities with many cross-modal features has reached perhaps its highest level of refinement in the wine-tasting field. To communicate the qualities of a wine—both taste and smell—to the reader, and to differentiate one from another, the great wine writers invoke association to a wide range of concrete and specific objects, using cross-modal references liberally in this endeavor. According to Parker (1990, p. 720), one 1983 wine "is quite rich, round and fruity, with a bizarre bouquet of rotting cardboard, smoke, and vegetal fruit. Yet the flavors are lush and intense. Drink it up." Another, from the same domain and the same year, "is less evolved and more obviously tannic, yet as it develops in the glass it reveals scents of rotten meat, toffee, caramel, and hickory. It has a velvety texture and very long finish" (p. 720). Another burgundy, from another domain and another year, is "rich, creamy, fat and loaded with fruit"; another is "supple, expansive and very complex in the nose (raspberries, new oak, and flowers)" (p. 725). The subtle distinctions among wines emerge, not from the general terms referring to abstract dimensions, such as rich or tannic, but from the specific, often cross-modal images—tastes that are round, velvety, supple, with associations such as rotting cardboard and smoke, as well as flowers and fruit. Such images permit articulation of this complex, primarily subsymbolic representational modality. The linkage to symbols, and ultimately to language, is made by this route. If the connections are effective, tastes and smells are evoked for the reader as well.

MOTORIC, TACTILE, AND SOMATIC REPRESENTATIONS

The functional division identified by Kosslyn is applicable for other spatially based modalities such as body movement, tactile representation, and representation of some types of bodily experience. The implicit, spatial coordinate system that Kosslyn has identified for vision is shared with these modalities. On the one hand, we need to make precise and flexible computations on a continuous, implicit metric when we attempt to grasp or position an object that is out of sight, or place our feet properly while climbing a steep rock. On the other hand, we learn to distinguish and identify objects by touch, and we develop an enduring image of our own bodies, inside and out, to be able to tell "what hurts," to distinguish a gastric pain from a muscular one. To enable such representation, stable, prototypic images of our external environment and internal systems must be formed.

For the blind, the system of touch is enormously versatile, organizing experience across other sensory modalities and providing organizing metaphors for abstract ideas and for emotion as well. The world of Helen Keller was built largely on her sense of touch—working for her as visual symbols and metaphors with visual reference work for the sighted:

> Through the sense of touch I know the faces of friends, the exuberance
> of the soil, the delicate shapes of flowers, the noble forms of trees, and
> the range of mighty winds. Besides objects, surfaces, and atmospherical
> changes, I perceive countless vibrations. (1908, p. 43)

Thus, she refers to continuous, spatial gradients (e.g., the variety of surfaces) and prototypic images (the faces of friends; the delicate shapes of flowers), as well as representations in which tactile or kinesthetic representations are integrated with properties of other modalities ("the range of mighty winds," "countless vibrations").

AUDITION

The functions of audition parallel those of vision and touch, operating in a sequential format with their own specific qualities. We respond to extremely fine gradations in recognizing variation in an auditory signal. We also register enduring, prototypic auditory images that permit us to recognize classes of sounds over contextual and other variation and to differentiate one class from another. Thus, on the one hand, we respond to continuous variation in pitch, timbre, and loudness, and to subtle differences in tone of voice, which tell us when someone is tired or angry or sad. We respond emotionally to differences in a baby's vocalizations, even when we cannot identify or articulate the meaning of these. On the other hand, we recognize and identify particular melodies or chords, and distinguish the sound of a violin from a cello or a clarinet. We can identify a friend's voice, whether in person, over the phone, or on a tape recorder, provided sufficient ranges of signals are retained. We distinguish our own baby's cry from all others—even in a crowded room—(or at least we think we do). Each of these identifiable entities constitutes discrete "objects" in the auditory domain. As for visual images, such auditory entities appear to be formed by auditory input processed on continuous dimensions funneling into functionally equivalent classes represented by prototypic images—a remembered melody, the sound of a violin.

Audition resembles vision and differs from olfaction and taste in that specific, coordinate systems may be identified, even for continuous processing dimensions. As for vision, the implicit coordinates that underlie computation in the auditory system can be specified both in properties of the stimulus (such as pitch and amplitude) and in the specific features of the receptors that register variations in these properties. There may also be audiospatial coordinates paralleling visuospatial ones and reflecting the ability of sound to represent distance and location.

While the computational basis for forming representations of objects and relations among them differs across modalities, the general bipartite processes of symbol formation occur in their own modality-specific formats in all of them. I suggest that the application of this approach to each, individual sensory modality is a fertile field of basic research that needs to be explored. In all modalities, people register very fine distinctions, which permit them to guide their movements, track changes in location and orientation, or differentiate shifts in the multiple sensory qualities of the stimulus. In all modalities, people also overlook such fine discriminations and form functionally equivalent ranges of representation and prototypic images. These representations of objects may be constructed within a specific modality for visual, auditory, or tactile representations, or they may be cross-modal images or concatenations of images in episodes, as is most likely to occur for odor, taste, visceral experience, and movement. However, the general transition from subsymbolic representation to prototypic imagery to words may be traced in each modality and forms the central model of the symbolizing process.

CHAPTER 8

Emotion and Cognition
A NEW INTEGRATION

The goal of this book is to develop a new model of emotion and cognition that is applicable to psychoanalysis. In developing this model, I lay the foundation on the information-processing approach that is central in cognitive science today. I have identified structures and functions of mind that are relevant in accounting for some of the basic processes with which psychoanalysis is concerned. However, psychoanalysis is concerned with emotional experience and emotional meanings in their somatic and sensory contexts, and the cognitive models are less specifically applicable in that respect. In this chapter, I will briefly review theories and research on emotion, its relationship to cognition, and its neurophysiological substrate, to develop a foundation for an integrated theory of emotion and mind.

Modern scientific psychology has, until recently, implicitly accepted a Platonic view of the human psyche as divided into separate functions of cognition, emotion, and conation or motivation. In this context, the study of emotion was focused largely on the qualities of subjective emotional experience. Cognitive scientists have attempted to study cognition independent of emotional factors, as reflected in much of the research outlined earlier. Also in the Platonic shadow, many theorists have assumed a view of emotions as processes that interrupt the coordination of ongoing cognitive and behavioral sequences and have distinguished emotion from motivation on this basis. Thus, Pribram (1984) defines emotion as "derived from processes that stop ongoing behavior," and defines motivation in terms of activation of readiness mechanisms, when the organism "is ready to 'go' and to continue 'going' " (p. 26). Taking a similar position, Simon (1967) has argued that emotions can be represented in computer simulations by an interrupt system that calls on corrective subprograms when difficulties arise in the major program.

Some emotion theorists have recently begun to question the Platonic distinctions and the focus on phenomenological aspects of emotion. The field of emotion theory has undergone its own paradigm shift, related to that of the cognitive revolution, from a focus on quality of emotional experience to an emphasis on the emotional meaning of events, which may be processed outside of as well as within awareness.

I will begin here by briefly reviewing several of the important early theories of the activation of emotion and its role. There are also a number of competing taxonomies of the discrete emotions that have been proposed during the past several centuries, from Descartes (1650) to the present day (see, e.g., Panksepp, 1982; Plutchik, 1980; Tomkins & McCarter, 1964); I will not attempt to cover these. Ultimately, I am concerned with developing a general theory that will account for how emotional processing occurs, rather than specifying the particular dimensions on which emotions may be differentiated, or the particular forms that emotions may take.

EARLY THEORIES OF EMOTION: IDENTIFYING THE PHYSIOLOGICAL BASE

Early theories have primarily sought to account for the experiential qualities of emotion and have formulated the account in physiological terms. Although I will discuss the neurophysiological substrate of emotion, my goal remains to formulate a psychological rather than neurophysiological theory. Building on Lange's "visceral theory" (1885), James (1894) argued that bodily changes, including emotional expression, determine emotional experience, rather than emotions preceding or determining bodily expressions, as in the commonsense view. According to James, the perception of an arousing event by sensory cortex leads to bodily changes, including changes in facial expression and muscular and visceral activity—shivering, screaming in terror, attacking, running away. This activation was understood as primarily of a reflexive or instinctual type. The experience of these bodily changes constitute the emotion state.

James's initial formulation incorporated complex patterns of somatic, visceral, and muscular events as differentiating the emotions. He characterized the physiological responses underlying and differentiating emotion states as "almost infinitely numerous and subtle" (1884, p. 250), "reflecting the infinitely nuanced nature of emotional life" (quoted in Ellsworth, 1994, p. 223). James's vivid descriptions of these responses include expressive movements, visceral feedback, actions, and "various 'pangs,' 'glows,' 'fullnesses,' and 'tingles' that are difficult to classify": "A glow, a pang in the heart, a shudder, a shiver down the back, a moistening of the eyes, a stirring of the hypogastrium, and a thousand unnameable symptoms besides, may be felt the moment the beauty excites us" (James, 1890, p. 470; quoted in Ellsworth, 1994, p. 225). James describes his experience of waking from a nightmare most vividly in terms of such combined bodily events: "On such occasions the horror within me is largely composed of an intensely strong but indescribable feeling in my breast and in all my muscles, especially those of the legs, which feel as if they were boiled into shreds or otherwise inwardly decomposed" (1894, p. 207).

The complexity and subtlety of these physiological responses were in principle sufficient to account for an infinitely nuanced range of emotional experience. However, James later retreated to a considerably simplified version of this theory, closer to Lange's more exclusive focus on emotion as determined by the operation of the vasomotor systems. The James–Lange theory has been generally understood and criticized in this simplified form, in particular, as postulating that different emotions are distinguished by specific patterns and qualities of autonomic nervous system activation.

Cannon (1927) argued that autonomic activation is too slow, too insensitive, and not sufficiently differentiated to account for the latency, dynamic range, and variety of emotional experience. In contrast to the James–Lange formulation, Cannon placed the critical emotion mediator higher in the diencephalon, in the subcortical forebrain. According to Cannon (1927, 1931), the brain possesses a special emotional system whose integrative structure is the hypothalamus. Papez (1937), building on Cannon's work, postulated a circuit theory of emotion, centering on the hypothalamus. Sensory stimuli activate the hypothalamus, which then discharges to the periphery to produce emotional responses and to the cortex to produce emotional experience. According to this approach, emotions are generated within the central nervous system by the hypothalamus, prior to activating the cortex.

A role for temporal lobe functions in emotional processing was first shown by Klüver and Bucy (1937). They discovered that large lesions of the temporal lobe of monkeys produced a syndrome that they described as "psychic blindness." The animals were not blind to the sensory characteristics of stimuli but failed to compute their affective significance, so that their behavior became maladaptive in specific ways. For example, they were no longer threatened by the presence of previously feared stimuli, attempted to copulate with members of different species, and did not distinguish edible from inedible objects.

MacLean (1949, 1952) postulated the existence of a specific group of cortical and subcortical structures, a visceral brain or limbic system, as constituting the emotion processing system of the brain. According to MacLean, the limbic system is made up of phylogenetically ancient structures that constitute a unified and dedicated anatomical system for emotion. Some aspects of MacLean's model have since been questioned and modified (Swanson, 1983; Brodal, 1982). Limbic areas, particularly the hippocampus, are not dedicated exclusively to processing of emotion but contribute as well to other cognitive operations, including spatial behavior (O'Keefe & Nadel, 1978) and the forms of memory characterized as declarative, as discussed earlier. However, MacLean's basic claim concerning the role of limbic mechanisms in mediating emotion is generally accepted today (LeDoux, 1989; Buck, 1988). Current neurophysiological research on the emotions may be seen as building on the basic limbic system hypothesis and as elaborating, extending, and qualifying this, as will be discussed.

Attribution and the Cognitive Appraisal Controversy

A major problem that arose for early theorists such as James–Lange and Cannon was a failure of correspondence between emotional experience and physiological changes. The same emotional experience and emotional expression were found to be associated with different organic symptoms; conversely, variation in emotion occurred without change in organic events. Chemically induced organic or visceral responses alone do not produce emotion, and surgical isolation of the viscera does not prevent their occurrence. In a series of experiments, Schachter showed that the emotional meaning or attribution of the same chemically induced physiological states varied as a function of experimental context (Schachter, 1959; Schachter & Singer, 1962). This differentiation of emotions depends on complex cognitive factors, not directly on neurophysiological changes only. Once a person is in a state of arousal, he then tries to account for his state in the context of his understanding of his current situation; thus, he defines the nature of the arousal on the basis of the meaning of particular events.

Other cognitive theorists, going beyond Schachter's approach, argued that the capacity of a stimulus to arouse a physiological response must itself be determined by a prior mental analysis. Rather than operating to attribute an ongoing physiological event to an element in the stimulus situation, the emotional experience begins with an appraisal of the significance of the stimulus event. Such cognitive appraisal occurs in several stages: first, the initial evaluation of the significance of a situation, followed by additional evaluations of the situation that now may encompass the physiological activation, then followed by selection of appropriate responses (Lazarus, 1984).

In opposition to theories of cognitive appraisal, Zajonc (1980) argued that cognition and affect are separable and at least partially independent systems. The major evidence for independence of affect and cognition came from studies of "exposure effects" (Zajonc, 1980) in which liking or preference for stimulus objects was induced by repeated exposures, without recognition of the object or awareness of its familiarity. Thus, the subject shows liking for an object, which is based on its familiarity but without cognitive appraisal of the familiarity having occurred. A long-standing controversy between Lazarus and Zajonc as to whether affect precedes or follows cognitive appraisal remains unresolved (Lazarus, 1984; Zajonc, 1984a, 1984b).

Facial feedback theorists (e.g., Tomkins, 1962; Ekman, 1984; Izard, 1977) argue that feedback from the facial musculature has the specificity that is lacking in the physiological arousal, and the immediacy that is lacking in cognitive appraisal, and that interconnected patterns of facial expression and somatic response are sufficient to account for the discrimination of emotional events. Recent research by Ekman and his colleagues has demonstrated a relationship between specific facial expression and differentiated autonomic events (Ekman, 1984). However, the question remains as to where in the system the emotional meaning that determines the change in facial expression may be computed for other than instinctual responses.

NEW EMOTIONAL
INFORMATION-PROCESSING MODELS

In recent years, the field of emotion theory has moved away from the earlier emphasis on accounting for emotional experience, toward a focus on emotional information processing. This provides the needed perspective concerning the intrinsic integration of emotion with cognitive functions. Many researchers today define emotions as essentially adaptive, motivational mechanisms, which interact with or are aspects of cognition. Scherer (1984) characterizes emotion as "the interface between an organism and its environment mediating between constantly changing situations and events and the individual's behavioral responses" (p. 295). From this perspective, emotions are seen as particular types of information-processing schemas, which enable evaluation of the meaning of events for an individual's well-being and provide the basis for directing action. This does not deny the subjective experience as a component of the emotion construct but avoids restricting emotion to its pheno-menological aspect. In a survey of theoretical positions on emotion, Scherer (1984) states:

> There now seems to be a growing consensus among emotion theorists that emotion is best treated as a psychological construct consisting of several aspects or components: a) the component of cognitive appraisal or evaluation of stimuli and situations, b) the physiological component of activation or arousal, c) the component of motor expression, d) the motivational component, including behavior intentions or behavioral readiness, and e) the component of subjective feeling state. (p. 294)

Within the framework of current work, researchers can move forward from controversies concerning cognitive versus physiological factors to development of a more comprehensive, integrated formulation of emotional information processing. From this perspective, the crucial question that a theory of human emotion must answer is how differential emotional meanings are assigned to different events, and how emotional meaning is assigned for some stimuli and not for others. The essential question is how the emotional *meaning* of an event—its significance for the well-being of the organism—is computed, not how the emotional *experience* is determined. This new approach also permits a formulation of the concept of unconscious emotion, which has seemed paradoxical from the standard Platonic perspective.

In lower mammals and nonmammalian vertebrates, the computation of stimulus significance is, to a considerable extent, genetically built in. Key environmental stimuli have the power to trigger or release instinctive, reflex-like emotional responses that direct behavior. However, primates and higher mammals need to process and evaluate the differential significance of sensory input (a snake, a picture of a snake, a shadow in a doorway) in order to determine, in a flexible manner, whether—or to what degree—emotional significance will be assigned. To do this, they must be able to learn the emotional significance of stimuli, transfer this to other, related stimuli, discriminate among stimuli, and change values that have been assigned.

Consider an individual walking in the woods. A long, thin object coils its way into peripheral vision. What is the nature of the response that may be expected? The theories of James–Lange, Cannon, and more recently, Zajonc and Ekman appear to focus on responses that are largely hardwired, reflexive, and innate. When one perceives such a coiled object, one tends to get excited, or scream, or jump, or flee (or some combination of these). The feeling of fear then emerges as a function of the expressive, or motoric, or autonomic response. On the other hand, as the attribution theories emphasize, the somatic and motoric reaction of an American hiker walking for the first time in the Tuscan hills above Sienna, who has just seen a sign warning of vipers, will be different from that of the same individual walking in a familiar park on Long Island, where there are no known poisonous snakes, and where he has walked many times before, even if the perceptual images as seen in peripheral vision are highly similar. An adequate theory of emotion must mediate this difference in response, in effect, must account for both the swift and immediate response that is characteristic of many such situations in which one moves away before one is aware of having recognized the threat, and also for the cognitive evaluation that modulates this response to varying degrees.

I will address this question in this chapter in terms of current theories of the neurophysiological substrate of emotion to complete our survey of these approaches. In the formulation of the multiple code theory of the emotion schemas, in Chapter 12, I will then provide the emotional information-processing model that is compatible with the emotional circuitry that will be outlined here.

The Thalamo-Cortico-Amygdalar Circuit

The current neurological theories of emotion can account for cognitive computation that differentiates systematically among stimuli depending on their adaptive significance for an organism, but that may also occur with immediacy and outside of awareness. The amygdala has now been identified by many researchers as the critical emotion mediator, performing the functions attributed to the vasomotor centers of the brain stem by James–Lange, and to the hypothalamus by Cannon and Papez, and accounting for connections to cortical functions. Weiskrantz (1956) and others have shown that lesions of the amygdala, located deep within the temporal lobe, impair the positive motivational value of visual stimuli. Whereas damage to temporal neocortex disrupts visual discrimination and object perception, amygdalar neurons are more sensitive to the affective significance of stimuli than to their sensory characteristics. The amygdala receives afferents from the visual, auditory, somatosensory, gustatatory, and olfactory areas of the cortex. Interruption of connections between modality-specific cortical areas and the amygdala produces a modality-specific psychic blindness, as in the Klüver–Bucy syndrome (Downer, 1961; Horel & Keating, 1969).

Pathways of Emotion

Neurophysiological models now generally converge on the following pathway for processing the emotional significance of a stimulus. Input received at sensory receptors is transmitted to the sensory thalamus, then to the sensory neocortex, the cortical association areas, the hippocampus, and portions of the olfactory cortex, among other structures, and to regions of subcortical forebrain, which include the amygdala, hypothalamus, anterior thalamus, and other components. The efferent pathways from the forebrain then descend to determine activation and regulation of musculoskeletal, autonomic, and endocrine systems, which underlie the expression of emotions in its bodily forms, including facial expression, action, and somatic effects. The autonomic component may involve projections to neurons in the lateral hypothalamus as well as other brain areas involved in autonomic regulation.

The operation of the hippocampus–amygdala circuitry speaks directly to the question of how the emotional significance of stimuli is computed on the neurophysiological level. Connections between the hippocampus and the amygdala permit the amygdala to receive integrated cognitive information processed through the cortex. Such information contributes to the amygdala's computation of the emotional significance of sensory information from the environment or from within the body, thus accounting for varying degrees of emotional response for different stimuli.

The definition of "stimulus information," as this figures in emotional circuits, is broad and includes stimuli that originate in the external environment (exteroceptive stimuli) as well as stimuli that originate within the body (interoceptive) and the brain (thoughts and memories). The amygdala has been shown to be involved in evaluation of the emotional significance of viscerosensory inputs as well as information about the external world (Kapp, Pascoe, & Bixler, 1984). For example, the vagus nerve, made up of afferents from tissues of the abdominal cavity, including gut, heart, and blood vessels, projects onto a nucleus of the medulla, from which neural fibers then project onto the amygdala. Electrical stimulation of the vagus nerve affects the activity of amygdalar neurons (Radna & MacLean, 1981). Interruption of vagal activity disrupts performance in emotional tasks (Albiniak & Powell, 1981). Current research on the effects of emotional arousal on memory also support the role of the amygdala in processing viscerosensory input. Secretion of the hormones adrenaline and noradrenaline, which prime physiological reactions in emergency situations, also act on pathways in the amygdala to boost memory for certain emotionally loaded events. Drugs that block the usual effects of these hormones impair emotional memory specifically, without affecting memory for neutral details (Cahill, Prins, Weber, & McGaugh, 1994).

The amygdala also assigns emotional significance to information retrieved from memory and to images and thoughts. Activation of the emotional circuitry may be generated entirely within the central nervous system without requiring the participation of peripheral sensory systems. Images arising in memory and activating cortical networks may arouse emotion, with all its efferent concomitants, as may information from bodily, motoric, or external receptors. Thus, motivation is affected by somatic needs, or drives, and also by environmental factors, but not dependent on these.

Information from all sources, feeding into the amygdala, then impact upon efferents that determine the expression of emotion through somatic, autonomic, and behavioral channels. These efferents may feed back to cortical projections as well, so that somatic and motoric information may contribute to the ongoing evaluation and reevaluation of emotional meaning.

Cognitive information may be brought to bear to modulate efferent activity through the hippocampal projections onto the amygdala. The hippocampus blocks irrelevant stimuli from eliciting arousal and permits differentiation of stimuli on the basis of perceptual features and associative connections; thus, we may not jump for the same stimulus on Long Island as in Tuscany, or we may jump less. Hippocampal lesions interfere with the modulation of conditioned emotional responses by cognitive (contextual) information, as shown in experimental studies. Whereas the amygdala is required for conditioning of affective significance, the hippocampal projections are required to prevent the amygdala from assigning affective weight to irrelevant stimuli (Solomon, 1977; Rickert, Bennet, Lane, & French, 1978).

In the absence of hippocampal modulation, any stimulation is more likely to acquire the power to increase or induce the physiological effects of stress. This is supported by a study of the contrasting roles of hippocampus and amygdala in gastric pathology. Whereas amygdalar lesions have been shown to reduce the development of ulcers following stress, hippocampal lesions aggravate such stress-induced ulcer formation (Henke, 1982).

The circuitry outlined here is bidirectional. The amygdala projects directly to the hippocampus; thus, ascending circuits may be activated, which project back to the same areas that initially contributed to activation of the amygdala. Through these projections, emotional evaluations mediated by the amygdala influence perception, memory, and thought. Thus, the hippocampus–amygdala complex provides a neurophysiological basis for the bidirectional interaction of emotional evaluation and cognitive processing, involving sensory, motoric, and somatic processing systems, which is central to the evaluation of emotional meaning, as this figures in an emotional information-processing theory.

Alternate Circuits: The Thalamo-Amygdalar Bypass

In addition to the thalamo-cortico-amygdalar (T-C-A) circuitry outlined here, LeDoux has also identified an alternate route for emotional computation of a more primitive and immediate sort, bypassing cortical structures. Relay nuclei of the sensory thalamus send projections directly to the amygdala, as well as projecting onto sensory areas in the neocortex. The thalamo-amygdalar (T-A) projections are monosynaptic and thus more rapid than the T-C-A route, in which at least three additional synapses intervene (LeDoux, 1989). The two circuits differ also in that direct T-A projections arise primarily in thalamic areas with cells that are characterized as relatively nonspecific and weakly tuned, contrasting with highly integrated inputs from modality-specific and multimodal association areas processed through the hippocampus.

In contrast to the cortico-amygdalar projections that account for evaluation of complex stimuli, the thalamic system is probably not capable of object recognition, so that the T-A projections appear to be involved in processing the affective significance of relatively simple sensory cues and in conditioning paradigms. For example, these mechanisms appear to be necessary and sufficient for the conditioning of simple fear responses (LeDoux, Sakaguchi, & Reis, 1984; LeDoux, Sakaguchi, Iwata, & Reis, 1986; Iwata, LeDoux, Meeley, & Arneric, 1986).

As outlined by LeDoux, the T-A circuitry has its roots in evolutionarily earlier processing systems. In primitive vertebrates, which lack a well-developed neocortex, subcortical sensory structures provide the primary inputs to subcortical forebrain areas, such as the amygdala. Thus, the thalamo-amygdalar circuit may play an important role in the processing of emotional information in human infants prior to the full maturation of the neocortex and its anatomical connections. The T-A pathways may also mediate emotional reactions in adults, occurring prior to recognition of specific perceptual features or recognition of objects.

The T-A pathway, providing the amygdala with "quick and dirty" representations of peripheral stimuli, may have an additional adaptive function in preparing the amygdalar neurons to receive complex information, following more slowly via the T-C-A route, for example, by informing the amygdala of the sensory modality that is being activated and of basic stimulus properties. This could enable selection and tuning in of appropriate neuronal ensembles in the amygdala and facilitate processing of information received shortly thereafter via the cortical projections (Le-Doux, 1989).

The T-A circuitry is thus able to account for immediate, defensive responses based on crude stimulus information and directed through efferent connections of the amygdala. The types of stimulus features identified by Zajonc (1980) as mediating preference formation, and Zajonc's finding that object preference precedes object recognition, are compatible with the crude processing capacities of the T-A pathway. While such responses may be initiated inappropriately in some situations, false-positive responses to threat are likely to constitute less of a problem for the survival of the organism than failure to respond to real danger, as LeDoux has argued. Furthermore, the defensive reaction can generally be halted if more detailed perceptual analysis (provided by way of cortico-amygdalar connections) indicates that the threat is not real.

On the other hand, there is increasing evidence that unchecked activation of the amygdala and its efferent outputs may, in some cases, be a danger in itself, triggering aggressive responses or activating visceral systems in inappropriate situations. Excessive and prolonged visceral arousal of this nature is associated with hypertension and gastric ulcers, as well as breakdown of immune defenses (LeDoux, 1986).

In addition, the T-A sensory pathways, if not coordinated by cortical processing, might lead to learning and activation of conflicting responses to the same stimulus. Similarly, associations to specific sensory features might, in later situations, be generalized inappropriately to other features by activation of topographically weak thalamic neurons with limited sensory coding and discriminating capacities.

This analysis of the underlying neurophysiological circuitry brings us back to our hiker in Tuscany or Long Island. The image of an object coiling along the road is transmitted from the retina to the thalamus and then to the visual cortex. Through T-A pathways, affective responses with efferent autonomic and motoric components may be directly activated. Heartbeat may increase; the person may call out and prepare to run; visual receptors may be tuned. At almost the same time, through cortical (including neocortical–hippocampal) networks, properties of the stimulus are computed and integrated; these also activate affective representations via cortico-amygdalar connections. Through these pathways, the particular affective responses that occur will be modulated to varying degrees and in varying ways by the person's knowledge of snakes in general, and of the fauna of the region in which he is hiking, and his motoric and somatic responses will be determined by this. For the hiker on Long Island, the T-A activation of heart rate and motor response will be modulated through T-C-A circuits by his knowledge that no poisonous snakes have been identified there. For the same American in Tuscany, the information processed through the cortex will serve to intensify the initial T-A-instigated response. The evaluation of emotional significance determines which descending efferents are activated and which autonomic, humoral, and behavioral responses occur.

A PSYCHOLOGICAL MODEL OF EMOTIONAL INFORMATION PROCESSING

I am concerned in this book with the development of a psychological, not a neurological, theory. However, in building a psychological model, it is important to show that its claims are compatible with what is know about the neurological and somatic substrate. The development of a psychological or information-processing model of emotion is informed, and constrained, by our knowledge of the neurological structures and processes that have been outlined here. The complex, bidirectional circuitry of the emotion system, which incorporates information from sensory and somatic systems, and from the cortex, as reflected in the current neurological models, is compatible with the interactive organization of emotional information processing in the multiple code theory that is proposed in this book. The basic position, which is largely in agreement with current emotion research, as with neurophysiological findings, is that emotional information processing may best be accounted for as following the same basic processing rules as all information processing. The differences between emotional information processing and other forms lie in the components of the informational system that are dominant, not the basic structures or functions themselves. We need to develop the broader concept of information as incorporating many types of somatic and sensory events; we cannot restrict the concept of information to visual imagery and language only. This is important not only for building a psychoanalytic theory of emotional information processing, but also for the long-range development of general models of human cognitive functions.

In the new information-processing perspective, emotions incorporate cognitive, behavioral, and physiological functions of many types, and the study of emotion needs to include all of these. Given the complexity of the components of emotion, the categorization of the emotions must be complex as well. Development of prototypes through chunking of experience into functionally equivalent classes must occur for emotion as for all other types of experience. Within a category characterized as anger, for example, there will be a wide range of exemplars, with variation both within and across individuals. A theory of emotion, like theories of perception or cognition, must be able to account for the complex range of variation of the emotions, with their multiple components, as well as for their classification and their representation in verbal form. While we will not talk about the nature of specific, discrete emotions or the possible dimensions of differentiation that have been proposed, we will address, in Section Four, some of the general issues of how general categories of emotion schemas—adaptive and maladaptive—may be formed.

We may note that the new formulation of the emotion networks essentially bypasses the long-standing cognitive appraisal controversy. It is not that affect necessarily precedes or is independent of cognition, as Zajonc (1980, 1984a, 1984b) would argue, or that cognitive appraisal is always necessary in the generation of emotional meaning, as in the formulation of Lazarus (1984). Rather, many different forms of information input will participate in the generation of emotional meaning, dominated in some cases by subsymbolic, and in others by symbolic, including verbal, forms. As I have also emphasized, both cognition and emotion have a wider range of functional operation than has been recognized in earlier views, and these domains of operation overlap to a considerable degree, as I will elaborate in the formulation of the multiple code theory in Chapters 11 and 12.

THE ROLE OF AWARENESS

Like all information processing, emotional information processing goes on to a large extent outside of awareness. The complex of responses that characterizes an emotion is usually associated with particular subjective feelings but may be defined independently of this. As LeDoux (1989) points out, "The end-products of both affective and cognitive processing may reach conscious awareness, but neither affective nor cognitive processing is synonymous with or require the participation of phenomenal experience" (p. 281). Awareness or lack of awareness of emotional information processing is a variable that needs to be studied in its own right.

Attention and awareness are themselves understood as theoretical constructs, defined in terms of other constructs within a model of mind and inferred from a range of observable events (Posner & Rothbart, 1989). In physiological terms, information processed by sensory and emotion cortex, including feedback from the body, or information from the social or physical environment, along with feedback information from the efferent pathways of the amygdala, may become conscious by projection to the central attentional system, which is anatomically related to the frontal lobes (Shallice, 1982). The continuous, multifaceted processing that occurs outside of focal attention constitutes the core of the cognitive and emotional unconscious. The dynamic unconscious, or the concept of representations that are "warded off," involves a subset of these, with its own specific etiology and its own features, as will be discussed. Thus, the new approach accounts for the "computation" of unconscious as well as conscious emotional experience that is necessary for a psychoanalytic model.

CHAPTER 9

The Infant's Cognitive and Emotional World

The interaction of perception, action, and visceral experience, which determines the emotions, has its roots in earliest infancy in the context of the mother–infant interaction and continues to develop in increasingly complex form throughout childhood and throughout life. The development of emotional information processing needs to be understood in the context of the child's developing cognitive and linguistic competence, and the particular interpersonal frame in which this development is played out.

James (1890) described the infant's perceptual world as a "blooming, buzzing confusion." Similarly, Piaget (1950) also viewed the early mental life of the infant as relatively undifferentiated with respect to basic parameters such as time, space, and causation. He characterized the infant in the first year and a half of life as unable to represent the world of objects in its absence, to have memory of the past, or to generate anticipations of future events. According to Piaget, the infant's knowledge of the world during that period of life is based on development of sensorimotor schemas, sets of perceptual and motoric skills, which enable recognition of objects and appropriate behaviors in response to them, and which are developed through imitation of increasingly complex and precise motoric activities. The sensorimotor schemas are not concepts in the symbolic sense. Conceptual or symbolic representation is attained, according to Piaget, when these complex sensorimotor schemas develop fully, and become internalized in the form of images freed from physical

138

interactions with objects. This occurs in the preoperational phase, usually beginning at about a year and a half. The work of both Winnicott and Mahler rested on views of the early mental life of the infant as characterized by lack of differentiation of its own experience and of self from other.

The cognitive functions of the infant have recently become accessible to systematic observation in a new way. It is now generally recognized that the perceptual world of the infant is far more articulated than was assumed by Piaget, Winnicott, or Mahler. Using the general approach of cognitive psychology, researchers such as Fagan (1974), Fantz (1964), and Eimas (1975) have developed experimental procedures for investigation of infant perceptual organization and memory. These techniques include measurement of attentional preference through length of fixation and procedures based on habituation patterns. For example, when an infant has been habituated to a particular stimulus, perceived change or novelty will elicit specific measurable effects (e.g., changes in eye fixation or learned motoric responses such as foot kicks). The child's capacity to discriminate stimuli can then be assessed by measuring the amount of change on a specified stimulus dimension that is sufficient to elicit a novelty response. Such techniques now provide observable indicators that enable systematic inference into the infant's inner life.

The empirical infancy research has provided considerable evidence that the timetable and order of development of cognitive functions are considerably different from the sequence postulated by Piaget. The perceptual world of the infant is now seen to be organized to a large extent in a manner similar to that of adults. The type of perceptual organization that Piaget associated with concept formation is now seen to be in place well prior to the complex motoric organization that underlies the sensorimotor schemas. Thus, concept formation cannot be said to depend on sensorimotor schemas, as Piaget assumed.

The findings show that infants, even in the first half-year of life, live in a world of solid, permanent, predictable objects—human and otherwise—that interact and affect one another (Spelke, 1985; Leslie, 1982, 1988). They are born with the capacity to perceive time durations and have considerable capacity for spatial perception. Infants are able at birth to discriminate slight differences in rhythmicity, intonation, frequency variation, and phonetic components of speech, measured by behavioral indicators of discomfort and sucking rate (DeCasper & Carstens, 1980; DeCasper & Fifer, 1980). By 3 to 4 months of age, they understand that objects are permanent and continue to exist when out of sight (Mandler, 1991). There is also considerable evidence for recall of past events, over periods of at least 24 hours, at 9 months of age (Meltzoff, 1988), and even some evidence for recall as early as 4 months of age (Baillargeon, 1987).

Five-month-old infants recognize and remember patterns over periods as long as 2 weeks (Fagan, 1974; Fantz, Fagan, & Miranda, 1975). Three-month-old infants can remember specific objects in a training mobile and detect small changes in its composition (Greco, Hayne, & Rovee-Collier, 1990). DeCasper and his colleagues have even provided evidence for memory and learning *in utero.* Babies at birth preferred a tape recording of their mothers reading a Dr. Seuss story initially heard *in utero* over another story by the same author, also read by their mothers (DeCasper & Spence, 1986).

Other experimental studies have provided direct evidence for the development of prototypes in infant perception. Strauss (1979) showed 10-month-old infants a series of schematic drawings of faces that differed as to physical features such as placement of eyes and ears, or length of nose. Using the habituation paradigm, which assesses perception of novelty, infants were then "asked" to "select" the single drawing that best represented the series; in other words, the drawing was identified for which lowest average novelty responses were shown. The drawing that the infants identified in this way was the one that was most representative in the sense of averaging the features previously shown, but that they had in fact never seen before; that is, the averaged prototype.

CONTINUOUS VERSUS CATEGORICAL PROCESSING IN THE INFANT'S PERCEPTUAL SYSTEM

The separate functions of continuous versus categorical perception, operating in modality-specific ways, which are seen as central to the adult's cognitive and perceptual world, appear to be in place for the infant as well. In many studies using habituation and preference techniques (summarized by Bornstein, 1979, 1985), the infant's capacities for these bipartite functions within the auditory and visual systems have been found to be similar to those of adults.

The Infant's Auditory System

The perception of phonemes depends on differences in pitch and voice-onset time. The physical parameters underlying both pitch and voice-on-set time vary continuously, and infants from birth onward show acute sensitivity to changes in these parameters (Weir, 1976). While the underlying physical variation is continuous, phonemes are perceived categorically by adults, generally in three phonetic categories, characterized as prevoiced, voiced, and voiceless. Eimas, Siqueland, Jusczyk, and Vigorito

(1971) showed categorical processing of phonetic perception in 4-month-old infants in a way that paralleled that of adults. The infants were able to distinguish sounds corresponding to adult phonemic contrasts but did not respond to differences of equal acoustic magnitude within phonemic category ranges. These findings have been replicated with both synthetic and natural speech stimuli, and extended to other speech contrasts, as reviewed by Bornstein (1979, 1985).

Eimas and others have argued that the categorical perception of phonemes in early infancy constitutes evidence for the status of speech as innate in the human species (Eimas, 1975; Liberman, Cooper, Shankweiller, & Studdert-Kennedy, 1967; summarized in Bornstein 1979). However, several studies have also demonstrated categorical perception of phonemes in primates and other mammalian species, including the monkey and chinchilla, whose auditory systems are similar to those of humans (Morse & Snowdon, 1975; Waters & Wilson, 1976; Kuhl & Miller, 1975, 1976).

Visual Functions in Infants and Infrahuman Species

The work of Kosslyn, as discussed earlier, focused on the fundamental bipartite capacity for discrimination on continuous dimensions, and categorical perception, in the visual system of adults. Similar bipartite visual functions have also been found in infants and species other than man. All infrahuman species that see color have been found to partition the spectral continuum into categories of hue (Bornstein, 1979). Categorical organization of the perceptual field—such as perception of discrete phonemes and discrete hues—seems to be a matter of basic perceptual functioning, together with modality-specific processing. Such categorical processing, which provides the fundamental groundwork for the symbolizing function, is neither a specific, innate function associated with language, nor one that is specific to human adults or human infants, but is an aspect of perceptual processing that is shared across species and across modalities.

This is not to deny the potential effect of differential life experience in effecting reorganization of the perceptual field in each modality. While subjects from different cultures may show differences in placing category boundaries within the color spectrum, they show uniformity when the organization of the color field is assessed in other ways, such as through psychophysical studies of color scaling. Similar results have been found with adults from a wide range of language and cultural communities and in studies of perception with infants and infrahuman species. As Bornstein points out, wherever such categorical forms of perception have been sought "—in bee, pigeon, monkey, and chimpanzee, as in man—they have been found" (1979, p. 54).

Experience has its effects, and differential organization of the perceptual field occurs to some extent, as determined pragmatically by individual cultures. Nevertheless, the findings—in infant research, adult psychophysical studies, research with infrahuman species, and cross-cultural studies as well—provide evidence that this relativism is more precisely characterized as *reorganization* of a fundamentally organized field in which categorization has initially occurred based on perceptual principles and then been reorganized or refined based on experiential events. In no instances do we see experience as imposing a primary organization on what has been until then a buzzing confusion or homogeneous, undifferentiated field.

DEVELOPMENT OF THE LANGUAGE–THOUGHT INTERFACE

The bipartite nature of the *nonverbal* perceptual and cognitive systems, including continuous and categorical processing, is in place from the beginning of human life and has been found in other species as well. The categorical function, by which the continuous gradients of perceptual experience are chunked into discrete prototypic images, is the core of the symbolizing process as this operates in the nonverbal system, well prior to the acquisition of language. While this and other major cognitive capacities are developed prior to language acquisition, it is also the case that major advances occur when language is acquired. The advent of language is of basic importance in permitting new means of organization and direction of the self, and new forms of communication and sharing with others.

Researchers and theorists in the area of cognitive development have generally looked at early, nonverbal processing without addressing the cognition–language interface. In contrast, developmental linguists have generally identified the kinds of concepts that are represented in language acquisition without relating these to prior or ongoing cognitive development. As Mandler (1992) points out, neither field has contributed an adequate theory linking the two. Just as the work of Piaget does not provide an adequate basis for conceptual or symbolic development, it also does not account for the process of linking nonverbal experience and words. The sensorimotor operations that characterize the first year and a half of cognitive life, in Piaget's theory, are pattern-matching and motor control devices that deal with complex, continuous, analog information and are thus ill suited for mapping into the symbolic system of language, as Mandler (1992) has argued. The general failure of developmental theorists to address the language–thought interface parallels the corresponding failure throughout cognitive psychology and linguistics, with few exceptions, as will be discussed further in Chapter 11.

A major exception was the pioneering work of the Russian psychologist Vygotsky (1934). Vygotsky's work predates the recent breakthroughs in infancy research by about half a century. However, his conceptual contribution to our understanding of the language–cognition interface in the child's development is still uniquely valuable today. In his seminal analysis of the concept of "word meanings" and their development, Vygotsky (1934, p. 83) draws the following major conclusions:

1. Thought and speech have different roots in ontogenetic as in phylogenetic development.
2. We can identify a prelinguistic stage in the thought development of the human child, as well as in other species that do not develop language. We can also identify a preintellectual stage in the speech development of the human infant.
3. Up to a certain point in the child's development, the two functions develop along different lines and independently of each other.
4. At a certain point, these lines meet, whereupon thought becomes verbal and speech rational. The two functions reciprocally influence one another from that time.

The preintellectual roots of speech in the child's development include babbling, which may be characterized as practice with the sounds of speech, crying, vocalizations of many types, even the infant's first words; all of these are predominantly emotional and social functions and forms. The prelinguistic forms of thought include purposive actions, problem solving, and tool use. Both lines of development proceed separately to a relatively high level before they can be joined:

> At a certain moment at about the age of two the curves of development of thought and speech, till then separate, meet and join to initiate a new form of behavior. . . . The child "makes the greatest discovery of his life," that "each thing has its name" [Stern, 1914, p. 108]. . . . At this point, the knot is tied for the problem of thought and language. (Vygotsky, 1934, pp. 82–83)

The complex psychological unit of "word meaning" is the crucial product of this union of thought and speech. "It is in the internal aspect, in word meaning, that thought and speech unite into verbal thought. . . .

Word meaning is both thought and speech" (Vygotsky, 1934, pp. 5–6). Vygotsky has identified a mode of representation that he terms "inner speech," which is an internalization of the communicative speech forms that are learned by the child. Inner speech, which is speech for oneself, differs from external speech forms in relying on predication only, rather than including the subject–predicate structure required for communicative language. According to Vygotsky, such inner speech is the format of thought, the means by which the child represents all knowledge about the world, and which he uses to control and direct himself.

Vygotsky's work was seminal in identifying the separate lines of development of thought and speech, prior to acquisition of verbal thought, and their integration in a new conceptual form. However, his theory leaves out of account the continuation of these separate functions throughout life. His theory is an elaborated form of a verbal mediation theory and is vulnerable to the objections that have been raised to that class of theories. His notion of inner speech can account for processing within the symbolic domain, perhaps including discrete, symbolic imagery within the construction of inner speech, but does not incorporate the wide range of information-processing functions that we have identified as figuring in the emotions.

Vygotsky (1934), in fact, explicitly excludes the domain of emotional expression from the integrative union of vocalization and thought:

> The higher, specifically human forms of psychological communication are possible because man's reflection of reality is carried out in generalized concepts. In the sphere of the emotions, where sensation and affect reign, neither understanding nor real communication is possible, but only affective contagion. (p. 8)

Vygotsky thus relegates the expression of emotion to the preintellectual roots of speech, differentiated from thought, and restricts the powerful notion of developing word meanings to more neutral cognitive domains. This is particularly surprising in view of his familiarity with the great Russian authors, who were masters of expressive and evocative verbal forms.

PRELINGUISTIC PRIMITIVES: MANDLER'S APPROACH

Mandler's investigation of "prelinguistic primitives" is a recent attempt to account for the interface of language and thought as this develops in the second year of life. Her work brings current research to bear on the thought–language interface that Vygotsky studied. Mandler has addressed the relationship between conceptual development and language acquisition in terms of the nature of the organization of the infant's world that is necessary to provide a basis for words to be attached.

> Language is unlikely to be mapped *directly* onto sensori-motor schemas. There is a missing link: a conceptual system that has already done some of the work required for a mapping to take place. One of the functions of this early conceptual system, I believe, is to redescribe sensori-motor information into a form that is more compatible with the mapping process; that is, it forms an interface between analog sensori-motor functioning and the discrete symbols of language. . . . To illustrate, it would be extraordinarily difficult to go directly from the continuously varying physical parameters of the movement involved in picking up one object and placing it in another to the statement, "The marble is put into the cup." (1991, pp. 414–415, emphasis in original)

While Piaget viewed early concept development as dependent on sensorimotor functions, and Vygotsky characterized the cognitive world of the infant as first based on purposive activity and then organized by inner speech, Mandler argues that concepts are formed by a mechanism of "perceptual analysis," a reduction and redescription of information coming into sensory receptors that can take place "on line." Mandler's notion of perceptual analysis may involve comparison of one object with another, or attending to aspects of an object that have not been previously noticed. According to Mandler, such perceptual information initially may have a largely global, holistic character of the type that we have characterized as continuous or subsymbolic processing. Analysis of the categorical features (e.g., "green," "has legs," etc.) that might be expressed in a linguistic or propositional format is a separate, perhaps in some cases, a later intellectual achievement.

Mandler has proposed that the characteristics of infant concept formation, as carried out through perceptual analysis, are consistent with the notion of *image-schemas,* as formulated by cognitive linguists (e.g., Johnson, 1987; Lakoff, 1987; Langacker, 1987). Image-schemas consist of mappings from spatial structures, which include general aspects of the trajectories of objects and their interactions in space, to conceptual structure, the meanings of objects, and the kinds of events they participate in. The infant has the capacity to encode the spatial structure it perceives into schematic form; this allows formation of concrete memory images and provides the conceptual format onto which language may subsequently be mapped. The development of image-schemas is dependent on perceptual experience only and does not require the physical manipulation of objects that was required in Piaget's theory; thus, it can account for concept formation prior to emergence of highly developed motor skills.

Mandler has identified several types of concepts that may be formed in infancy through image-schemas based on spatial structures; these include Animacy, Agency, Containment, and Support. *Animacy* refers to the distinction between objects that engage in biological motion and those that do not. According to Mandler, infants register perceptual information concerning the beginning of a trajectory, as well as information concerning its course. They notice that objects that start up on their own move in a different way from objects that are caused to move, for example, things with self-motion may respond to the infant or to other objects from a distance and take irregular or unpredictable paths. Infants may thus distinguish a class of animate objects on this basis. There is evidence that infants can distinguish these types of motion as early as 3 months (Mandler, 1992).

A concept of *Agency* would be built by combining image-schemas of animate motion and caused motion. Four-month-old infants show evidence of surprise at a film of a hand picking up an object without making contact with it, indicating violation of expectations already formed and suggesting that a schema of Agency is already in place by this time. The image-schema of *Containment* represents objects in a space that is at least partially enclosed. The schema of *Support* represents an object above and in contact with a surface; 5½-month-old babies are surprised when containers without bottoms hold things, indicating presence of the Support schema.

Perceptually determined image-schemas provide the basis for acquisition of many basic grammatical notions, including modals (Sweetser, 1990; Talmy, 1988), prepositions (Brugman, 1988), and tense (Langacker, 1987). The concept of Agency is directly related to the subject–predicate distinction that underlies grammatical structure. The prepositions "in" and "on" are explicated in perceptual form in the image-schemas of Containment and Support. As Mandler notes, these are the earliest prepositions to appear in child speech and are learned in errorless fashion (Clark, 1977; Johnston, 1988). The perceptual image-schemas enable spatial representation of quite abstract concepts and serve as a bridge to language by this means.

On the basis of her analysis of the development of the image-schemas and their operation, Mandler proposes the following three-tier processing architecture as developing during infancy to account for concept development and the mapping of language onto thought:

1. Perceptual as well as sensorimotor procedures, which are largely global in structure—such as the perceptual experience of containment and support, the perceptual experience of movement and

how it is caused—provide the basis for the recognition of objects and the relationships between them.

2. The perceptual information so encoded is redescribed into image-schemas, in which spatial structure is used as the basis for conceptual structure, including the basic concepts of Animacy, Agency, Containment, and Support. These image-schemas include analysis of features in nonverbal, imagistic form, which is potentially amenable to propositional format, and "provide the earliest meanings available to the infant for purposes of thought" (Mandler, 1992, p. 8).

3. The image-schemas may then be redescribed in language.

NEW VIEWS OF THE INFANT'S EMOTIONAL WORLD

Mandler's formulation focuses on cognitive rather than emotional development. Changes have also taken place in our understanding of the infant's emotional development, which parallel the revision in our understanding of the infant's cognitive world and depend on this revision. The new findings concerning infant perception and memory, as well as recent studies of emotional development, now raise considerable questions concerning psychoanalytic views. Mahler's (1968) formulation of autistic and symbiotic phases as characterizing the early life of the infant has come into question from this new perspective. According to Mahler, the newborn infant in the autistic phase screens out external stimulation, particularly social stimuli. This is followed by "normal symbiosis," which lasts approximately from the second month to about 8 or 9 months. The infant in this phase is seen as experiencing a state of fusion or "dual-unity" with the mother, from which a separate self and other gradually emerge. In contrast to Mahler's formulation, recent research has shown that young infants are able to discriminate the emotional expressions of others, have expectations concerning others and goals for engaging in interactions with them, and are able to evaluate whether these goals are being met, based on their own emotional state. These evaluations then lead to further emotional and behavioral effects.

The emotional competence of infants as young as 3 months has been shown dramatically in the "still-face" experiments of Tronick and Cohn (1989). In this paradigm, mothers are instructed to remain still-faced when looking at their infants, rather than to respond in their usual manner. Tronick (1989) describes the results of this maternal behavior as follows:

> Confronted by these manipulations, most three-month-old infants initially signal to their mothers with facial expressions, vocalizations, and gestures in an attempt to get their mothers to resume their normal behavior. The infants' message is that their mothers should change what they are doing. When these other-directed behaviors fail to achieve that goal, the infants express negative emotions and use self-directed regulatory behaviors in an attempt to control their emotional responses. They look away and self-comfort. These reactions occur even when the mothers are still-faced for only a few seconds. Moreover, the infants' negative affect and utilization of self-directed regulatory behaviors do not end simply upon the resumption of normal behavior by their mothers. Rather, there is a continuation of the infants' negative mood and reduction in visual regard of their mothers for the next few minutes. This finding suggests that even three-month-old infants are not simply under the control of the immediate stimulus situation but that events have lasting effects, that is, they are internally represented. (p. 114)

The traditional assumptions concerning the undifferentiated nature of infant mental life have also been questioned by Stern (1985). He argues that infants have organization in their experiential field, including some sense of self and other from birth:

> They are predesigned to be aware of self-organizing processes. They never experience a period of total self/other undifferentiation. There is no confusion between self and other in the beginning or at any point during infancy. They are also predesigned to be selectively responsive to external social events and never experience an autistic-like phase.
>
> During the period from two to six months, infants consolidate the sense of a core self as a separate, cohesive, bounded, physical unit, with a sense of their own agency, affectivity, and continuity in time. There is no symbiotic-like phase. In fact, the subjective experiences of union with another can occur only after a sense of a core self and a core other exists. (p. 10)

According to Stern, the period from about 9 to 18 months is devoted not only to the developmental tasks of individuation and autonomy, but also equally to the seeking and creating of closeness and sharing, "learning that one's subjective life—the contents of one's mind and the qualities of one's feelings—can be shared with another" (p. 10). It is not that humans necessarily begin with autism and symbiosis, and must seek separation and autonomy; the developmental task in the emotional and interpersonal domain is more complex. Human infants experience themselves as separate and alone, and are motivated to seek closeness. This motivation is intrinsic to emotional organization, not secondary to satisfaction of bodily needs.

In Stern's formulation, the infant's organization of the core self and the complementary representations of core others are based on the discovery of fundamental invariants of experience—sequences of events involving one's self in interaction with objects and people, which recur and provide order to experience. Stern has specified four basic experiential invariants that operate within the nonverbal system and contribute to the development of an integrated sense of self and has discussed the specific capacities that the infant requires to identify these. These four basic emotion structures by which the self is organized—Agency, Coherence, Affectivity, and Memory—are defined by Stern as follows:

1. *Agency* is defined in the sense of having volition and control over self-generated actions, as distinguished from the actions of others. Volition is represented in the form of motor plans; such plans are guided by proprioceptive feedback. The consequences of actions are then experienced in varying ways. For actions upon the self, there will be felt consequences; for actions upon others, there will generally be systematic, contingent responses by them.

2. *Coherence* refers to the sense of being a single, bounded physical entity. This is dependent on factors such as unity of location, for example, the sound of a voice comes from the same direction as the image of a face. The self and others also show coherence of motion, temporal structure, form, and intensity gradients.

3. *Affectivity* refers to characteristic constellations of self-events associated with separate emotional states. These include proprioceptive feedback, patterned sensations of arousal, and qualities of feeling specific to the emotions.

4. *Memory* involves continuity of experience that maintain a core self-history. In addition to the motor memories, which figure in Piaget's notion of a sensorimotor schema, there is now considerable evidence of perceptual memory systems that operate from the first months of life, as shown in the research by Mandler and others outlined earlier.

INTEGRATION OF THE FEATURES OF EXPERIENCE

Stern (1985) then raises the question of how the repeated, invariant features of experience that have been identified—the experiences of Agency, Coherence, Affectivity, and Memory—become integrated into the organizing perspectives that are characterized as the sense of self and, complementarily, of others. He proposes that memory for repeated episodes provides the basis for such integration. As defined by Stern, episodes are small but coherent chunks of experience, which include "sensations, perceptions, actions, thoughts, affects and goals," and "which occur in some temporal, physical, and causal relationship" (p. 95). He gives the example of a "breast-milk" episode, with the following atttributes: "being hungry, being positioned at the breast (with accompanying tactile, olfactory, and visual sensations and perceptions), rooting, opening mouth, beginning to suck, getting milk" (p. 95). As specific episodes repeat, the infant begins to form a generalized memory, which Stern characterizes as

> an individualized, personal expectation of how things are likely to proceed on a moment-to-moment basis. The generalized breast-milk episode is not in itself a specific memory any more; it is an abstraction of many specific memories, all inevitably slightly different, that produces one generalized memory structure. It is, so to speak, average experience made prototypic. (pp. 95–96)

These prototypic memory structures involving actions, sensations, and affects, all occurring in a temporal, physical, and causal relationship in an interactive, interpersonal context, then form the basis of the nonverbal representational schemas that Stern terms Representations of Interactions that have been Generalized (RIGs). The studies concerning feature abstraction in the domains of phoneme, color, and form perception, which have been described earlier, support Stern's view that the infant is able to represent such categorical and prototypic experience from the beginning of life.

Lewis and Brooks (1975) and Beebe and Lachmann (1988) have provided evidence that very young infants are able to represent distinctive features of interactions, to construct prototypes that are composites of experience, and to apply these capacities directly to interpersonal and emotional experience. Beebe and Lachmann argue that early, repetitive, interaction structures organize evolving nonverbal representations within the first year. According to these authors, the infant "represents the distinctive features of social interactions before they are abstracted and before they are symbolized." These features include characteristic temporal and spatial patterns of behavior carried out by both participants in an interaction, as well as facial affective patterns. The interaction structures are represented as "patterns of mutual regulation, as they are organized by time, space and affect" (1988, pp. 310–311). The capacities necessary to develop these structures of cognition and social interaction are in place in the first year of life, long before language is acquired.

Affects, with their multimodal structures, are particularly well suited to contribute to the continuing sense of a core self.

The self-invariant constellation belonging to each discrete emotion occurs, for any infant, in a number of contexts and usually with different persons. Mother's making faces, grandmother's tickling, father's throwing the infant in the air, the babysitter's making sounds, and uncle's making the puppet talk may all be experiences of joy. What is common to all five "joys" is the constellation of three kinds of feedback: from the infant's face, from the activation profile, and from the quality of subjective feeling. (Stern, 1985, p. 90)

The expression and, presumably, the experiencing of basic affects change very little throughout life. The infant uses the same muscles to smile or cry as the adult, and the proprioceptive feedback from these expressions will thus also correspond. Emde (1983) has referred to the continuity of affective experience, beginning in infancy, as constituting an invariant affective core to what he terms the "prerepresentational" self. There is also evidence that infants remember conditions associated with particular affective experiences. Six- to 7-month-old infants, who had seen and laughed at a hand puppet performing amusing actions, smiled when they were shown the puppet in a quiet, unmoving state a week later; infants who had not initially played with the puppet did not respond with positive affect at the still presentation (Nachman & Stern, 1983).

CONVERGING DATA ON THE SYMBOLIZING FUNCTION

As we can see from this brief review of organizing schemas in cognitive and emotional development, Mandler's concept of perceptual analysis, leading to the development of image-schemas, parallels Kosslyn's analysis of the means by which perceptual information in continuous processing systems is chunked or funneled through functionally equivalent classes of representation to prototypic imagery, including representations of relations as well as objects. These concepts converge also with Stern's formulation of emotional organization through development of abstract, prototypic experiential schemas. The implications of this convergence will be discussed in detail in the presentation of the referential process and the verbalization of emotion in Chapters 11 and 13.

CHAPTER 10

Multiple Coding on the Neurophysiological Level
LATERALIZATION AND MODULARITY OF FUNCTION

The multiple code theory, which will be presented in Section Three, is a psychological model, a theory of mind, not a neurophysiological model or theory of brain. The elements of the multiple code theory are psychological constructs, defined in terms of other psychological constructs and inferred from observable behaviors within the theoretical framework of a nomological net, as I have discussed in Chapter 4. Mental constructs are not *reducible* to neurophysiological ones. As the two levels of theory become increasingly well developed, however, we would expect that constructs of mind and constructs of brain would be potentially *translatable* to one another. We may also expect that neurological data, like behavioral, linguistic, and other observations, will provide evidence that will contribute to the support, or disconfirmation, of psychological theories.

From this perspective, considerable neurophysiological evidence was reviewed in Chapter 7, showing that imaging occupies the same processing channels as are used by perception in visual and other modalities, thus supporting the modality-specific nature of imagery, as postulated in the multiple code theory. Considerable neurophysiological data have also been reviewed concerning the division of function in the human visual system. The various studies, discussed in Chapter 7, converge generally in differentiating a ventral system that underlies identification of objects, and associations among these, from a dorsal, parietal system that is specialized for spatial functions, and in placing the site of integration of these systems in the hippocampal formation. The difference in function between olfaction and vision, and the close correspondence of olfaction to processing of emotional experience also have correlates in the physiological system. Previous chapters have also included neurophysiological findings related to the new research on cognition and emotion, and their integration in a general theory of emotional information processing.

A discussion of neurophysiological evidence related to multiple coding and the referential process would not be complete without some reference to the studies of cerebral specialization and lateralization by Gazzaniga and others during the past several decades, as well as the more recent research on modularity rather than lateralization of function. From this perspective, the major importance of the findings that will be presented in this chapter is not so much to demonstrate the localization of specific processes, but to provide additional evidence from neurophysiology concerning the basic psychological division of function between categorical and continuous processing, and the integration of these processes.

I will first review some of the basic research concerning lateralization of mental functions, including lateralization of emotion, then look at the neurophysiological evidence for modality specific processing, then examine more closely the important distinction between categorical and continuous processing and its modality-specific applications. I will also show how the major classifications of mental functions are retained in the new modular or componential accounts, but in a more complex form.

HEMISPHERIC LATERALIZATION OF VERBAL AND NONVERBAL FUNCTIONS

Studies of patients with unilateral brain lesions have provided evidence, accepted for almost a century, indicating left-hemisphere specialization for language functions. Damage to the left cerebral hemisphere can cause severe disruption of language functions, while damage to the right produces little, if any, such disruption. While some left-handed persons may have right-hemisphere dominance for language, current data indicate left-hemisphere specialization for over 95% of the general population (Rasmussen & Milner, 1977). Evidence based on focal brain lesions also supports right-hemisphere specialization for some nonverbal perceptual functions (Milner, 1974).

These findings, based on localization of lesions, correspond in large part to results based on the commissurotomy or split-brain technique. The procedure of surgically severing the two cerebral hemispheres at the corpus collosum was developed in the early 1960s, in an effort to treat severe and otherwise intractable epilepsy. In the intact brain, information is continually exchanged between the two hemispheres across the corpus collosum. The surgical isolation of the hemispheres permits independent evaluation of the functions of each. The split-brain studies have focused primarily on the visual system and to a lesser extent on studies involving tactile stimuli.

In commissurotomized patients, it is possible to direct visual input selectively to the left or right hemisphere by projecting the visual image to the opposite half-field of the retina, and thus to study the capacity of each hemisphere in relative independence of the other. Vision is the only modality that allows for such strict lateralization. Touch information is also lateralized to a considerable extent, and there is some lateralization for auditory information. However, for touch and sound, there is evidence that somatic and sensory cues are registered ipsilaterally, thus raising questions concerning findings in these modalities.

The main tenor of the findings concerning localization of function in commissurotomized patients is well known. Such patients easily name visual stimuli flashed into the right visual field (reaching the left hemisphere). When stimuli are flashed to the left visual field, patients report seeing nothing. Similarly, patients, while blindfolded, can easily name objects held in the right hand but not the left. Conversely, right-hemisphere specialization has been found for some nonverbal processes, including facial and other pattern recognition, perceptual memory for stimuli that are not readily named, and visuomotor, tactile–spatial, and a variety of geometric and other mathematical tasks.

The evidence for isolation of function in commissurotomized patients can be dramatic. In one series of studies, a commissurotomized patient is shown a simple design, such as a cube, and asked to draw it. His left hand, which receives its major motor control from the right hemisphere, has no problem with this task; his right hand, directed by the left hemisphere, cannot do it. Similarly, the left hand can assemble blocks to match a pattern; the right hand cannot. The left hand may try to intervene and help the incompetent right hand. If the patient is told he may use either hand, the two hands become engaged in a struggle. The left makes progress, and the right comes in and undoes this (Gazzaniga, 1985, 1988).

In the years since the lateralization research began, the findings of this paradigm have been elaborated, qualified, and also questioned in many ways. The basic findings of the split-brain research have been expanded by some researchers to a more general view of the left brain as controlling analytic processes and the right brain as functioning in an analogous and holistic way. Some writers have also proposed broad characterizations of right-brain functioning as dominant in creativity and in synthetic (as opposed to analytic) thought. General characterizations of left- and right-brain cognitive styles have been popularized by Ornstein (1972).

Along these lines, several writers (Bogen, 1969; Galin, 1974; Hoppe, 1977; McLaughlin, 1978) have proposed an association of the primary and secondary processes of thought with cerebral lateralization. Bogen noted a loss of dream reports as well as loss of visuospatial memories in split-brain patients. Galin discussed the development of separate streams of consciousness attributed to the two hemispheres; in a conflict situation, for example, the left hemisphere might process and communicate a neutral or positive verbal response, while the right hemisphere processes a nonverbal experience of anger, which is then communicated through facial expression. As Galin also notes, the type of knowledge processed by one hemisphere may not translate well into the "language" of the other. Hoppe has noted impoverishment of dreams and fantasies in split-brain patients, as well as in a patient with a right hemispherectomy. He suggests that psychosomatic patients, who show lack of access to primary process thought, and dull and stiff verbalizations, may be suffering from what he terms a "functional commissurotomy."

PROBLEMS IN LATERALIZATION RESEARCH

A number of methodological problems have been identified, particularly in the early phases of this work, that raise questions concerning some aspects of the lateralization findings. First, the completeness of the commissurotomy varies among split-brain patients, so that some degree of connection between the two hemispheres may remain. There are now tests to verify the completeness of the surgery, but these were not used in the early phases of the research. Furthermore, even where the commissurotomy is complete, the commissural separation does not create isolation at the midbrain level, and there is possibility for interaction there. In addition, the subjects of this research are patients who have suffered severe seizures for many years, so that their overall capacity might be reduced. As Gazzaniga (1985) points out, preoperative testing is absolutely necessary to make sense of the split-brain results, that is, to show how the whole brain carried out these tasks, but such testing was not rigorously applied in much of the early research. Not the least of the problems in this field, according to Gazzaniga and other empirical lateralization researchers, has been the speculative proliferation of notions concerning hemispheric specialization, and particularly concerning right-hemisphere function, without systematic evidence being provided. The broader the claims concerning lateralization of function, the more problematic the evidence for them.

RIGHT-HEMISPHERE FUNCTION: DOMINANCE OR DEFAULT?

The nature of right-brain function has emerged as a major source of question and controversy in recent years. In a series of experiments with split-brain patients, Levy and her colleagues (Levy, Trevarthen, & Sperry, 1972; Levy, 1983) found experimental evidence for right-hemisphere superiority for a number of perceptual tasks. In these studies, competing stimuli were presented simultaneously to the two visual half-fields of split-brain patients, and the patients were asked to point to a matching choice from among alternatives displayed in free vision. Right-hemisphere dominance, indicated by the subjects' matching stimuli shown to the left visual field, was found for many types of objects and patterns, including faces, nonsense shapes, common objects, and geometric figures. Right-hemisphere dominance was also found for orientation of objects and for direction of motion of moving stimuli. The left hemisphere dominated in matching words with pictures, matching pictures according to rhyming names, selecting color patches named by color words, and matching pictures according to functional association (e.g., hat and gloves). These left-hemisphere-dominant tasks are characterized by Levy as involving word–image or word–percept connections.

The right hemisphere has also been shown to be superior in a variety of other perceptual and geometric tasks, including matching irregularly shaped wire "nonsense" figures by touch (Gazzaniga & LeDoux, 1978); deciding whether tachistoscopically presented arrays of dots are aligned in rows or columns, as defined by relative dot distance (Nebes, 1973); matching solid geometric shapes to two-dimensional drawings (Levy, 1970); and matching arcs of circles to whole circles of the same diameter (Nebes, 1972).

In a study examining the relevance of right-hemisphere function to aspects of mathematical reasoning, Franco and Sperry (1977) showed patients a set of objects related by some geometric or topological invariant and then asked them to select by touch the one, from among three other objects, belonging to the set. The task requires understanding of set-defining characteristics in the geometric and topological domains, and the capacity to relate these properties to new exemplars in a different modality. For all patients, mean right-hemisphere accuracy was greater than for the left hemisphere, and the right hemisphere completed the task with greater speed. These findings indicate that the right hemisphere is superior to the left for geometric and topological functions, even in the relatively complex types of reasoning tapped by this task.

ALTERNATE VIEW OF RIGHT-HEMISPHERE FUNCTION: GAZZANIGA'S CRITIQUE

Gazzaniga (1983, 1985) has questioned many of the findings concerning right-hemisphere superiority for visuospatial functions and has offered alternate explanations for some of the apparent differences in performance that have been reported. While strong, right-brain superiority was initially demonstrated for performance on spatial-manipulation tasks such as Kohs Block Design, recent results employing more careful examination of both pre- and postoperative capacities have suggested that both hemispheres, in interaction, were contributing to performance of these tasks. Gazzaniga has also suggested that the crucial difference for such tasks may be in the motoric rather than the perceptual component. Patients who demonstrate a right-hemisphere superiority for standard administration of the Block Design test may not show such differences when the task is transformed into a perceptual one, for example, to find a match between pictures of the designs.

The right hemisphere has been found in many studies to be superior to the left on facial-discrimination tasks; patients with right-hemisphere lesions show greater impairment in such tasks. However, Gazzaniga and Smylie (1984) found right-hemisphere advantage only for highly similar faces; there were no significant differences in performance between the two hemispheres for dissimilar faces. Similar results were found in a study using a set of subtly different, hard-to-name colors as stimuli. On the basis of these and other findings, Gazzaniga (1988) has argued that the two hemispheres, in fact, have equal capacity to solve perceptual tasks, rather than the right hemisphere being specialized for perceptual processing. The apparent right-brain advantage actually results because the right hemisphere proceeds directly with perceptual processing, rather than automatically operating to generate names, while the left brain automatically shifts into a verbal processing mode, regardless of whether this is the optimal way to perform a task. Thus, the left hemisphere automatically operates to assign names to things and can do this more readily for dissimilar than for similar stimuli. It will also continue trying to carry out its naming function, even when no clear and nameable distinctions are present, and no labels are available, rather than shifting into the perceptual mode. This, rather than diminished capacity for perceptual processing, according to Gazzaniga, constitutes its disadvantage in such task situations. Evidence for this argument also comes from studies of event-related brain potentials in which a component of the human brain wave that is associated with stimuli that are unexpected or unclassifiable was found to be generally larger in the right hemisphere. According to Gazzaniga, the left hemisphere reacts to a low-probability stimulus by naming or classifying it, thereby reducing or eliminating this brain-wave component, while the right hemisphere does not automatically operate in this way.

On the basis of a wide range of findings, Gazzaniga has argued that the left hemisphere is as well equipped to remember patterns as the right, but its verbal function automatically inteferes in some specialized task situations. He goes even further to speculate that in developing a lateralized specialization for language in the left hemisphere, the human organism pays the price of arrested development in the right: "It could well be argued that the cognitive skills of a normal disconnected right hemisphere without language are vastly inferior to the cognitive skills of a chimpanzee" (1983, p. 536). This position is of course highly speculative and controversial, and Gazzaniga himself has qualified this in some ways: "The right hemisphere does appear uniquely capable of certain kinds of visual, tactile, and auditory processing, and it is of interest to elucidate the nature of such specialization" (p. 547). As he notes, the nature of hemispheric function will emerge only by fully controlled testing of commissurotomized patients.

LINGUISTIC CAPACITY IN THE RIGHT BRAIN

Adding to this complexity was the finding, during the mid-1970s, of linguistic capabilities in the right hemisphere of some split-brain patients. When words are flashed to the left visual field, the patient typically states that he doesn't see anything. However a commissurotomized patient with some right-hemisphere linguistic capability can correctly select an object based on a word shown to his right hemisphere. Thus, his right hemisphere could understand the meaning of the words, although it was mute and could not report this; his right hemisphere also responded to verbal commands. Another subject could write out messages about information presented to her disconnected right brain, although she could not speak from it.

Some of the earlier findings of right-brain language function may have been ambiguous in that the necessary controls, as described earlier, were not fully applied. However, capacity for right-hemisphere language has also been found for some patients for whom full commissural section, including the anterior commisure, has been verified, and where strict controls over lateralization of question and mode of response have been applied. In cases where actual right-brain language capability has been verified, Gazzaniga argues that this may have developed in a compensatory manner as a result of left-hemisphere damage occurring prior to commissural section. This issue remains controversial, and the source, nature, and limits of right-hemisphere language capacity remain unclear (Zaidel, 1983). Further complicating these findings, Gazzaniga and his colleagues have demonstrated presence of some interhemispheric interaction, even in fully commissurotomized patients (Holtzman, Sidtis, Volpe, Wilson, & Gazzaniga, 1981; Gazzaniga, 1988); thus, the actual localization of the observed language function may itself be open to doubt.

The findings of the lateralization research remain unclear in many ways. The studies of patients with unilateral brain lesions and commissurotomized patients generally converge in demonstrating left-hemisphere specialization for language. Considerable evidence has also been found for right-hemisphere superiority for a number of perceptual tasks. However, there is at least some evidence (and considerable speculation) concerning left-hemisphere capacity for perceptual tasks, as well as some right-hemisphere language capacity. All of the lateralization findings are confounded by questions such as failure to test for completeness of commissurotomy in the early work; the possibility of interaction at the midbrain level, even where the commisural separation is complete; failure to establish preoperative levels of function in much of the research; and considerable individual variation among subjects. What we can conclude with some certainty, based on the findings to date, is that the simple dichotomy of function postulated in the early research has been disconfirmed, and that the situation is far more complex than was initially believed.

GENERATIVITY AND RIGHT-HEMISPHERE FUNCTION: EVIDENCE FROM EVOLUTION

Another perspective on the difference between right- and left-hemisphere function has been introduced by Corballis (1989). This work, based on evidence from evolution and focusing on the normal brain, throws new light on the distinctions of function with which we are concerned. Corballis has focused on the feature of *generativity* as the central and crucial characteristic of human cognition; according to his approach, it is generativity, rather than language per se, that is the essential function of the left cerebral hemisphere. Generativity is the power to produce novel assemblages by combining elements in a rule-governed way; these new composites may be words, sentences, multipart manufactured tools, or multipart images.

The faculty of generativity is an essential component of the symbolizing process, as discussed in Chapter 5. As Corballis has shown in his evolutionary analysis, generativity emerges with *Homo erectus* and the Acheulean tool culture about 1.5 million years ago and reaches its full form with *Homo sapiens,* the development of complex tool use, and rapid, flexible speech in the last 200,000 years. The capacity to form multipart entities from elementary parts in a rule-governed manner was intrinsic to the early construction of complex tools. While naturally occurring objects were used as tools in earlier times, the manufacture of tools for specific functions appears to be unique to hominids (Foley, 1987). The evolutionary progression of tool use follows the same course as the emergence of language.

The analysis of Corballis provides a different source of evidence concerning the fundamental distinction between analogous or subsymbolic processing and symbolic processing, characterized by generativity. This distinction has emerged in many different ways in the research reviewed in this section. Corballis discusses pattern recognition as a process that must be accounted for outside of the generative or symbolic domain. It might be possible, in principle, to conceptualize pattern matching or pattern recognition as generative tasks. However, to recognize a face, or differentiate one individual's face from another's using a generative process, would require a parsing or decomposition of the overall pattern into its perceptual elements by reverse application of the rules of their composition, followed by comparison of this to a pattern stored in memory to which a similar decomposition into elements has been applied. Furthermore, the differentiation and computation would need to be carried out within the time frame in which humans actually carry out such recognition; there is evidence that these conditions are not met. The same constraints arise, perhaps even more strongly, for discriminations within the other sensory modalities. We can see that PDP or subsymbolic systems are designed precisely to account for the type of analog processing that cannot be carried out in generative or symbolic modes. The distinction identified by Corballis provides an interesting evolutionary perspective on the major distinction between symbolic and subsymbolic processing that has been discussed in previous chapters, and some evidence for lateralization on this basis.

LATERALIZATION OF EMOTION

Early research seemed to indicate general right-hemisphere lateralization of emotion. There is now considerable evidence, however, demonstrating differences in lateralization for positive and negative affects. Left-hemisphere specialization has been shown for processing of certain forms of positive affect, particularly interest and curiosity, while the right hemisphere shows specialization for negative affects (Davidson, 1984). Data from patients with cerebral lesions and patients with affective disorders, experimental studies with normal subjects, developmental findings with infants, and phylogenetic data, are all consistent with this conclusion.

Galin (1974) suggested that repression may involve a functional disconnection between certain regions of the two cerebral hemispheres. In these terms, repression of negative emotional information might mean that such information, represented in certain right-hemisphere regions, does not get complete access to verbal centers in the left hemisphere. Davidson and his associates have identified individuals whom they term "repressors," who characteristically show little verbal response to negative information. "Repressors" show heightened autonomic and muscular activation in response to mildly stressful stimulation, while producing verbal reports of little anxiety. Both of these formulations reflect certain assumptions concerning the role of verbal processing that are not seen as viable today. It is also clear that Davidson's concept of repression, based on a generalized notion of negative affect, needs to be distinguished from the psychoanalytic concept, which concerns events that are conflictual or threatening in specific, individual ways. Nevertheless, Davidson's findings concerning the characteristics of "repressors" are suggestive and of interest for a psychoanalytic model.

Along these lines, Davidson has made the further suggestion that the classification of emotions, as this relates to cerebral dominance, may depend on an *approach–avoidance* rather than negative–positive dimension. Thus, the left hemisphere may be specialized for emotions associated with approach, including anger and interest as well as desire, while the right hemisphere is dominant for avoidance. Experimental studies of facial affect recognition have found left-hemisphere localization for angry as for happy faces. As Davidson points out, approach behavior involves voluntary, sequential execution of actions, including fine motor behavior; the left-hemisphere fine motor region is specialized for the control of fine manual behavior and sequentially executed movements on both sides of the body. The nature of action associated with withdrawal tends to be more automatic and reflexive, and less differentiated; the right hemisphere may be specialized for this. Thus "repressors," in Davidson's sense, might produce verbal reports associated with approach, while executing more undifferentiated behaviors associated with withdrawal. Davidson also suggests that depression may interfere with spatial cognitions involved in exploration and approach, while positive feelings may enhance these cognitions.

LATERALIZATION OF ODOR PROCESSING

Ideas concerning neurophysiological organization and its relation to psychodynamic processes also emerge from research on the lateralization of modality-specific functions such as odor. Little is known about cerebral localization for odor processing. Overall, there is some evidence favoring right-hemisphere dominance for odor processing, although a left-hemisphere role may also be present. Several studies (Rausch, Serafetinides, & Crandall, 1977; Abraham & Mathai, 1983) found more pronounced deficit in odor memory in patients with right temporal lobe damage. However, there remains considerable controversy among researchers in this field, and the neuroanatomical organization of the brain for odor processing is not yet systematically understood. Eskanazi, Cain, Novelly, and Matson (1986) found significant impairment of odor recognition associated with damage in both hemispheres; they suggest that the disparity with previous findings may have resulted from their using environmentally realistic stimuli, presumably previously encoded by the subjects, in contrast to the pure chemical odorants used by the other investigators. The suggestion of Eskanazi et al. is consistent with the conclusion, reached in Chapter 7, that odor memories are often represented as complete, unitary episodes. We might expect that episodes that incorporate a wide range of cross-modal imagery, language, and emotion would be represented in both hemispheres. The realistic nature of the stimuli used by Eskanazi et al. would facilitate their representation in episodic form.

In the light of the analysis of odor processing in Chapter 7, we may hypothesize that olfaction, like emotion, incorporates a range of functions that are not readily classifiable in relation to lateralization. Thus, while pure odor representations, and even the odor prototypes that have been postulated, might be primarily right-hemisphere functions, the differentiation and organization of odor incorporates specific images of people, events, and places such as are associated with left-brain function.

MODALITY-SPECIFIC AND COMPONENTIAL DIVISIONS OF FUNCTION: THE MODULAR ACCOUNT

Overall, the data suggest that there is indeed some consistent lateralization of function, but this is far more complex than was envisioned in the early days of the lateralization research. This greater complexity is in line with the new and continuously changing understanding of brain function in general. There is much redundancy and much parallel processing in human sensory systems, as well as multiple functional systems, operating differently in various regions of the brain. An obvious but important point, which may sometimes be overlooked in reviewing the lateralization research based on split-brain studies, is that both hemispheres generally participate in information-processing tasks in the normal, intact brain. Gazzaniga, Kosslyn, and others have argued that the earlier view of lateralization should be replaced by a modular account, which is not simply tied to hemispheric differences. The modular approach enables a more precise account of the neurophysiological substrate of continuous and categorical forms of information processing.

Componential Function in the Visual System

Using largely anatomical and electrophysiological techniques, visual processes such as motion detection, color detection, and other primary features of visual perception have been localized to different brain structures, with the different channels beginning to be identified in the retina and continuing into the association cortex. According to Kosslyn (1987), visual processing that generates explicit representations of objects and parts of objects, as in the categorical set of subsystems, and that operates independent of language, may become dominant in the left rather than right hemisphere. These would include (1) subsystems that process categorical representations to arrange parts in their appropriate locations in an image; (2) shape-encoding subsystems that produce representations of easily categorized shapes; and (3) subsystems that access and interpret categorical representations to shift attention to a particular element or class of elements. On the other hand, no such left-hemisphere dominance would be expected for imaging functions involving continuous processing of spatial relations, such as (1) subsystems that encode location for purposes of navigation or search; (2) subsystems encoding shapes as they appear from varying times or points of view; (3) subsystems that access stored coordinate representations to position attention at a specific location. Thus, Kosslyn sees the processes of image construction and the generation of language as left-hemisphere functions, while no left-hemisphere dominance is expected for nongenerative, analogic imagery functions. This distinction is supported by considerable empirical research.

Several predictions emerging from Kosslyn's model have been tested using the experimental techniques of the split-brain paradigm. One series of studies was carried out with a patient whose corpus collosum had been fully sectioned about 3 years before. This patient had previously been extensively tested, and his right hemisphere was known to be capable of comprehending verbal instructions and making simple deductions and classifications (Sidtis, Volpe, Wilson, Rayport, & Gazzaniga, 1981). In these studies, the patient was given several tasks differing in the degree to which they require processing of categorical information versus information based on continuous, implicit metrics.

The categorical tasks involved processes such as generating images composed of multiple, discrete parts in particular relationships to one another. Thus, the patient was asked to decide whether particular animals (e.g., cat, mouse, ape, or sheep) have ears that protrude above the top of the skull. Assuming this particular information has not previously been verbally encoded, the patient needs to generate images of the animals in order to answer the question. A significant left-hemisphere advantage was shown for this imaging task. The patient answered correctly with left-hemisphere presentation on 87.5% of the trials, while the right was correct on only 45%.

In contrast, size-comparison tasks require analog functions rather than generative imagery construction. In one set of tasks, the patient was asked questions such as which of two similar-sized objects is larger, or whether named objects are taller than they are wide. The stimulus materials and general procedures were the same as those that had been used in the multipart image tasks, and only the questions were different; no left-hemisphere advantage was found for such size-comparison tasks. Thus, as Kosslyn's formulation would predict, the localization of imaging functions differs depending on whether categorical processing or processing on continuous, implicit metrics is required.

Additional evidence for a left-hemisphere advantage for categorical perception has also been provided in neurological research. Damage to the posterior left hemisphere is strongly correlated with loss of discrete imagery (Farah, 1984). Several cases have also been reported of specific deficits in generating multipart images following left-hemisphere damage (Deleval, De Mol, & Noterman, 1983); Grossi, Orsini, & Modafferi, 1986). Experiments with normal subjects, employing rapid tachistoscopic presentation of the stimulus to one visual field, also support the left-hemisphere localization of generative imagery and categorical functions (Kosslyn, 1987). This division of function is compatible as well with Corballis's hypothesis concerning generativity as the underlying defining feature of left-hemisphere function.

Componential Division of Function and the Coconscious Mind

The focus on componential division of function, rather than distinctions based on lateralization, brings us closer to the types of functional dissociations with which analysts are concerned and the relationship of these to unconscious mentation. One of the most striking aspects of split-brain research is the extreme dissociation of function shown by these patients. As Gazzaniga has pointed out: "There is a certain eerie quality to watching a hand draw or point to places when the left brain of the patient does not in fact know under what command the left motor system is responding" (Gazzaniga, 1988, pp. 446–447). Given the notion of modularity, Gazzaniga suggests that such observations may be extended to functional as well as surgical dissociation. Thus, Gazzaniga has presented a view of the normal human brain as organized into relatively independent functioning units, or modules, that work in parallel; this organization accounts for shifts in awareness and the operation of unattended thought.

Many processes occur in independent modules outside of awareness in parallel with conscious thought. These modules can discharge and produce ideas, images, even behaviors:

> At the level of conscious experience, we frequently ask ourselves where particular ideas come from when they appear in our consciousness. For example, when we write, we suddenly think of the exact way to phrase an idea. Where does such an insight come from? We don't seem to know. We seem only to have access to the product of these brain modules and not to the process itself. (Gazzaniga, 1985, pp. 4–5)

In Gazzaniga's terms, behaviors that have no origins in our conscious thought processes are characterized as "capricious":

> For example, we just happen to eat frogs' legs for the first time or we decide to read a different kind of book. But as we shall see, we humans resist the interpretation that such behaviors are capricious because we seem to be endowed with an endless capacity to generate hypotheses as to why we engage in any behavior. (1985, p. 5)

When behaviors occur that are instigated by one of these modules, operating out of consciousness, a special brain component, which Gazzaniga calls the "intepreter," then is activated and generates hypotheses for this. The "interpreter" is a brain component found in the left-dominant hemisphere of right-handed humans.

> The emerging picture is that our cognitive system is not a unified network with a single purpose and train of thought. A more accurate metaphor is that our sense of subjective awareness arises out of our dominant left hemisphere's unrelenting need to explain actions taken from any one of a multitude of mental systems that dwell within us (Gazzaniga and LeDoux, 1978). These systems, which coexist with the

language system, are not necessarily in touch with language processes prior to a behavior. Once actions are taken, the left, observing these behaviors, constructs a story as to the meaning, and this in turn becomes part of the language system's understanding of the person. (Gazzaniga, 1983, pp. 535–536)

In this sense, behavior guides beliefs; we act, observe ourselves acting; then the left hemisphere constructs a belief to account for this.

Gazzaniga and his colleagues refer to empirical research with split-brain patients as supporting this position. In an experiment with LeDoux, different pictures were presented to each hemisphere, for example, a picture of a claw to the right visual field (left brain), a snow scene to the left visual field (right brain). Cards with pictures on them are set up in front of the patient, and he is instructed to select the card that goes with the picture he sees. The correct selection for the left hemisphere, which received a picture of a claw, is a picture of a chicken; for the snow scene, the correct selection is a picture of a shovel. A typical response for a commissurotomized subject is to point to the picture of the chicken with the right hand and the shovel with the left. When asked to explain the response, the subject replies, for example, that the chicken claw goes with the chicken and one needs a shovel to clean out the chicken shed. Thus, Gazzaniga argues, the left brain does not know why the left hand points to a shovel, but sees it happening and therefore works to supply a theory to make sense of what its own body is doing.

Other versions of this experiment, which are quite relevant to psychoanalytic issues, have examined effects of emotional activation in commissurotomized patients. In one experiment, a frightening movie of a fire, lasting over a minute, was shown to a subject's right hemisphere. (The verification of lateralized presentation for relatively long exposure times was made possible by an eye-tracking device; this precisely measures the movement of the eyes and stops the presentation of the stimulus at the slightest eye movement.) The subject reported seeing only a white flash. She also reported feeling kind of "scared" and "jumpy," although she didn't really know why: "I think maybe I don't like this room, or maybe it's you. You're getting me nervous." She then turned to an assistant in the room and said: "I know I like Dr. Gazzaniga, but right now I'm scared of him for some reason." The opposite result was obtained for pleasant filmstrips.

According to Gazzaniga, the language system of the left hemisphere is "intimately linked to a cognitive system that strives for consistency and order in the buzzing chaos of behaviors that are constantly being produced by the total organism" (1983, p. 536). The crucial distinction between the psychoanalytic model and Gazzaniga's position is that, in his view, the operations of both the nonverbal and the interpreter modules are capricious and undetermined. Thus, he characterizes actions such as the patient's pointing to the shovel and the anxious response following the fire movie as capricious in this way. In the same sense, he speaks of the "exact right way to phrase an idea," which "comes into awareness without our knowing where this came from," as emerging accidentally.

It seems apparent, however, that the empirical studies with split-brain patients carried out by Gazzaniga himself and his colleagues make the opposite point; they provide evidence, not for capriciousness, but for the psychoanalytic claim that behavior is determined. The experimental design is such that we know specifically how the responses are determined, although the patient does not. The processing that goes on in the coconscious modules is constructed and organized by motivated processes, as Gazzaniga's own results makes clear. The exact right way to phrase an idea does not emerge accidentally but is determined by motivated processes of thought of which we are unaware. As Gazzaniga says, without exploring the implications of this formulation, each of the actions that go to make up the "buzzing chaos" arises from one of the "multitude of mental systems that dwell within us" but may be dissociated from one another and from language. The patient is frightened because she has seen frightening filmstrips accessible to one of her mental systems but not to the one that interprets and talks.

FUNCTIONAL DISSOCIATION IN THE INTACT BRAIN: TOWARD A PSYCHOLOGICAL MODEL

In an intact brain, the separate modules are part of the total, more or less integrated functioning of the emotional information-processing system. It is important to recognize the partial and inadequate nature of this interaction, even in intact individuals. Nonverbal modules, particularly modules with subsymbolic forms, are likely to be experienced as outside of oneself, or to remain out of awareness. A theory of emotional information processing must account for such dissociation and also account for the interactions that do occur. The story that is constructed to make sense of the meaning of behavior may not be the true story. It could take considerable work to find the actual trigger of the behavior or affect, either in current experience or in the emotion schemas that have been previously constructed. However, one story is not as good as another; there are determining factors that can be discovered.

The psychoanalytic position is that these phenomena, which have been demonstrated in split-brain patients, play themselves out continually in all individuals. Thus, Gazzaniga (1985, p. 78) gives an example of spending an enjoyable evening with friends and feeling that all is well with one's life, then waking up the next morning feeling anxious and depressed. Obviously, nothing has happened in the intervening 12 hours to change one's good fortune. In Gazzaniga's terms, a nonverbal module, with negative emotional associates, has somehow randomly or "capriciously" been activated, so that a negative mood is felt. This just happens; then the verbal module, reflecting or talking about the event, looks for some explanation for it.

It is but a short step to reformulate this in terms of some psychoanalytic speculations. For example, something happened at the gathering with friends, or after the gathering, that triggered the anxiety or depression, something that presumably registered in the coconscious nonverbal modules and not in verbal ones. This is likely to be an event that is manifestly trivial, not registered as important, but associated with earlier, anxiety-producing events, including threatening or dreaded experiences that the individual is motivated to avoid. The association may be made analogically (through the strong pattern-matching capabilities of the right brain), without implicating the symbolic processing mechanisms of the left hemisphere. Perhaps his wife spoke to him in a slightly ridiculing way, moved slightly away when he put his arm around her in a moment of affection, or smiled a bit too warmly at his best friend. None of this registers in the left hemisphere (or symbolic, or verbal systems), perhaps at most as a "white flash." However, the pattern-matching capacities of the right brain (or subsymbolic, or implicit processor) then may operate and activate an anxiety-producing memory or image and associated feelings. He has memories of being rejected when he showed affection to someone he loved; he feels rage at that person; he expects to be abandoned again. This pattern-matching process, which activates the anxious memories and negative expectations, may not happen at the moment of the event—it may happen only later, or may begin at the moment, just enough to be registered, and then radiate along networks of associations, eventually arousing anxiety or depression that has no apparent source.

The left hemisphere then operates to provide an acceptable explanation of why he wakes up feeling upset. He may not have a direct association to the actual events that occurred, or to the feelings of anger or fear of abandonment that are activated, but he will have some associations that are related to these, that share features or emotional patterns. Perhaps he remembers that his boss spoke to him in an offensive way. Later, his analyst seems to have a cold expression as he opens his office door. These associations may be drawn from aspects of the emotional memory that remain accessible to awareness, while the core of the memory is warded off. The events that determined the depressed or anxious feeling with which he awoke are as systematic and real as the anxiety-arousing film of the fire in the experimental situation; the difference is that the former are private, not known to observers, as well as not accessible to oneself. The triggering events, and the memories associated with them, are in fact generally identifiable only under special circumstances, as in psychoanalytic work. In treatment, the determining factors, which are not accessible to the patient, may eventually emerge in memory and in the shared experiences of the relationship. The assumption of determinism, as this operates in free association, is based on the premise that the associations that emerge are driven by the underlying emotional state.

Gazzaniga (1985) himself recognizes the close similarity between the modularity of mind as he formulates it and Freud's concept of unconscious mental functioning:

> One can quickly adapt Freud to the theory of modules by changing his concept of "unconscious process" into the idea I present here of "coconscious but nonverbal mental modules." A response tendency, a decision for action on the part of a nonverbal mental module, is not unconscious. It is very conscious, very capable of effecting action. One of its features, that it cannot internally communicate with the dominant hemisphere's language and cognitive system, should not find it being characterized as "unconscious." With that single correction in Freud's formulation, much of what else he claims as important in mental life can be viewed in modern mechanistic terms. (pp. 117–118)

Gazzaniga appears to assume the dominance of the verbal system as the cognitive organizer. This assumption is seen in his formulation of modularity, as in his view, referred to earlier, of the cognitive skills of a disconnected right hemisphere without language as "vastly inferior to the cognitive skills of a chimpanzee." One might adapt Gazzaniga's notion of modularity to a psychoanalytic view, and potentially to a multiple code theory, as we shall see, with a qualified definition of "modern mechanistic terms," which incorporates systematic nonverbal processing, including subsymbolic and symbolic formats, and with the substitution of a notion of emotional determinism for the misplaced formulation of capriciousness. With those changes, we can then see Gazzaniga's results as providing new empirical support for the concepts of psychoanalysis on a neurophysiological level. The individual may not be aware of the sources of his emotion or his behavior; the goal of the psychoanalytic process is to uncover the reasons for these. In Gazzaniga's research, these reasons do certainly exist; they are built in to the experimental designs. The assumption of psychoanalysis is that the reasons exist in an individual's life as well.

THE MULTIPLE CODE THEORY AND THE REFERENTIAL CYCLE

The multiple code model is a general theory of psychological organization that has been constructed on the basis of the diverse fields reviewed in Section Two. I have covered models of cognitive architectures and theories of cognitive functions. I have also covered research on the functions of specific sensory modalities, as well as research on emotion, and on cognitive and emotional development. In presenting this basic research, I have included evidence from neurophysiological as well as behavioral observations. As I have emphasized, however, the multiple code theory is a psychological, not a phenomenological or a neurophysiological, theory. The theory—like all modern psychological theories—is formulated on the level of hypothetical constructs, defined in terms of other constructs and inferred from observable indicators within a nomological network.

In this section, I bring together the research reviewed thus far to develop a summary formulation of the multiple code theory as this applies generally in adaptive as well as maladaptive functioning. Once the components and concepts of multiple coding are in place—including the concepts of the referential process connecting all systems and the emotion schemas—I will go on to apply this model to pathology and its repair in treatment. I will also trace the operation of the referential process in a wide range of functions, including emotional development, scientific invention and discovery, dreams, and free association. In the final two chapters, I outline a research agenda based on this theoretical foundation and present an empirical study of a long-term, fully recorded psychoanalysis. I then discuss promises to be fulfilled and challenges to be met in developing the psychoanalytic method in modern dress.

CHAPTER 11

Basic Concepts of
the Multiple Code Theory

The emotional information processing system incorporates multiple diverse components, as I have shown in detail in the preceding section. Multiple functions and processing formats have been identified. No single code model can account for the range of functions that have been observed. It is also the case that people must act in relatively integrated ways in organizing behavior, working toward complex, long-term goals, and communicating experience to others. The multiple code theory provides an account of emotional information processing, using the basic architectures of the subsymbolic and symbolic systems. In the first part of this chapter, I will describe the basic components of the multiple code theory; in the second, I present the pivotal concept of the referential process, which accounts for their integration. The theoretical framework enables the development of empirical measures that serve as operational indicators of the nature of the underlying structures and their integration or dissociation; the basic measures of referential activity (RA) developed in the context of the multiple code theory, will be presented in the third part of the chapter.

COMPONENTS OF THE MULTIPLE CODE THEORY

Subsymbolic Formats

As outlined in Table 11.1, subsymbolic processing systems (modeled by connectionist or parallel distributed processing [PDP] systems) are

173

global and analogic processors, operating on continuous dimensions without discrete elements or specified metric units. The subsymbolic system is massively parallel, with multiple synchronous operations, and is characterized as content rather than structure determined. Dimensions, coordinates, units, and processing principles are intrinsic to each processing component and each type of content. Subsymbolic processing applies, in different ways, in all sensory modalities and is dominant in olfaction and taste. It is the essential mode of operation of visceral and kinesthetic systems, and is, by its very nature, represented primarily in private codes, which are not readily amenable to being communicated or shared.

Subsymbolic processing accommodates infinitely fine variations; this processing is not represented by standard metric systems or computational rules. We recognize changes in the emotional states of others based on perception of subtle shifts in their facial expression or posture, and recognize changes in our own states based on somatic or kinesthetic experience; we carry out this processing without being able to specify the basis on which the judgments are made.

In operating without explicit intention or direction, subsymbolic processes and representations may be experienced as, in a sense, "outside of oneself," outside of the domain of the self over which one seems to have intentional control. As an outside agent, subsymbolic processing may appear to act in some instances in benign, in some instances in malevolent ways. On the one hand, we long for a visit of the muse, which enables the creative process to flow; on the other hand, we often feel at the mercy of our emotional or physical processes and feel unable to direct them intentionally. That is why we sometimes call upon outside agents—alcohol, coffee, pep pills, tranquilizers, sleeping pills, antidepressants—to regulate these functions.

TABLE 11.1. Properties of Multiple Coding Formats

	Symbolic codes	
Subsymbolic codes	Nonverbal	Verbal
Analogic processing on continuous dimensions	Discrete, specific imagery or analogic patterns	Words with phonological, syntactic, and semantic features
Modality-specific; sensory, visceral, kinesthetic	Modality-specific; all sensory modalities	Amodal
Modeled by parallel distributed processing (PDP) systems	Sequential or parallel; modeled by classical symbolic systems	Sequential, single-channel format

Symbolic Processing Systems: Images and Words

In information-processing terms, as outlined in Table 11.1, "symbols" are defined as discrete entities with properties of reference and generativity. Symbols may be verbal or nonverbal.

Imagery: The Nonverbal Symbolic Code

Images may be characterized as transitional in format, combining some features of both subsymbolic representations and verbal symbols. Images, like words, are discrete entities that represent other entities and may be combined in rule-governed ways. (The type of symbolic imagery that has been identified as having psychoanalytic meaning constitutes a subset or special case.) Images may look like or depict the entities they represent but may also be analogic patterns, or may even represent other entities in an abstract or arbitrary way, as stars and stripes in a particular configuration represent the United States. Images can be processed and combined both sequentially and in parallel, and sequences of images can represent episodes and events. In contrast to subsymbolic systems, which operate without explicit identification of elements, dimensions, or metrics, symbolic processing depends on identification of explicit parameters and is more amenable to intentional control. We can intentionally construct images or recall images of objects in their absence, although images may also come into mind in an unbidden way.

As in the processing of subsymbolic information, the processing of imagery is modality specific, occupying the same channels as are used for perception in a given modality. Images, like percepts, are registered within individual modalities and may also have cross-modal features. We perceive, or remember the ballerina's leap and glide, and also remember the quality of its integration with the accompanying music. We can imagine the sound of someone's words as he speaks—in anger, or fear, or love—modulated, or intensified, by the expression of his face. Discrete images, including sequences of images in episodes with cross-modal features, provide an intrinsic basis for the organizing and symbolizing of subsymbolic experience, operating within the nonverbal system outside of language, and also provide the basis for connecting nonverbal experience to words.

The Verbal Code

Words are the quintessential symbolic elements, embodying the central features of symbol systems in most direct form. Words, like images, may be represented in a range of different formats in long-term memory. The underlying representation of language is likely to be some kind of logical or propositional structure, rather than the surface forms of language. I do not take a position as to the particular nature of the format underlying either words or images; my fundamental claim is only that these formats must be different, and that the nature of each underlying format is such as to fit the criteria outlined in Table 11.1. A number of different models of underlying structures might be proposed that meet these criteria, as I discussed briefly in Chapter 5.

Words have arbitrary reference, with few exceptions, as in onomatopoeia, and the information carried by words is largely neutral as to modality. A string of words has the same syntax and meaning when it is heard or read, or taken in by touch, as in braille, although the emotional impacts of the various formats are likely to differ.

Every spoken, verbal message may be characterized in terms of its phonemic features, its morphological and syntactic organization, and its semantic meaning; thus, language may be viewed as multiply encoded on several different levels. The multiple coding of language is perhaps most obvious in poetry and in the transmission of emotional experience, where sound and semantics both contribute to the message that is sent. Here, we see the operation of what might be termed a "subsymbolic verbal code." The paralinguistic features of speech, including vocal tone, pausing, loudness and pitch, that may express emotion most directly are processed in subsymbolic format; however, these features may be classified, to some extent, as vocal rather than verbal. Paralinguistic features of language may be but are not necessarily connected to symbolic language, and may also carry communicative information in their own channels. These features are particularly dominant in emotional communication. One may cry, laugh, or groan, in loud or soft tones, along with language or in place of it. Dissonance in communication of emotional meaning occurs when the information carried in the linguistic and paralinguistic tracks do not correspond. The role of such subsymbolic verbal (or vocal) processing, which might constitute a fourth processing format, is not considered as such in this formulation of the multiple code theory and needs to be addressed further in subsequent work.

While language has multiple levels of form, it operates, in its dominant information processing function, as a sequential, single-channel symbolic device, sending or receiving only one message at a given time. We do not listen and speak and read at the same time; we have difficulty understanding speech when interruptions or cross talk occur (as parents, teachers, and moderators of scientific meetings know quite well). In some cases, we may appear to follow two messages or participate in two conversations simultaneously; however, the processing is not genuinely concurrent but involves brief and intricate sequential attentional shifts (Broadbent, 1958).

Humans, like all species, are capable of multiple, complex functions outside of the guidance of language, and continue to carry out such functions throughout life, as we have seen. On the other hand, we also recognize that humans took a giant leap forward with the acquisition of language and the nature of this leap needs to be understood. Language is the medium that is most directly and obviously amenable to intentional control. It is the code that humans invented, the code we use to regulate and direct ourselves, to manipulate others, to communicate, and to lie. Language is the code in which the knowledge of the culture is preserved and transmitted; many—but not all—types of inner experience may be represented; many types of logical relationships can be expressed. We use language to indicate inclusion into categories and exclusion from them, to negate propositions, and to make generalizations and distinctions, although it is also the case that the symbols of natural language and logic do not precisely correspond. We require language to place events in a time sequence and to develop concepts of past and future. Language is the primary medium of psychoanalysis, although it is not the primary medium of thought, and certainly not of emotion.

The Attribute of Consciousness

The dimension of consciousness is not uniquely associated with any of the three coding formats. While subsymbolic processing is generally characterized as implicit, automatic, and unintentional, it may also in some cases occur within awareness. Balanchine focused his dancers' attention on a particular sequence of moves by physically enacting or guiding them. Master teachers in music and the arts work in corresponding ways. Learning by apprenticeship in crafts or trades, as well as in the arts, depends on the focusing of conscious attention on subsymbolic processes: how to hold a saw, how to put an even coat of paint on a wall, how to know—see, or feel, or smell—when sugar has reached the correct stage of caramelization or the egg yolks have thickened to the desired consistency. Psychoanalytic training involves learning through experiencing to identify one's own sensory, motoric, and visceral experience, to "read" the cues that others send out concerning their internal states, and to work on these intentionally and within awareness. The elusive concept of "empathy" may be defined as ability to understand and be aware of subsymbolic information transmitted by others on the basis of a variety of cues, including one's own subsymbolic response.

The relationship of symbolic processing to consciousness is also complex. Imagery and language may both be processed within and outside of awareness. Imagery is the central medium of dreams, according to current dream research, as in Freud's model. We "attend to" dream imagery when we sleep but may or may not then be able to retrieve these images when we awake. People are also able to construct imagery intentionally, in waking life, and to examine their images. Language is generally understood as operating within attentional focus; this relates to the status of language as a sequential, single-channel device. However, verbal processing has also been shown to occur in dreams and otherwise off-line. The poet who awakens with a phrase that has eluded him has carried out verbal processing outside of the conscious domain.

The important point to be kept in mind here is that the attribute of consciousness is itself complex, perhaps varying in quality with different contents. Like other aspects of inner experience, the attribute of consciousness needs to be developed and studied in relation to other variables, and by inference from observable events.

CONNECTING THE SEPARATE SYSTEMS: THE REFERENTIAL PROCESS

Our accounts of subsymbolic and symbolic processes have demonstrated a world of diverse processing modes operating alongside the "logical" organization of the verbal mode. To account for the overall organization of the human information-processing system, connections among all representational systems are required. Nonverbal representations, including subsymbolic components that are processed continuously, synchronously, and in parallel, must be connected to one another and to the discrete symbols of language processed in single-channel, sequential format. The distinct formats must be interconnected to allow integration of functions, organization of goal-directed behavior, and establishment of a unified sense of self. On the most obvious level, there must be integration of systems to enable us to talk about what we experience and to connect the words of others to what we know and feel. In my research, I have introduced the concept of referential activity and the referential process as the function of integration of the multiple, diverse components of the human information-processing system, connecting the disparate modality-specific representations and processes of the nonverbal system to one another and to words (Bucci & Freedman, 1978; Bucci, Kabasakalian-McKay, & the RA Research Group, 1992; Bucci & Miller, 1993).

While the existence of multiple, disparate representational formats has been widely recognized in cognitive science in recent years, the problem of how these systems are linked has been largely ignored outside of our own research. The issue of integration of systems is left essentially unresolved within the PDP approach. The PDP models developed thus far are restricted to highly specific tasks, as we have seen. Each unit forms its own pattern of activity through learning, and the activity pattern learned by one network is generally indecipherable to another. Some researchers within this paradigm have the hope that PDP formats may eventually be developed to account for the integration of systems; however, no such models have been produced thus far. Many researchers now recognize the need for hybrid models incorporating symbolic as well as subsymbolic formats to account for the overall organization of separate systems, the integration of experience in memory, and the direction of information processing or action in relation to specified goals, as we have seen in Chapter 5.

Within the symbolic formats, propositional or common code models incorporate modality-specific representation at the input level and in short-term memory, while assuming a single, common representation at the underlying level of long-term memory. According to these models, all verbal and nonverbal meanings are derived from the same abstract, amodal representation. From this perspective, there is no problem of integration of long-term memory systems; there is only one system to which all input refers and in which all meaning is represented. Full translatability between nonverbal and verbal representations, via the common code, is necessarily assumed:

> What is the relation between the meaning that is extracted from the sentence "There is a cat in this room" and the meaning that is extracted from seeing a cat in the room? The relation must be quite intimate because a person who sees the cat will immediately (that is, in a few hundred milliseconds—see Chase and Clark, 1972) conclude that the sentence is true, and a person who hears the sentence may form some expectation of seeing a cat (unless the room is supplied with the kinds of crannies in which cats love to hide). (Simon & Kaplan, 1989, p. 16)

As we have seen in Chapter 5, however, the assumption of a single common code is questioned within its own domain of studies of symbolic architecture and is further questioned by findings concerning the multiplicity of function in memory systems, as well as by neurophysiological findings. On the basis of these observations, multiplicity of function appears to be the more verdical, if less parsimonious, approach to modeling human information processing in general; the operation of multiple functions is even more apparent in accounting for the emotional information processing that concerns us here. The inherently partial and limited possibilities for translation between nonverbal experience and words constitute a central problem for the common code approach, which has been overlooked by researchers in that paradigm. There are many experiences that cannot be spoken in a sentence; many sentences are spoken that do not lead to corresponding experiences in a hearer, and there are many reasons for failures of correspondence other than the habit patterns of cats.

The dual code approach, as formulated by Paivio (1971, 1986) and his colleagues, recognizes separate verbal and nonverbal codes, not only at the input level but also at the level at which meaning is assigned, and postulates a system of referential connections linking the verbal and nonverbal codes. Dual coding accounts for gradations in the degree to which nonverbal experience may be connected to words, as the common code theories cannot. This variation has been demonstrated in many experimental studies. Paivio, Clark, Digdon, and Bons (1989) have provided evidence for the referential process as a distinct function that may vary independently of verbal and nonverbal processes. However, dual as opposed to multiple coding focuses on symbolic, primarily visual, imagery, as the nonverbal component, leaving out of account the vast domain of subsymbolic functions in all modalities, and the far more complex mechanisms that would be required to integrate such processes with language. Thus, the dual code model as formulated by Paivio and his colleagues fails to provide a specific account for the mechanism of the referential process, or to account for the limitations on its operation.

Freud's model of the psychical apparatus emphasized the operation of two distinct modes of thought, the primary and secondary processes. In psychoanalysis, however, the separation of systems is understood largely as dissociation determined by pathology and defense, and the difficulty of finding words for experience is treated primarily as a matter of conflict or resistance. Repair of the dissociation is seen as occurring through dominance of one system over another: the unconscious becoming conscious, ego taking over where id has been. The Freudian model does not account for the continued operation of multiple information-processing systems throughout normal, conscious mental life, or for the inherent difficulties of translation among representational systems, which apply for all human information processing, not painful or threatening emotional experience only.

Freud's emphasis on integration by dominance of the ego or the conscious system reflects his implicit verbal dominance position. The major developmental theories also emphasize abstract verbal processing, leaving out of account the crucial role of language in connecting to other modes of nonverbal thought. Logical verbal processing—as in the symbolic mode of Bruner (1966), or Piaget's stage of formal operations (Inhelder

& Piaget, 1958)—is assumed to be the developmental goal, the optimal mature mode, replacing earlier, more primitive systems of cognitive organization. Only Werner, of the major developmental theorists, has incorporated the possibility of dual lines of processing, reflecting different functions for some individuals throughout life. However, Werner does not incorporate this as a necessary and central part of mental life for all individuals, and also fails to address the issue of the integration of the separate processing tracks (Werner & Kaplan, 1984).

Prototypes and the Referential Process: Converging Research

While the cognitive and developmental fields have generally not addressed the question of the integration of disparate representational systems, there is a body of converging evidence, gleaned from a number of diverse areas, that does have bearing on this question. Kosslyn, Rosch, Mandler, and Stern, whose work has been reviewed in Chapters 5, 7, and 9, have been concerned with the issues of integration of systems, each in a different way. From quite diverse perspectives, their work converges in recognizing construction of prototypic imagery as the mediating mechanism linking global, implicit, subsymbolic processes with more discrete, symbolic images that may then be mapped into a verbal code. I will apply these converging findings to formulate an account of the basic mechanisms of the referential process, the means by which subsymbolic and symbolic representations are linked to one another and to words.

According to Kosslyn (1987), perceptual information varying on continuous gradients is chunked into ranges that are experienced as equivalent for the functioning of the organism. Kosslyn's concept of continuous stimulus variation is comparable to the multiple code formulation of subsymbolic representation, as modeled by PDP systems. These functionally equivalent classes of stimuli, constructed as chunks of continuously varying sensory experience, are represented as prototypic images. The prototypic images figure in symbolic processing and are the type of discrete elements to which words may be attached. This provides the basic mechanism of symbolizing, outside of, and independent of language, and is the core mechanism on which the referential process is built. Kosslyn's formulation of the construction of prototypic images was developed specifically for the visual modality. I have extended his basic formulation to account for construction of prototypic imagery in other sensory modalities, in ways determined by their specific features, and for cross-modal imagery as well.

Like Kosslyn, Rosch (1975) has investigated the basic process of prototype formation as operating in nonverbal systems, independent of language. Rosch's notion of the "fuzzy" categorization of prototypes, like Kosslyn's notion of functionally equivalent classes, provides a basis for chunking nonverbal information into discrete, symbolic representations. Rosch's system incorporates prototypes built on functional as well as perceptual equivalence: for example, prototypic representations of an object to sit on, or an object with legs and a surface on which we place other things. Rosch has also applied her concept of natural prototypic structure to the organization of the flow of experience in terms of episodes or events; thus, her formulation accounts for event structures as themselves having prototypic form.

In her concept of image-schemas and their mapping into language, Mandler (1992) has identified two basic stages of concept development in infants that parallel the visual functions identified by Kosslyn and provide the necessary basis for the child's symbolic development. According to Mandler, the infant begins with encoding of perceptual and sensorimotor information, which may have a global, analogic character. The perceptual information is then redescribed into image-schemas in which spatial structure is used as the basis for conceptual structure. The image-schemas that represent the basic conceptual structures—Animacy, Agency, Containment, and Support—include specific, discrete features that might be mapped into language and expressible in words.

Stern's (1985) formulation of the child's prototypic emotional memories, which he has termed Representations of Interactions that have been Generalized (RIGs), parallels the cognitive processes as described by Rosch and Mandler. In contrast to Mandler's focus on the cognitive, particularly the visuospatial domain, Stern's notion of the RIG is far more broad, including actions, sensations, and affects occurring in an interactive, interpersonal context. Repeated episodes incorporating actions, experience in all sensory modalities, and visceral experience, and involving other people in relationship to oneself, form the prototypic memory structures that provide order to experience, including emotional experience, and are the basis for the development of a sense of self.

The Mechanism of the Referential Process

The basic mechanism of the referential process, through which all manner of nonverbal experience, including emotional experience, is connected to words, is derived from these converging approaches. Within each sensory modality, the continuously varying subsymbolic representations that make up the functionally equivalent classes of representation are connected to and represented by specific images that function as symbols or prototypes. The chunking of continuously varying ranges of representations into discrete prototypic representations is the fundamental process of symbolizing within the nonverbal domain. Only after discrete prototypic images and features have been thus constructed can mapping of experience into language occur.

The chunking of continuous representations into prototypic images based on equivalence of structure, or function, or association in time or place may occur across as well as within modalities, as I have discussed in the characterization of the nonverbal symbol system. By this means, cross-modal symbols and concatenations of images in prototypic episodes are formed. The formation of prototypic episodes is discussed by Rosch (1978) in her formulation of event structures, and by Stern (1985) in his characterization of RIGs. As we will see in the next chapter, the prototypic episode is a central, organizing feature of the emotional information-processing system. Repeated episodes provide the basis for the construction of the emotion schemas, from the beginning of life, well prior to the acquisition of language, and also determine the process by which emotional experience may be symbolized and communicated to others, as we shall see in subsequent chapters.

Based on these convergent formulations, the stages of the referential process, the mechanism of transformation from subsymbolic information to nonverbal and then to verbal symbols may be outlined in simplest form as follows:

1. Continuous stimulus variation (subsymbolic representations).
2. Chunking into functionally equivalent classes of representations.
3. Construction of prototypic images (nonverbal symbolic forms) that operate at varying levels of abstractness.
4. Representation in verbal form.

Operations of different sorts within the verbal system may then occur, including descriptions of images or episodes, the formulation of abstract ideas, the operations of logic, and the examination of concepts in the shared discourse. The referential process is bidirectional; the listener translates verbal messages into all manner of nonverbal representations by this means. The process is also recursive; new verbal connections feed back to activate new nonverbal ones, as we shall see in subsequent chapters.

The basic symbolizing function of the referential process occurs in the ontogenetic development of concepts and symbols, as Mandler and Stern have discussed, and occurs repeatedly throughout cognitive life as new images are constructed and communicated, as shown by Kosslyn and Rosch. The infant forms an image of mother on the basis of multiple, ever-changing appearances chunked as functionally equivalent to produce the enduring prototypic image. This enables recognition of mother in the many, varied contexts and forms in which she appears. We form prototypic images of objects, people, and all entities in this way. We may also form prototypic representations of concepts that appear abstract by this means, such as spatial relationships (on top of, inside, underneath), as Kosslyn has pointed out.

Prototypic images and episodes constitute the "lingua franca" of the nonverbal representational system, enabling the connection of multiple, disparate representations to one another, within and between modalities, and also enabling the connection to words. The referential process underlies the processes of discovery and invention in science and the arts, by which subsymbolic analog representations are organized in new ways, and new categories are formed. Metaphoric expression can be understood in such terms, symbolizing what has been largely subsymbolic, and enabling its connection to words. Writers—and analysts—know and use the power of such metaphoric means. In its etymological origins, in Greek, metaphor is the figure of speech that "carries beyond." Metaphor carries the meaning beyond the object that is named to a network of associated images and events, and beyond the subjectivity of one individual across to another's. The symbols build the meaning of the subsymbolic states and enable these to be shared.

With her intuitive understanding of these processes, Helen Keller describes a progression from tactile to verbal representation that is strikingly like the symbolizing transformation proposed here: "But I know that my physical ideas, that is, ideas derived from material objects, appear to me first in ideas similar to those of touch. Instantly, they pass into intellectual meanings. Afterward, the meaning finds expression in what is called inner speech" (1908, p. 118). The "ideas derived from material objects," which Helen Keller describes as appearing in forms similar to those of touch, may be characterized as modality-specific subsymbolic representations. The "intellectual meanings," not yet verbal, are her version of symbolic prototypes. "Afterward," these lead to verbalization for oneself, which Keller (like Vygotsky, 1934) refers to as inner speech. Given certain transformations within the verbal system, these ideas may then be spoken (or signed). The referential process applies in this way for expression of emotion, as for all types of thoughts and ideas, as we shall see in the next chapter.

THE DIMENSION OF REFERENTIAL ACTIVITY: EMPIRICAL RESEARCH

The referential process organizing nonverbal experience and connecting it to words is a cognitive function in its own right, like verbal, or imagery, or performance abilities, and may vary independently of any of these. Just as people may differ in verbal ability and in nonverbal performance abilities, they may also differ as to their capacity to integrate nonverbal systems and connect them to language. The capacity to express all manner of nonverbal experience, particularly emotional experience, in verbal form has been termed referential activity (RA; Bucci & Freedman, 1978, 1981; Bucci, 1984). Level of RA varies among individuals as a relatively stable trait or level of competence, determined by genetic and experiential factors. RA also shows considerable trait or performance variance, fluctuating within an individual over time, as a function of interpersonal context and physiological or emotional state. This is the aspect of language function that is central to the talking cure. Variation in level of RA serves as both an indicator of capacity to engage in psychoanalytic treatment and a means of tracking the effectiveness of the treatment process.

Just as the referential process has not generally been studied in cognitive or developmental research, it has also been neglected in the psychometric field. Most verbal intelligence tests, such as the Similarities or Vocabulary subtests of the Wechsler Adult Intelligence Scale (WAIS; Wechsler, 1981), focus on the dimension of abstract verbal processing. For a Similarities item, asking in what way two entities—for example, an apple and an orange—are alike, the response that achieves the highest score is that they are both fruits. This is a response that calls on organization within the hierarchies of verbal semantic memory. Responses that call on concrete, sensory qualities—they are both sweet, or juicy, or round—receive a lower score. The same type of scoring criteria applies for Vocabulary items.

In our research (Bucci & Freedman, 1978, 1981; Bucci et al., 1992; Bucci & Miller, 1993; Bucci, 1995), we have extensively developed the construct of Referential Activity (RA) as a significant cognitive function in its own right, with measurable trait and state variation. RA has been shown to vary independently of standard measures of verbal intelligence, as of performance and imagery measures, and to have significant emotional, interpersonal, and clinical implications. We have developed a wide range of measures to assess RA variation. These include features of language style and other measures that indicate more active and direct connection between all manner of nonverbal experience and words. The RA construct and its measurement are pivotal in our application of multiple coding constructs to empirical work, including our work on the psychotherapy process.

Features of Language Style Related to RA

A major focus of this work has been the identification and validation of features of language style associated with the RA dimension. How do people talk when they are connecting to imagery and emotional experience, as differentiated from the way they talk when they are in a state of dissociation from such experience and have access only to intellectual processes or thoughts in linguistic form? Can we find systematic indicators in the language that is produced that reflect these differences in underlying state?

The identification of linguistic features associated with RA is supported empirically by the dual coding research, as outlined earlier. As Paivio and his colleagues have shown, referential connections are most active and direct for specific and concrete images, and words referring to them, less direct for abstract concepts and words. This principle applies for all sensory and somatic dimensions, not vision only, as we have discussed, in introducing our multiple coding approach. As Helen Keller has shown us so beautifully, a statement about a slice of lemon that causes the mouth to pucker, or about the velvet of a ripe peach, the velvet of a rose, or of a baby's dimpled cheek, is far more closely connected to nonverbal experience than general statements about flowers or fruits (Keller, 1908).

Our understanding of RA language style variation is also supported by the research on representation of prototypic forms. The basic category, as defined by Rosch—such as "apple," "rose," "chair"—is the most general level for which prototypical images of objects can be constructed, and the most general verbal level for which direct referential connections are available. While there are, of course, many different types of apples or chairs or roses, people do construct images of such entities in prototypic form, as Rosch has shown.

Prototypic images cannot be constructed for terms on the next level of abstraction, such as "fruit," "flower," or "furniture," and the referential connections are correspondingly less direct for such terms. There is no prototypic image that would be capable of representing "fruit," for example, representing, in *a single perceptual entity*, a banana, a lemon, a tomato, a bunch of grapes, a strawberry, a watermelon, and an olive. Such entities are recognized as members of the same category primarily on the basis of particular properties and classification systems present in one's general knowledge store, rather than on the basis of immediate and direct sensory experience. We can establish referential connections from the word "fruit" to imagery only by working down the verbal hierarchy to exemplars for which prototypic images can be formed, for example, by imagining a bowl of fruit.

Higher order category terms such as "food," and abstract terms such as "human needs," "truth," or "justice," are even less closely connected to nonverbal experience and require more intervening associations. Organization of elements into hierarchical category systems is a function of the verbal system, reflecting the logical organization of semantic memory. The higher level, like the lower level, category terms can be connected to nonverbal imagery through working down the categorical hierarchies to the concrete and specific level. The difference is that more intervening steps are required. Power, beauty, and truth can be found in the tangible properties of things, as Helen Keller has told us, mediated by their associations to specific objects and events, but the connection is indirect, going through a sequence of representational levels before concrete reference is found.

In the converse direction, subsymbolic nonverbal experience, including taste, smell and visceral experiences, are most difficult to connect to words; such representations are dominant in the emotion schemas, as will be discussed. To express such experiences in words, the speaker must be able to move from the analogic and global representations of the emotion schemas to representations of objects or features that are amenable to being named, as illustrated in the discussion of the verbalization of smell and taste.

Measurement of RA Language Style

Given the theoretical framework of multiple coding and the referential process, qualities of language may then be used as operational indicators of connection to nonverbal, particularly emotional experience. The RA measures have been developed to assess these qualities of language and have been extensively validated in our research. The measures tell us whether or to what extent nonverbal, including emotional, experience is likely to be activated in the speaker's (or writer's) mind as he generates his discourse, or whether his language is being generated within the verbal hierarchies of semantic memory, dissociated from nonverbal experience. Here, I will introduce briefly the nature of the RA language dimension and some of the methods of RA measurement that play a central role in our research.

High RA—active and direct connections between imagery and words— is reflected in language that captures a quality of immediacy in the speaker's representations and that is likely to evoke vivid, specific, and immediate experience in the listener as well, as in the following example[1]:

> "I can't stand fruit with bad spots in it. It gives me the creeps. So I picked up that pineapple and it looked so nice, and then my finger went right through inside it, into this brown, slimy, mushy stuff, and my stomach just turned over."

In contrast, low RA language is general, abstract, and vague. The speaker appears not to be connecting to his own experience and fails to connect to the listener:

> "I can't really think of too many times when he forced me to do something when I didn't want to. I mean, there's a lot of times he didn't do stuff that I wanted him to do. The other way around. He was . . . if I didn't understand something, he would tell me what was going on, stuff like that."

RA may also be low where emotions are talked about, but in a general and abstract sense:

> "I love people and I like to be with people. And right now I feel very bad because I can't be with them and do the things I would like to do. But I'm looking forward to a happier and healthier future and—I don't know what else to say. What else can I talk about? Well—I've had a very eventful life, I think. I've worked practically all my life and I love people."

In our research, we have developed systematic procedures for assessing the qualities of language style associated with the RA dimension. The methods for scoring RA include qualitative rating scales and objective measures based on quantifiable linguistic features. I will describe some of the methods of RA measurement here and apply this approach to verbatim transcripts of psychoanalytic sessions in Chapter 17.

The RA Scales

The RA rating scales measure the Concreteness, Imagery, Specificity, and Clarity of speech. Concreteness is based on degree of perceptual or sensory quality, including references to all sense modalities, action, and

---

[1]Examples are taken from Bucci et al. (1992).

bodily experience (not cognitive concreteness in a regressive or deficit sense). Specificity refers to amount of detail; a highly specific text involves explicit descriptions of persons, objects, places, or events. Clarity refers to clarity of an image as seen through the language; how well-focused the linguistic image is judged to be. Imagery refers to the degree to which the language evokes corresponding experience in the reader or hearer. A manual has been developed that gives instructions for scoring the RA measures and applying these to psychotherapy sessions and other texts (Bucci et al., 1992).

The four scales are generally significantly intercorrelated and may be combined to yield an overall RA score. The scales of Concreteness and Imagery are generally more highly intercorrelated with one another than with either of the other two scales; an average of these two, termed CONIM, may be used as reflecting level of sensory imagery expressed in language. Similarly, Specificity and Clarity scales show relatively high intercorrelation and may be combined to provide an indicator of discourse organization, termed CLASP. The RA measures have been applied to many types of texts, including brief monologues, early memories, and thematic apperception test (TAT) protocols, as well as transcripts of therapy sessions (Bucci, 1988, 1989, 1993, 1995, 1997).

In addition to the scales, a number of specific linguistic features have been identified as related to the RA dimension. These include linguistic features that impart a quality of immediacy to spoken language, such as direct quotes and stylistic use of the present tense in describing past events: "So he comes into the room and he sits down, and he says to me. . . . " Metaphors, which represent abstract thought or emotional experience in concrete and specific form, are quintessential indicators of the RA dimension, as will be discussed further in the Chapter 13.

Computer-Measured Referential Activity

Computerized referential activity (CRA) measures have now also been developed (Mergenthaler & Bucci, 1993; Bucci, 1995). These have the obvious advantage of efficiency in application to large samples and studies of long-term psychotherapy and psychoanalytic treatments. Beyond that, the new computerized procedures bypass the problem of reliability of judges' scoring and have the benefit of imposing a consistent standard across diverse populations. Whereas judges' scores tend to be determined to some extent by the general level of a given sample, the computer measures necessarily impose the same standards on all. The computerized procedures have now become our primary linguistic tools for study of the treatment process; the empirical study to be presented in Chapter 17 uses these techniques.

The development of computerized content-analysis procedures is based on the premise that features of language style may be assessed through analysis of specific lexical items, and categories of these, independent of their sequential ordering or grammatical construction. This premise has been thoroughly validated in the computerized content-analysis field, and computer dictionaries assessing particular content areas are in wide use in clinical and other fields (Stone, Dunphy, Smith, & Ogilvie, 1966; Martindale, 1975; Mergenthaler & Bucci, 1993).

The CRA dictionary was formed empirically by modeling the RA scales as scored by expert judges. Details of the construction of the CRA dictionary were presented by Mergenthaler and Bucci (1993). The method and its application to psychoanalytic transcripts are outlined in Chapter 17. The CRA list now in use includes approximately 100 each high- and low-RA words. Overall CRA is computed as the difference between scores for words matched by these two dictionaries. Thus, the number of words matched by the low-CRA list is subtracted from the number matched by the high-CRA list to yield the overall CRA score.

The CRA measure is unusual among computerized language-analysis procedures in focusing on the style rather than the contents of language. The items in both lists are primarily function words with high frequency in language use. While there are fewer than 200 words (types) altogether in the two lists, they account for *approximately half* of the words (tokens) spoken in normal discourse. Thus, this is an exceedingly powerful measure that remains a reliable indicator of language style even for small segments of text.

While empirically derived, both the high- and low-CRA lists turn out to be consistent with the theory of the referential process, as outlined earlier in this chapter. The high-CRA list consists of highly frequent function words, including particular classes of prepositions and pronouns, that people tend to use when describing images and events. These would include prepositions and adverbs representing spatial relations, such as "in," "on," and "outside."

Such function words, which appear abstract and without specific concrete reference, are actually rooted in basic nonverbal representational concepts. They are the type of words that Kosslyn (1987) has identified as referring to prototypic imagery of spatial relations. Similarly, Mandler (1992) refers to spatial terms of this nature as a means by which children map perceptual concepts onto language.

As we would expect, based on our analysis of the referential process, the high-CRA list also includes third-person-singular pronouns. Speakers use such pronouns in describing the persons who figure in specific events.

The following excerpts from monologues[2] by two student nurses describe the same type of event, a visit to the hospital delivery rooms, but show the differences in use of imagery and focus on other persons that are associated with the RA dimension.

1. "So I walked into this other room and there's this lady laying there and she's all by herself. There was nobody even there with her from her family or anything. So I went into the room and I was holding her hand and I was teaching like the deep breathing, to try to relieve the pain. And she—all of a sudden she says to me, 'Oh my water just ruptured.' And I just—I looked and I had to look really close. It was hard to tell. It wasn't a big gushing; it was just a little trickle. And I said, 'All right, just hold on a second and I'll get the doctor.' "

2. "It's very interesting seeing women you know going through labor and birth. And I always wondered like if I wanted to have children or not and I don't know. It just posed a lot of questions in my mind because like I don't want to have children but then when I see how happy they are after the birth I thought, 'Oh, it must be nice.' But then when you think about what comes after—all the work and all the sacrifices and responsibility. And I don't think I'm—I could handle it."

The first student nurse captures her experience on the maternity ward through a specific episode centering on a patient, as reflected in many occurrences of third-person-singular pronouns. The experience seems to be alive in the speaker's mind and comes alive for the reader. The second ruminates on her own reactions; she does not tell about any specific event or specific person who may have figured in her visit, and she fails to connect to the reader as well.

Other items on the high-CRA list include articles ("a," "an," "the") that are used with specific nouns, as well as other specific indicators of time and place.

In contrast to the high-CRA list, the low-CRA items include words that figure in logical reflection and rumination, including conjunctions and logical terms ("or," "although," "but," "not") and general, nonspecific modifiers and terms ("all," "very," "more," "most," "something," "sometimes"). Such usage indicates processing dominated by the verbal mode rather than by reference to imagery and emotional experience.

The CRA measure currently in use represents overall RA, the average of the four individual scale scores. In current work, my colleagues and I

---

[2]Examples from Bucci et al. (1992).

are also attempting to develop separate word lists that will model the individual RA scales. The application of the computerized procedures to psychoanalytic sessions will be described in Chapter 17.

Construct Validity of the RA Measures

Measurement of RA in patient and analyst language style is central to our empirical work on the psychoanalytic process. From variation in RA language style over the course of treatment, or within a session, we make inferences to changes in the patient's—or the analyst's—inner state. Increase in RA is interpreted as indicating increasing integration of nonverbal representations, including perception, kinesthetic processes, and emotion schemas, with each other and with language, and also as indicating increasing connection of the speaker to the listener. Decrease in RA indicates the converse. The inference to the meaning of the measures is based on the nomological network within which the RA construct is defined.

Both basic and clinical research studies have been carried out to develop convergent and discriminant validation for the RA measures. The RA measures have been validated as indicators of cognitive–linguistic–affective integration and as associated with adaptive interpersonal functioning in a meta-analysis of RA by Samstag (1996). Construct validation of the RA language style measures is also provided by the experimental research within the dual coding paradigm, as discussed earlier. Studies contributing to the construct validation of RA have been summarized by Bucci (1993, 1995) and Bucci and Miller (1993). I briefly describe several of these studies here.

In basic studies of the RA construct, we have found that individuals with high-RA language style show relatively rapid naming speed when naming sequences of familiar colors or objects. Such simple naming tasks provide direct measures of individual variation in the basic function of connecting images and words. This correlation between naming speed and language style holds after correction for general personal tempo, which may affect all measures, so that naming speed variation due to differences in the peripheral functioning of the speech apparatus, or motor performance in general, may be ruled out. Individuals with high-RA language are also likely to use more hand movements integrated with the rhythms of speech, indicating connections of linguistic and motoric functions. In a study asking for characterizations of subtle color differences, high-RA subjects were more likely to generate descriptions by using metaphoric associations (green, like fir trees in a dense forest) rather than using implicit metrics or dimensions (very dark green, almost black, somewhat shiny). These functions tap aspects of the integration of systems, connecting images and other nonverbal experience to verbal representations, moving back and forth flexibly among systems. The correlation of individual differences in these functions with individual differences in RA language style contributes to the convergent validation of the RA measures.

The construct validity of RA is supported through discriminant as well as convergent validation. Performance on standard verbal intelligence tasks, such as the Similarities and Vocabulary subtests of the WAIS, is not correlated with differences in the RA measures. The standard intelligence tasks primarily reflect connections within the hierarchies of the verbal system rather than links between nonverbal representations and words (Bucci & Freedman, 1978). Tests of verbal fluency, based on phonological features, are also unrelated to RA. In contrast, scores on the Comprehension subtest of the WAIS, which requires "commonsense" knowledge and integration of systems, do show a significant positive relationship to RA measures (Bowen, 1988; Bucci & Freedman, 1978). Some performance tasks, for example, tests of spatial relations such as the Block Design subtest of the WAIS, are also referential tasks, depending on the logical verbal system to guide manipulation of visual designs (Rapaport, Gill, & Schafer, 1968; Bowen, 1988).

Many empirical studies have been carried out to examine the relationship of RA to clinical concepts. Some of these are summarized in Bucci and Miller (1993), Bucci and Mergenthaler (1993), and Bucci (1995). RA levels in the patient and therapist have been shown to predict to success of psychodynamic treatment. We have found level of RA to be significantly related to aspects of object relations, measures of physical health, nature of interactions between mothers and their children, and the effectiveness of psychodynamic treatment. RA is low in depressive illness and in flat-affect schizophrenia (Bucci & Freedman, 1981; Dodd & Bucci, 1987). Interestingly, Morey (1992) found a positive correlation between RA and positive symptoms of schizophrenia, measured by the PANSS (Positive and Negative Syndrome Scale) developed by Kay, Fiszbein, and Opler (1987).

Validation studies have also been carried out for the CRA measure that assess its relationship to RA as scored by judges, as well as its direct relationship to clinical judgments of spoken material. CRA has consistently shown significant, relatively high correlations with judges' ratings of RA for many different types of spoken language, including psychoanalytic transcripts. Interestingly, CRA also tends to show somewhat more variability than RA for the same language samples; to be less influenced by certain types of contents, such as dramatic or violent material; and to be more affected by the speaker's style of describing an event regardless of its nature. The computer can score language style independent of particular content type in a way that human judges cannot. Thus, the CRA procedure not only is useful as a matter of efficiency, but adds interesting information and sources of variance of its own. In validation studies with clinical judges, we have seen that CRA peaks are highly likely to be characterized as narratives, including descriptions of memories, fantasies, and dreams (Kalmykova, Mergenthaler, & Bucci, 1997).

Different patterns of RA and CRA fluctuation have been identified as characterizing various aspects of the treatment process. RA and CRA peaks are found in the type of language that represents the emotion schemas, as will be discussed in detail in Chapters 12 and 14, and such language is the medium of transmission of private emotional experience in the shared discourse. These measures and other computerized and judge-scored measures allow us to track the course of treatment and to evaluate the effect of the analyst interventions in a new way, as will be discussed in Chapter 17.

CHAPTER 12

The Emotion Schemas
and Their Vicissitudes

The referential process, which I have just discussed, and the emotion schemas, to be covered in this chapter, are theoretical constructs distinguishing the multiple code theory from other information-processing models in the cognitive science field. The emotion schemas account for our construction of a self and our knowledge of the interpersonal world, and lay the groundwork for an emotional information-processing—rather than a cognitive information-processing—theory.

The emotion schemas begin to develop in nonverbal form, including subsymbolic processes and symbolic imagery, from the beginning of life; later, linguistic components are incorporated as well. "Emotion schemas" are defined as prototypic representations of the self in relation to others, built up through repetitions of episodes with shared affective states. The affective states consist of clusters of sensory, visceral, and motoric elements, which are largely subsymbolic, and which may occur within or outside of consciousness. Such affective states are activated repeatedly and regularly in response to particular people and events. Stimuli and situations that may be manifestly quite disparate are associated through activation of similar affective states. In the same sense that repeated observations of an object form functionally equivalent classes and prototypic images, so repeated episodes with a common affective core, involving other persons in relation to the self, also form functionally equivalent classes from which prototypic images of episodes are generated.

The prototypic episodes themselves, laid down in memory, constitute the structure of the emotion schemas. They are concrete events made abstract, metaphors of the contingencies of one's life, incorporating what is likely to happen when one has a desire or need, what other people are likely to do, how one is likely to feel. They include images of the object of the emotion, the person we hate or fear or desire; patterns of visceral or somatic experience associated with arousal of an emotion state—what we feel, or expect to feel, viscerally, when we are angry or afraid or in love; and patterns of activation associated with such arousal—to attack, to flee, to caress. The images of people who figure in the prototypic episodes give symbolic interpersonal meaning to the subsymbolic constellations of the core affective state.

Stern's (1985) concept of the Representations of Interactions that have been Generalized (RIGs), which was discussed in Chapter 9, refers precisely to the type of prototypic episodes that characterize the emotion schemas. The organization of each person's emotion schemas depends on the child's interactions with the central figures in her life and the emotional valences associated with them. Repeated episodes may be defined for every type of significant interaction from the beginning of life—feeding, weaning, toilet training, being put to sleep alone. The infant forms prototypic schemas on the basis of multiple occurrences of such events in different contexts but with similar sensory and visceral and motoric activation. The multiple occurrences of a particular type of episode, chunked as functionally equivalent, with a common affective core, produce the enduring prototypic forms. The prototypic schemas with their players, times, and places, are formed first in the nonverbal system, then may be described in words. Different schemas may also be linked in multiple ways in more general prototypic emotion categories. In the mixed events of life, mixed and interconnected schemas are formed. Thus, schemas of weaning are associated with feeding but may also be associated with anger or abandonment or exploration or a sense of mastery or some combination of any of these. Memories of repeated prototypic episodes provide the basis for the general organization and integration of experience that underlies one's sense of self in relation to others, according to Stern.

An early childhood memory may be best understood as a representation of a prototypic episode, rather than one particular event, and represents an emotion schema in this way. The notion of prototypic episodes provides at least a partial explanation for the psychoanalytic concept of the screen memory: a stable, consciously accessible memory of an early, affectively charged experience, which both conceals and reveals the underlying emotional contents. The dual function of such prototypic episodes—to represent and to conceal—as these emerge in clinical work, will be discussed in detail in the sections that follow.

EMOTION SCHEMAS AND MEMORY SCHEMAS

The construct of the emotion schema builds on the basic notion of the memory schema (Bartlett, 1932). As defined by Bartlett, memory schemas are organized representations of past knowledge and experiences that are activated and altered by new experience and determine interactively how new experience is perceived. The basic concept of the memory schema has continued to be applied in many different and elaborated forms as underlying the organization of long-term memory and its role in information processing (Rumelhart, 1980; Neisser, 1976). Other investigators have formulated related structural concepts, such as scripts (Schank & Abelson, 1977) or frames (Minsky, 1975). Central to the concept of the schema is a view of memory as an active process of recategorization and reconstruction, not a simple repetition of images fixed once and for all in the mind. Memory schemas incorporate, within the structures themselves, the potential for development and change, contingent on environmental input to varying degrees.

Every activation of a schema generates new input that has the power to alter the schema in some way. New sensory input entered into organized, interacting schemas provides the basis for specific perceptions and responses in novel and unique situations. The trained naval gunner retrieves general schemas of space and movement, and enters the specific immediate parameters into these. The schemas enable him to determine for each new situation the specific angle of firing to a moving target from a moving source. The tennis player brings established perceptuomotor structures to bear in a similar way in making his contextually contingent computations. The scientist's knowledge determines his perception of all new events, so that he sees meanings in events that are meaningless to persons not so trained; the new input then further elaborates and refines the scientist's internal representation of the world.

Like all schemas, emotion schemas are active and dynamic, constantly reforming, not registered as fixed or static structures. The repetition of episodes that form the prototypic emotion schemas is not a simple replaying. The expectations and beliefs built into our emotion schemas determine how we perceive other people, what we expect, and how we act. Each person sees all interpersonal experience in the context of the emotion schemas that have been constructed in his life to that point. Events of the past, retrieved as memories, are also viewed and reconstructed in the context of the intervening events of one's life; in this sense, the present changes the past as it is remembered.

While the emotion schemas resemble other memory schemas in basic structure and mode of processing, they differ in contents, in particular the dominance of sensory and somatic components, and the importance of the interpersonal context in which the schemas are registered and retrieved. Each occurrence of an emotion schema in a new interpersonal context has the potential to alter its form, depending on whether a match or mismatch occurs between the expectation generated by the schema and the stimulus situation; and most crucially, on the extent to which the mismatch is recognized or is avoided in some way. The contents of the emotion schemas themselves affect the degree to which new input can be registered so as to bring about change. The dominance of certain types of subsymbolic input has the potential to make the emotion schemas particularly resistant to change, as we shall see in the Chapter 13.

The work of the neuroscientist Edelman (1989) suggests a neurological basis for the construct of the schema, which corresponds closely to the psychological formulation, and which applies to the emotion schemas as well. According to Edelman, the brain organizes information, including sensory and motoric representations, as interacting "maps" or collections of neuronal groups; these are connected to the sensory receptors as well as to one another. The maps sort incoming stimuli by similarity and other experiential properties. They interact so as to create categories of things and events, and constantly recategorize information in their interaction with one another. Thus, memories affect our perceptions as well as being affected by them. The maps are systematically organized, but are also amenable to reworking and recategorization on the basis of new input, so that a given perception as stored in memory will be affected by its temporal and spatial context—what has preceded it, the context in which it occurs, and what comes after as well.

The construct of the emotion schemas is compatible with the current approach to emotion theory, which incorporates a view of emotion as emotional information processing (Bower, 1981; Lang, 1994; Mandler, 1984). Thus, as discussed in Chapter 10, cognition, emotion and motivation are seen as interacting in the individual's adaptive organization, not as separate and competing processes. According to Lang:

> A memory of an emotional episode can be seen as an information network that includes units representing emotional stimuli, somatic or visceral responses, and related semantic (interpretive) knowledge. The memory is activated by input that matches some of its representations. Because of the implicit connectivity, the other representations in the structure are also automatically engaged, and as the circuit is associative,

any of the units might initiate or subsequently contribute to this process. (1994, p. 218)

Any component that is activated has the potential to activate other elements, so that language or imagery may activate traces of sensory or visceral experience or action, or the converse may occur. As Lang further argues, such emotion networks may be modeled as parallel, interlinked neural subnets, with properties of parallel distributed processing (PDP) or connectionist systems. The interactive operation of the emotion schemas is also compatible with what is known today about the neurophysiology of the emotions, as outlined in Chapter 10. The multicomponent nature of emotions is reflected in their complex cerebral patterning and in the nature of the circuitry linking sensorithalamic, cortical, and midbrain structures.

The structure of the emotion schemas is also compatible with the definition of affects by Kernberg (1990) as incorporating symbolic representational, motoric, and visceral components. Kernberg is using the term "affect" here in essentially the same sense as the term "emotion" has been used by the theorists cited earlier:

> I define affects as psychophysiological behavior patterns that include a specific cognitive appraisal; a specific expressive facial pattern; a subjective experience of a pleasurable, rewarding, or painful, aversive quality; and a muscular and neurovegetative discharge pattern. The expressive facial pattern is part of the general communicative pattern that differentiates each particular affect. (p. 118)

However, multiple coding diverges from Kernberg's inclusion of discharge phenomena and his corollary conception of affects as the "building blocks" of drives (p. 117), and adds a theoretical framework that accounts for affect (or emotion) in a broader information-processing context.

We may now also see that the concept of the emotion schema is in central and fundamental respects a restatement of Freud's concept of the transference, in more general, cognitive terms:

> Let us bear clearly in mind that every human being has acquired, by the combined operation of inherent disposition and the external influences in childhood, a special individuality in the exercise of his capacity to love—that is, in the conditions which he sets up for loving, in the impulses he gratifies by it, and in the aims he sets out to achieve in it. This forms a cliché or stereotype in him, so to speak (or even several), which perpetually repeats and reproduces itself as life goes on, in so far as external circumstances and the nature of the accessible love-objects permit, and is indeed itself to some extent modifiable by later impressions. (1912, p. 99)

FAILURES OF THE SYMBOLIZING PROCESS
AND MODES OF REPAIR

The emotion schemas are the basis for the organization of the self that defines what we know as personality and determines our goals and choices throughout life. The concept of the emotion schemas casts a wide net, accounting for adaptive as well as maladaptive functions. In psychoanalysis, we are particularly concerned with maladaptive schemas, how they are formed, and how to bring about change. The theory thus potentially provides a basis for an account of pathology in a broader context of psychological organization. At the same time, an understanding of the many different ways in which emotional information processing may become disordered can help to refine and elaborate the basic concepts of the emotion schemas and their organization. The formulation to be presented here is intended as a general outline that needs to be filled in, not a comprehensive theory of psychopathology or of specific pathological entities. The application of multiple coding concepts to specific pathological entities constitutes a project of its own. Even in this initial formulation, however, some of the clinical implications of the theory may be seen to diverge from standard psychoanalytic assumptions, and contrasting propositions can be stated and tested, as we will see.

The Formation of a Pathological Schema

Just as "every unhappy family is unhappy in its own way" (Tolstoy, 1939, p. 3), so the initial formation of maladaptive schemas may come about by many different means, the many ills to which the human psyche is heir: conflictual desires, feelings of despair, destructive impulses toward others or the self, anticipation of attack or abandonment. We should note that the description of maladaptive structures, as proposed here, is based on general concepts of personality organization, not any particular clinical theory. Specific clinical approaches—such as object relational, drive or ego psychology, Kleinian, or self psychology—might in principle be translatable into such general concepts, and the differences between them might thus become stateable and potentially even empirically testable. In formulating a general, essentially ecumenical level of personality organization, the approach proposed here is similar to the attempt of Wallerstein (1993) and his colleagues to identify " 'psychological capacities' that adherents of all prevailing psychoanalytic perspectives will agree to be attributes that comprehensively describe personality functioning" (p. 309). The multiple coding approach adds the perspective that the development and definition of such a set of constructs requires a general theory of psychological organization, a nomological network, that encompasses adaptive as well as maladaptive functioning, and within which constructs on varying levels of abstraction may be defined in relation to one another and to observable events.

In adaptive functioning, memory schemas are continually open to change. Each playing out of a schema has the potential to enter new information into it and thus to change it in some way. The change in emotion schemas, which are dominated by subsymbolic components, are generally more difficult to achieve than for other memory schemas. Subsymbolic processes work immediately and effectively as long as they fit; where the fit is not good, the subsymbolic processor may not be able to carry out the redirection that is needed. The tennis player knows he is not hitting well but is generally not able to figure out why. The symbolic processor needs to swing into action at this point; the player needs to identify specific elements of his footwork, or his timing, to see what is not working and to develop a new pattern of action. He may need a professional to help him recognize what is going wrong and what changes are needed.

Changes in emotion schemas present all the problems of cognitive and sensorimotor schemas and more. It is the nature of emotion schemas, as for all memory schemas, that any element of a schema—a word, an image, an action, a smell—may activate any other. When a negative emotion schema is activated by any of its elements, the affective core and the behavioral response associated with the schema will also be aroused. The schema may be aroused in ongoing experience or be activated by memory or imagination. In cases of negative and conflictual schemas, the sensory and visceral components, which cannot be intentionally regulated and controlled, are likely to incorporate pain. In this sense, the anticipation of a dreaded event is a partial replaying of it, with its painful somatic components, in some kind of trace form. The power of anxiety may be understood in those terms. It is *pain itself*—titrated and diluted—but pain. The individual feels it now, expects to feel more; his goal is then likely to be to reduce or avoid the pain.

Some people may have developed schemas of protection or soothing, perhaps incorporating internalized images of the caretaker, which are activated in response to painful expectations and enable some regulation of the affect. If the affect is not overwhelming, or if the schemas of self-soothing are effective in modulating the affect, the individual may be able to examine the validity of the expectation as this plays out in reality or in imagination. The individual may be able to take in new information in new situations and to examine the match or mismatch between an expectation and an event as it actually occurs. The expectations and beliefs that are associated with the threatening events may be changed, and the schema eventually reconstructed.

If the painful affect is overwhelming, a pathological emotion schema is likely to be formed. I will examine two aspects of the development and maintenance of neurotic emotion schemas that determine their painful and rigid nature: (1) defensive dissociation, which may be termed *desymbolizing*; and (2) dysfunctional attempts at repair, a *resymbolizing* process.

Dissociation and Desymbolizing

The individual in the grips of a painful emotion cannot directly control the subsymbolic components. Symbols are what we are able to regulate and direct to some extent. In neurosis, however, rather than using the symbol system to examine or evaluate the emotional meaning of a fantasy or anticipated event, or to test the veridicality of an expectation, the individual may attempt to avoid symbols by turning away from them or eliminating them in some way. Thus he retreats from, or acts destructively upon, the objects, images, sounds, and words that are linked to the schema and would serve to activate it. He may avoid such entities in reality or turn attention away from them as they are represented in imagery or memory. The operation of dissociation or desymbolization, in which the connections between the subsymbolic and symbolic components of the schemas are cut, works as the converse of the process of organizing the schemas. The operation of warding off and the construction of what we think of as the dynamic unconscious is accounted for by such dissociation.

This avoidance strategy is maladaptive in a number of ways. The painful subsymbolic contents continue to operate even if the symbolic object is avoided, but without being acknowledged or owned. Like all subsymbolic components not linked to symbols, they may be experienced as outside of oneself, outside of the domain over which one has control. At the same time, the individual has retreated from, turned away from, the symbols, the components of the emotion schemas that he may potentially intentionally direct. Thus, the infant, or the adult, carrying out this avoidance strategy would potentially be in a situation of experiencing high arousal of the somatic or motoric components of the emotion schema, which spreads over situations other than that in which it was evoked, without means of symbolic organization, communication to others, or regulation by the self.

This is the special nature of the emotion schemas that leads to their persistence and pervasiveness. The anticipation of the dreaded schema, with its affective core, is painful itself and thus self-validating. The strategy of dissociation or desymbolizing blocks the processes of ongoing evaluation and the possibility of self-regulation. The painful emotion schemas thus become self-perpetuating and encompass an increasingly wide range of situations other than those in which they were initially evoked. The individual feels aroused, without knowing the meaning of the arousal, and will feel this in many contexts where the arousal may not be adaptive.

Dysfunctional Repair: The Attempt to Resymbolize

To restore a sense of control over his bodily or emotional state, the individual generally attempts to provide some meaning for feelings that have been activated, to connect the subsymbolic processes to symbols once again. Since he is in a process of avoiding the actual source or meaning of the arousal, he needs to generate new scenarios, with new objects that account for the aroused affect. These are the kinds of processes that have been called "attribution" within cognitive theories of emotion, as discussed in Chapter 8. They may be understood in psychoanalytic terms as displacement and related defensive operations. The new object or new situation is likely to be similar to or associated with the dissociated symbolic elements of the schema but distant and different enough that the connection is not seen. The child in a state of rage at his mother feels the intense affective and somatic arousal but may not feel able to bear its emotional meaning and the possible consequences. He seeks for a different meaning, one that accounts for the arousal while warding off understanding of its real objectives. He may interpret the arousal as a feeling other than anger, may experience it in relation to someone other than the mother, or as directed against himself.

The construction of new schemas, unrealistic as they may be, constitutes attempts at symbolizing, spontaneous healing in the representational domain, while maintaining the initial defensive dissociation. Since the individual is still actively avoiding the actual emotional meaning of the schema, however, the regulation and control will be spurious. The schema remains maladaptive, persistent, and pervasive, but perhaps in a different way, with its own secondary effects. The attempted reconstruction is itself a component of the pathological structure, determining the particular form that the neurotic schema takes. The general need or wish for symbols, and for meaning, has potential positive impact, however, in retaining a basis for connection to objects and for cure.

The "Vicious Circle" and Its Repair

The dissociation of subsymbolic from symbolic functions is what blocks change and development in the emotion schemas from occurring in an adaptive way. This is the general core of neurosis, the essence of the condition that psychoanalysis is uniquely suited to treat, and also the condition that sometimes makes such treatment so difficult. Strachey's (1934) formulation of the neurotic "vicious circle" may be understood more simply in this context. The goal of psychoanalytic treatment, according to Strachey, is to make a breach in the vicious circle, so that the processes of development might proceed upon their normal course. He describes this process in metapsychological terms:

> If, for instance, the patient could be made less frightened of his super-ego or introjected object, he would project less terrifying imagos on to the outer object and would therefore have less need to feel hostility towards it; the object which he then introjected would in turn be less savage in its pressure upon the id-impulses, which would be able to lose something of their primitive ferocity. In short, a benign circle would be set up instead of the vicious one. (p. 341)

The constructs of the emotion schemas and the referential process account for the clinical observations associated with the neurotic vicious circle and its repair, without calling upon the failed conceptual machinery of the metapsychology. The vicious circle of neurosis involves the disconnection of subsymbolic components of the emotion schema from the organizing system of images and words, while the painful affect continues to be aroused and also becomes more pervasive. The structural change that is needed and that is so difficult to achieve is the connection of the dissociated affective core of an emotion schema to symbols that express its actual emotional meaning. This may require giving up displaced symbolic meaning, which may itself be causing difficulty and pain. Reorganization of the emotion schemas in lasting ways is what is meant by structural change. Such change is the essential goal of psychoanalytic therapy, distinguishing it from other treatment forms.

Psychoanalytic treatment is specifically designed to permit activation of old emotion schemas, with their affective core, in a new interpersonal context in which they can be tolerated, examined, and reconstructed, and where new emotional meanings can be developed. The change that is sought, and that is so difficult to achieve, concerns the subsymbolic sensory, visceral and motoric components of the schema, so that the individual actually feels different, sees the world differently. The activation of the schema itself, with its subsymbolic components, is necessary to permit such change. The old expectations need to be experienced, with their physiological and motoric, as well as imagistic components, in the treatment context. It is not sufficient to talk about the emotional expectations and beliefs; they must be experienced on a bodily level, in a sufficient range.

The activation of the subsymbolic components may occur through retrieval of memories of situations in which an emotion schema was played out and may also arise directly, in relation to the analyst. The power of the transference is understood most directly in this sense. The schemas laid down through repeated interactions with central figures in the individual's past now come to incorporate the new object, the analyst. The schema then plays out in the treatment, but, eventually, it is hoped, as a reconstruction rather than a repetition. By this means, new functionally equivalent classes of experience may be formed, enabling recategorization of the interpersonal field.

The treatment works in many different ways to enable activation of the schemas and to bring about change: by providing a new interpersonal context involving different, more positive responses; by fostering the development of new schemas of self-acceptance and self-care, and the patient's recognition of the reality of his current powers; as well as through interpretation, examination, and reconstruction of the experiences that are told or played out. The operation of this process will be illustrated in clinical material to be presented in Chapter 17.

A Componential Model of the Defenses

Given the formulation of maladaptive emotion schemas, a componential model of the defenses may be proposed, reflecting different levels of dissociation among systems, and different processes of attempted compensation and dysfunctional repair. I am not attempting to develop a comprehensive model of the defenses here, any more than I am attempting to develop a formulation of specific pathologies, but to provide a general framework that is clinically meaningful and also amenable to empirical study.

Defenses may be characterized as incorporating both dissociation and attempted repair, and may be distinguished in terms of their relative emphases with respect to these functions. I would suggest that defenses that are destructive of symbolic meaning are more likely to be considered low level or regressive; higher level defenses are those that carry some symbolic meaning of their own. The goals or effects of particular defenses, as of particular symptoms, need to be explicated specifically in each individual case. Various types of defense are likely to operate in individual ways in each case of neurosis; some operating to maintain the initial dissociation and others to repair it. The new symbols that are incorporated in the attempted repair may be adaptive or dysfunctional to varying degrees, as we have seen.

The construct of repression takes on an extended range of meaning within the multiple code formulation. Thus, at the simplest level, repression would involve breaking or blocking of referential links between nonverbal symbolic imagery and words, still leaving the connections between subsymbolic experience and images in place. In such cases, the basic symbolic organization of the emotion schema would remain within the nonverbal system, although, for a variety of reasons, the individual cannot—or does not—find words to communicate what he experiences.

It is not clear that dissociation is likely to occur in this simple form, or that, if it did, it would constitute an aspect of a neurotic defense. Instead, the desymbolizing process is likely to feed back to involve dissociation among the nonverbal components of the emotional schemas themselves, as well as between images and words. Thus, dissociations may occur among sensory, somatic, and motoric components of activation in subsymbolic format, and between these and images of "objects," the people who figure in the repetitive episodes that build the schema. In general, such desymbolizing is likely to be more severe to the extent that early organization is weaker, or trauma greater.

In a situation where relatively intact schemas have previously been formed and some connections to symbols remain in place, the affective core that is aroused, the feelings of rage or desire or terror, may be directed toward substitute objects that resemble the one that has been warded off, as in neurotic disorders involving displacement. The selection of new symbolic objects is driven by the nature of the schema, which the individual is striving both to symbolize and to avoid, as well as by the level of dissociation that has occurred. The principles of organization of the subsymbolic and symbolic systems operate to determine the choice of new objects and the new structures that are formed. This form of dissociation, in which the symbolizing function remains relatively effective, might be dominant in cases where the child has initially formed positive emotion schemas incorporating representations of the caretaker and then experiences conflictual feelings—anger or forbidden desires—directed toward the object of attachment.

If the central caretaking figures themselves have a more generally threatening rather than regulating or soothing effect, eliciting terror or anger, motivating withdrawal or attack, disruption of the basic organization of the emotion schemas and interference with the symbolizing process are likely to be correspondingly more severe. Some obsessions or compulsions may be understood in this way—as symbolic attempts to account for and control arousal whose real meaning is warded off. In other cases, the categories of object-symbols that are associated with the core painful affect may be rejected without being replaced by specific, substitute objects. The motoric components of attack, or fear of attack, may be turned toward the self, as in depression, or toward the body or parts of the body, as in various forms of somatization. The lack of capacity to substitute symbolic objects in the emotion schemas may reflect intensity of the painful components of the emotion schema or greater fragmentation of the emotion schemas in early development or in the course of life. It is just such structural weakness, leading to incapacity to use objects in a reparative way, that renders some individuals more vulnerable to posttraumatic stress disorder, or to disorders of somatization, and that makes psychoanalytic techniques seem less appropriate for such disorders.

The deepest dissociations involve failure to organize emotion schemas around symbols, rather than disruption of schemas that have previously been organized to some degree. This might result from absence of consistent, organizing human objects in the early life of the child, or from general, perhaps constitutional, inability to construct the symbolic forms. Such dissociations, in their most severe forms, perhaps with neurological determinants, might be associated with disorders such as autism and forms of schizophrenia.

LEVELS OF THE SYMBOLIZING PROCESS: IMPLICATIONS FOR TREATMENT

The model of pathology and defense that has been proposed here has specific implications for the treatment process, including cases where psychoanalytic treatment has not previously been seen as feasible. Where positive schemas incorporating the caretaker were initially constructed in the individual's development, the repair of emotional dissociation, as this occurs in treatment, may be expected to follow a somewhat parallel path. The caretaker was the primary object-symbol organizing the emotion schemas in normal development; in treatment, the analyst functions as a new object in the reconstruction of schemas that have been dissociated. The conflictual wishes that led to the original dissociation will emerge again in the new relationship, where they can be played out in a new way. The analyst provides a new object, and the treatment provides a new context; the old story is told in a new way. New schemas that are more veridical in current life, as well as schemas of soothing and protection, may be constructed.

In most instances, the process of transferring feelings from the displaced interpersonal object to the analyst will not proceed directly in this way. In many cases of dissociation or desymbolizing, the feelings are not organized in a form to permit such transference. According to the theory developed in Chapter 11, if the affect attunement described by Stern (1985) does not occur within some acceptable range, with a stable caretaking figure, the referential process itself will not develop, and the construction of emotional meanings will be blocked. Here, the symbolic role is not available for a new object to step into; the place is not reserved. A new role must be created, and the emotion schema must be organized in a more fundamental way.

In such cases, learning to be a patient will require development of the ability to symbolize, to enable the treatment to proceed. The development of the symbolizing process occurs alongside of development of new, interpersonal expectations; these types of learning must proceed in an interactive way. New connections to objects in the interpersonal context, in memory, in the person of the analyst, and in the patient's ongoing life facilitate the symbolizing process; development of the ability to symbolize facilitates further connections to objects.

The more severe the initial dissociation, the more difficult the problem of learning to symbolize. In some cases, the threat embodied in the dreaded schemas is experienced as so extreme that the individual turns against the symbolizing process itself in a more pervasive way. At the same time, the subsymbolic components—the potentially catastrophic and experientially annihilating terror and pain—are also most intense. The syndrome of alexithymia (being without words for feelings), as identified by Marty and de M'Uzan (1963), Nemiah and Sifneos (1970a, 1970b), and others, may be seen as reflecting such a crisis of symbolizing. Cases of this nature, as in posttraumatic stress disorder, somatization, and addictive disorders, have often been seen as not amenable to dynamic psychotherapy. As Krystal has pointed out: "Alexithymia is the single most common cause of poor outcome or outright failure of psychoanalysis and psychoanalytic psychotherapy" (1988, p. xi).

Where there is such a general state of rage or dread related to object-symbols, the repair process will be most complex. In these cases, the avoidance of symbols, or the attack on them, may be played out actively in the ongoing treatment relationship and also in the reexperiencing of the early relationships in memory. To enable the resymbolizing process to begin, in at least a minimal way, the treatment of traumatized or somatizing patients might require focusing on whatever discrete and specific entities are available to function as organizing symbols within the emotion schemas, before new connections to other symbolic objects, other people, can be built. This is one point at which implications of the multiple coding approach diverge from the psychoanalytic view. Symptoms and actions may operate in a progressive manner to further the symbolizing process, rather than being regressive, as the discharge model implies, and as has generally been assumed. The symptoms or actions themselves play a symbolizing role where other symbolic entities are feared and rejected. In cases of severe desymbolizing, a particular physical symptom or severe pain may constitute the only available discrete entity permitting entry of an emotion schema into the symbolic domain. That is one reason why patients hold on to their symptoms so fiercely—because they constitute a vehicle of meaning, rather than because they ward off meaning.

This formulation of the role of symptoms is compatible with Freud's (1895b, 1900) characterization of specific symptoms as carrying meaning, similar to the manifest content of dreams. However, we postulate a specific, facilitative role of somatic symptoms or actions in the symbolizing process, rather than viewing symptoms as alternate discharge modes. Our view opposes the widely accepted assumption of compensatory or substitute discharge, which is generally retained even where the connection to energic concepts may not be acknowledged. Thus, Kernberg (1984) has assumed an inverse relationship between aggressive action and verbalization. McDougall (1989) refers to somatization, as well as action, as substitutes for thought: "through which one disperses emotion rather than thinking about the precipitating event and the feelings connected to it" (p. 15).

The model of pathology and its cure that I propose yields a new delineation of the relationships between verbalization and acting out or somatization, including conditions under which a positive rather than inverse relationship might be expected, and leads to different implications for treatment as well. The first step of the symbolizing process, which is necessary for treatment to proceed, might be the patient making visceral or motoric experience discrete and bringing it into the domain of reflection. Talking about the symptoms or actions—connecting them to verbal symbols—then has considerable further powers, strengthening their symbolic operation and entering them into the shared discourse. The patient can focus on the symptom and provide associations to contexts and schemas in which it figures long before the role of any interpersonal objects in the emotion schema can be acknowledged. Eventually, through focus on symptoms in the shared discourse, the emotion schemas may be played out in the relationship to some degree, and new roles for new interpersonal objects may be created. By this means, schemas in which the analyst figures may ultimately be formed, and it may then eventually become possible to reach patients who have not previously been seen as reachable through a talking cure.

From the same perspective, and equally difficult to accept within a standard psychoanalytic view, the verbalization of specific, mundane details that is associated with alexithymia may be seen as an attempt to reconstitute a symbolic focus for a dissociated emotion schema, rather than an avoidance of symbols. The details of the psychosomatic narratives, like the specific symptoms in hysteria, themselves carry meaning, functioning as attempts at repair after defensive splitting, with potentially adaptive effects. The patient's focus on details of time and place may be an attempt to orient himself on a piece of solid symbolic ground in emotional memory, rather than a means of warding off memory (Dodd & Bucci, 1987). Speech loaded with specific, everyday details may be not merely a means of filling silence and avoiding primitive, chaotic anxiety, but an attempt to contain the chaos and render the anxiety less primitive, using the only symbolic means available. The basis for the fundamental rule—that the apparently irrelevant or trivial notions that come into focus are actually outliers of the warded-off schema that have escaped repression—may apply to such specific details, as well as to symptoms and viscerosensory experience.

SYMBOLIZING VERSUS SUBSTITUTE DISCHARGE: EMPIRICAL EVIDENCE

The implications of our symbolizing model have been supported in clinical work, and in empirical research. Rainer Schors in Munich (personal communication, 1993) has based his uniquely successful treatment of intractable pain on acceptance of pain as an *objective entity* to which the patient relates, and which is then worked with in the treatment. James Hull (personal communication, 1993) has described the treatment of a patient with borderline personality disorder, who experienced her tongue as being continually cut by the edges of her teeth. Only when Hull began actively asking her about the minute details of this, how it happens, which part of her mouth is affected, did the treatment begin to progress and an alliance begin to emerge.

The same principle has been supported in several experimental studies by Leventhal (1984) and his colleagues, in which subjects were exposed to pain and distress produced by cold water or blocking of blood circulation. Subjects who were explicitly instructed to attend to their painful sensations reported significantly lower pain levels, compared to control subjects who were given instructions intended to distract them from the noxious stimulus. The focus on pain actually reduced the *level* of pain as subjects reported this, although the subjects were more *aware* of their pain. The complex findings indicate that focus on pain may have adaptive effects in facilitating organization of emotion schemas, even though the experience may seem to be heightened by this means. People know they feel a stressor when they attend to it and consciously wish not to know; they are not aware of the beneficial effect of focusing attention in this way. According to Leventhal, focus on the painful stimulus facilitated its being experienced as an objective event and led to buildup of coping processes. In multiple coding terms, this corresponds to facilitation of the symbolizing process and its regulatory effects.

The effect of focus on somatic symptoms as facilitating symbolization, rather than avoiding it, was also supported in recent research using measures of RA, which assess activity of referential connections between nonverbal experience and words, as discussed in Chapter 11. The RA measures were applied in a study of the relationship between somatization, acting out, and verbalization in a sample of 50 female borderline inpatients (Okie, 1992). Based on the substitute discharge premise of the metapsychology, Okie initially predicted a negative correlation between verbalization of emotional experience as measured by the RA scales, and measures of somatization, injuries to the self, and acting out, based on coding of daily nursing reports. Contrary to her predictions, Okie found significant *positive* correlations between RA and symptoms. Patients who had more physical complaints, who incurred more injuries, either accidental or intentional, and who showed more acting-out behaviors, also made greater use of the type of language associated with access to emotional experience and successful psychoanalytic treatment, rather than turning away from such linguistic expression. Okie's results offer counterevidence to the general psychoanalytic assumption of substitute discharge and provide empirical support for a complementary relationship between symptoms and symbol formation. The borderline inpatients in her study may be understood as located emotionally or cognitively at a phase where some intrapsychic, nonverbal, symbolic organization focused on symptoms and actions may be needed before connections to other people, or to words, can be achieved.

Research by Hull (1990) further supports this formulation and its stage-specific implications. Hull found a positive correlation between measures of RA and symptom levels early in the treatment of a borderline inpatient with hysterical paralysis. Symptom levels were measured using the Symptom Checklist 90–Revised (SCL-90R; Derogatis, 1983), a self-report symptom checklist that was filled out weekly by the patient. The patient in Hull's study produced high-RA language early in treatment, associated with high symptom levels. We suggest that the florid, vivid, sometimes psychotic speech that she produced in this phase operated to enhance focus on symptoms as symbols, in the sense outlined above. This may be understood as the first step in symbol construction, reflecting the early stages in reparation of dissociation, as in Okie's findings.

At this early phase, however, Hull also found low levels of the type of patterning of RA scores that is associated with full operation of the referential process (Bucci, 1993). The vivid speech of the patient at this stage did not lead to periods of reflection and shared communication, which are needed for the recursive deepening of the process and the function of working through. Later in the treatment, as the patient improved (and symptom levels generally declined), the expected negative correlation between symptoms and RA was found, and levels of patterning reflecting occurrence of a systematic referential process increased. In the early phase, symbolizing was facilitated by the focus on symptoms. Later, the images expressed in the high-RA speech served more broadly as a basis for reflection within the communicative discourse and for connection to the therapist, the object now available in the interpersonal field.

Side Effects of the "Talking Cure"

The referential process is a powerful function with potentially significant emotional and bodily benefits, but also with potential risks. The "talking cure," like any powerful treatment, has its dangers. The florid, sometimes psychotic speech produced early in treatment by the borderline patient in Hull's study, which I believe to have constituted a first step in symbol construction and repair of dissociation, was also associated with higher symptom levels at that time. This symptom activation may be necessary to permit entry to the symbolizing process, before images and words can be retrieved; however, this raises the possibility of the individual being endangered by somatic conditions or acting-out behaviors in the transitional phase. For this reason, therapists may choose to avoid insight-focused treatments and to rely instead on supportive treatments aiming to bolster repression for patients with severe pathologies, such as schizophrenia or posttraumatic stress disorder (PTSD). In a study of Vietnam veterans with PTSD, Miller (1994) found that relatively successful outcome, measured by symptomatic change, in the type of psychotherapy used in a veteran's treatment program was associated with unchanged or lower rather than increased RA.

The meaning of symptoms—and by implication, the meaning of symptom alleviation—needs to be evaluated specifically in each individual case. There may certainly be instances that call for symptom alleviation, thus maintaining the dissociated state. There may be other instances where it is possible, and preferable, to work with symptoms and their meanings, so that deeper symbolizing transformations can occur. If the patient can bear the affect that is evoked, can move from symptoms to memories and images stored in nonverbal, symbolic form, and can connect to the therapist, he has a chance to bring the powers of the symbolizing process and the verbal system to bear in reorganizing his emotion schemas and making them more veridical and adaptive in his current life. If the patient cannot retrieve such memories or establish a therapeutic relationship, or if the memories or interactions evoke intolerable affect, further defensive dissociation, along with an increased reliance on symptoms, may result, with negative mental or physical health effects. In some cases, where long-term treatment is feasible, learning to symbolize, building the referential connections, itself becomes a major objective of the treatment, necessary to permit other changes in emotion schemas to occur. The interactive process, in which learning to connect to symbols and learning to connect to other persons develop together and facilitate one another, must occur to varying degrees in all psychoanalytic treatments. That is why psychoanalysis takes so long; that is also why it has power to bring about deep change.

CHAPTER 13

Linking Feelings and Words
THE REFERENTIAL CYCLE

The emotion schemas are dominated by subsymbolic experience. The essential feature of subsymbolic processing is not that it is nonverbal, although it usually is; not that it is automatic, unconscious or implicit, although it may be; but that it operates without the parameters of an action or a task having been explicitly defined, without discrete elements being identified, or explicit processing rules being required. This feature has several important, and in some senses opposing implications. On the one hand, the ability to operate without specific metrics and categories makes possible the ongoing functioning that is necessary in most areas of life, most of the time. In sports, in the arts, in everyday activities, and in our emotional responses to others, we are able to act in finely tuned ways, immediately and intuitively, without analyzing the elements of a task. The subsymbolic system is responsible for the implicit computations guiding such actions and responses.

On the other hand, the subsymbolic mode of response works only as long as the operative schemas are veridical and adaptive. This holds for emotional functions as for all the activities of life. When ways of thought, or acting, or feeling are fixed in a mode of operation that is maladaptive or destructive, implicit responses are likely to perpetuate the underlying distortion. To change the dysfunctional system evaluation of goals and reorganization of schemas are required. Such reorganization is likely to require intentional examination of the schemas in a way that subsymbolic processors cannot support. The individual must somehow "look at" his desires, expectations, and beliefs, not just permit them to play out in their usual patterns. Here, the power of the symbolizing system may be required.

According to the model proposed here, the process of change in psychoanalytic treatment depends on examination of dissociated schemas and, ultimately, their reconstruction in adaptive form. The general assumption underlying psychoanalysis, the talking cure, is that verbalization is necessary for such change to occur. However, language is not the optimal mode of representing or communicating emotion, as our model makes clear. The emotion schemas are dominated by subsymbolic information registered in sensory, visceral, and motoric form. The multiple, diverse lines of analogic experience, operating synchronously, must somehow be represented in a code that is composed of discrete lexical items, represented in discourse in the single-channel, sequential format of speech, and also registered in semantic memory in logical and hierarchical organization. We can see that the representation of emotions in words, and its interpretation in terms of word meanings, can be partial at best.

In this chapter, I discuss the operation of the referential process by which subsymbolic information, including emotional information, may be translated into verbal form, and the difficulties and limitations of this translation process. I then propose a stage model of the referential process and illustrate its general application in cognitive and emotional life.

THE LANGUAGE OF EMOTIONS

For most of us, it is extremely difficult to express strong emotion verbally. We often talk instead about what we are unable to express: "My heart is too full for speech"; "I was struck dumb with awe"; "My mouth hung open"; "I was absolutely speechless"; "My heart was in my mouth"; "All I can say is wow!" The lover stammers and is tongue-tied in the presence of the beloved; love songs are full of this verbal paralysis: "I can't begin to tell you how much you mean to me"; "You're just too marvelous, too marvelous for words." In grief, "the spirit intercedes with sighs too deep for words" (Romans, 8:26).

Both vocalization and facial expression are better suited than language to communicate emotion directly. The motoric and vocal expression of reactions and intentions involving face, posture, and voice constitute intrinsic components of the emotion schema itself. Such expression is innate and universal to some extent in humans and perhaps to a greater degree in other species. The view that facial expressions of emotion can be traced phylogenetically and are universal in humans, as part of our biological heritage, was put forth by Darwin and is held by many emotion theorists today.

It is not surprising, from an evolutionary perspective, that emotions are so difficult to express in words. The function of emotion in adaptation is similar to that outlined for odor. Emotions function primarily to mediate response to current situations rather than to evoke situations in their absence. They mediate between the constantly changing situations that impinge on an organism and its behavioral response, permitting flexible adaptation of the organism to the environment. The representation of entities in their absence, in image or word, is the domain of the symbolic; immediate response based on intuitive, implicit processing is the function of the subsymbolic mode, operating in human adults and infants, as in other species. Based on the theory of the referential process, as discussed in Chapter 11, we see that the subsymbolic sensory and somatic and motoric representations and processes that make up the emotion schemas are the components of the nonverbal system for which the referential connections are most distant and indirect. Humans, in this and other respects a rather transitional species, somehow try to generate verbal expression for a type of schema that has not evolved fully in symbolic form.

The symbolizing of emotional experience, for which most of us are ill-equipped, is the special domain of the artist or poet. Just as the wine writer turns the verbalization of the experience of taste into an art form, so the artist, musician, or poet does the same for emotion by contriving the construction of a symbolic context into which emotional experience may be embedded. The wine writer refers to specific images from a wide range of domains to capture the qualities of taste and smell; the artist or poet constructs a metaphor to capture emotion in a similar way. In the expression of emotion, as for taste or smell, metaphors may be understood precisely as concrete and discrete symbols for unnamed, subsymbolic feeling states.

The poet does not simply say "I love you" but describes images drawn from schemas of love and desire, and consummatory acts associated with these, which may be generally shared:

> How beautiful you are, how charming,
> my love, my delight!
> In stature like the palm tree,
> its fruit clusters your breasts.
> "I will climb the palm tree," I resolved,
> "I will seize its clusters of dates."
> (*Song of Songs* 7:9, ascribed to Solomon)

Subjective feelings are captured in tangible objects that have special power to activate a shared experience in another person, or to activate experience in memory. When the metaphor is transmitted to a listener or reader, it may serve to evoke the emotional experience with some of its subsymbolic components, permitting one to reconstitute elements of the experience that could be only partially represented in words. Poets use images whose emotional meanings are likely to be widely shared. The poets who speak to us most directly are those whose symbols activate our own subsymbolic, representational worlds.

Although verbalization is not the optimal means of expressing emotion, it is the optimal mode of communication with other people and of self-regulation and direction, as I have discussed. Verbalization is central to the work of psychoanalysis, bringing the power of symbol systems to bear on emotion schemas that have become maladaptive. Learning to be a psychoanalytic patient (or an analyst) depends on development of the referential process—building connections within an individual between emotional experience and words, and building connections between individuals in the shared discourse. In the context of the treatment, all participants must be poets, all must use metaphor, to some degree.

STAGES OF THE REFERENTIAL PROCESS

The basic mechanism of the referential process has been outlined in Chapter 11. The stages of this process, as they apply specifically to expression of emotional experience, are outlined here.

Subsymbolic Activation

The process begins with activation of an emotion, with its diverse components, including the affective core of sensory and visceral experience, tendencies toward actions represented as motor programs, and also including the objects of the emotion and other symbolic contents. The various components may operate within or outside of awareness; thus, the associated actions may be, but are not necessarily, represented as intentions, and the objects of the emotion may be recognized to varying degrees. In the phase of activation of the emotion, the subsymbolic components of the affective core are likely to be dominant; the person is aroused, sometimes without knowing at first "what is bothering him." This is the sense in which "affect precedes cognition," in Zajonc's (1980) terms. The dominance of the affective core is particularly marked for emotion schemas that are dissociated, where the objects and symbolic contents are largely outside of awareness. The subsymbolic sensory and visceral experiences that dominate in such schemas are most difficult to express in words.

The Symbolizing Phase

The phase of connecting subsymbolic experience to symbols may be divided into two substages, as follows.

Construction of Prototypic Imagery

Subsymbolic experience in all sensory modalities is chunked or categorized into functionally equivalent classes, which are then represented as prototypic images. This process holds for the emotion schemas as well. The emotion schemas are built through repetition of episodes that share a common affective core and are chunked as functionally equivalent in the organization of memory. Based on this formulation, I have developed the construct of the emotion schema as having the structure of a prototypic episode beginning, for example, with a wish or need and actions related to this, and leading to a complex sequence of reactions and counterreactions that may be expected to occur. Such episodes are the type of prototypic imagery that best facilitates the expression of the emotion schema in verbal form.

Narratives of Prototypic Images and Episodes

The writer or speaker—or the analytic patient—who wishes to communicate emotion does so most effectively by describing the specific images associated with an emotion, or an episode in which an emotion was activated. Narratives about other people, in relation to one's self, may be seen precisely as metaphors of the emotion schemas. The telling of a story—a narrative that expresses the subjectively constructed contingencies of one's life—is the closest one can come to communication of an emotion schema, or parts of a schema, in verbal form. In episodic form, the emotion schemas can be "told." These narratives may have the form of memories, including screen memories, fantasies, dreams, or events of current life. In treatment, the person of the analyst and the therapeutic context, as experienced by the patient in the here and now of the session, may be entered into the narrative in derivative or manifest form.

The Reflection Phase: Understanding and Verification

In telling the narrative, the person is able to communicate some of the symbolic contents of the emotion, in some cases, before he can explicitly characterize the nature of what he feels. Through this mechanism, he is able to characterize the emotion schema by describing a prototypic event associated with it and may evoke a similar feeling in the listener, even without being able to say what it is he feels, to give a name to it. Through verbalization of the episode, elaboration of connections and association within his own verbal system, and connection to a listener, the emotion may be explicitly identified ("I feel angry"; "I feel sad"). Eventually the basis for the emotion may be understood, and evidence for the new understanding may be brought to bear.

While the categorizing or identification of an emotion is an important function, it is likely to come at the end of a process of emotional exploration, as I have shown here. This is likely to be the case for all experience of any complexity; we feel some kind of arousal, may even act on it, before we identify what it is we feel. For most normal types of experience, where the symbolic contents are accessible, the phases as outlined here may operate smoothly, even outside of awareness. As for all operations of the referential process, the difficulty of the process comes to awareness most acutely when it is blocked, when we cannot find the words we seek. The process I have outlined here will operate in a particularly slow and limited way for emotional experience that has been dissociated or warded off. The account of the referential process that has been given here provides a basis for the power of the free-association process; the images and episodes, even those that may seem trivial and irrelevant, provide access to emotion schemas. Seemingly trivial events, whose emotional meaning is not explicitly recognized, are particularly effective for connecting to schemas where dissociation has occurred. If the referential process operates successfully, the new connections within the verbal system will feed back to enable change in the nonverbal ones. Examples of the bidirectional operation of the referential process and its effects in the interpersonal context of psychoanalytic treatment will be presented in Chapters 14 and 17.

DEVELOPMENT OF THE REFERENTIAL PROCESS: THE INTERPERSONAL BASE

Like the prototypic images of the self in relation to others, which are central to the emotions, the referential process by which emotional experience is expressed also begins to be built in earliest infancy, in the context of the mother–infant interaction. The development of the referential process begins well prior to the acquisition of language and continues in increasingly complex form throughout childhood and throughout life.

In addition to its function of linking subsymbolic systems to one another and to symbolic forms, the referential process has the further role of linking one individual's internal representations to another's, creating a new, shared referential space by this means. From its earliest development, the referential process, as applied to emotional experience, includes not only connections between one's own subjective state and overt expressions, but also connection between one's inner experience and the expressions of others. The mother's behavioral and facial reactions constitute the first external symbols that may be used by the infant as referring to his own inner state. Each of these reactions serves as a kind of "nonverbal metaphor and analog" for the infant's subjective experience. Emde, Klingman, Reich, and Wade (1978) and Campos and Stenberg (1980) refer to the notion of "social referencing," which concerns the infant's use of the mother's affect signals as external indicators that have reference to his own inner states. In a profound sense, the mother's expressions serve as nonverbal prototypic symbols for emotions, functioning as other prototypes to clump functionally equivalent classes of subsymbolic experience (classes of the infant's inner states) into discrete units that contribute as well to the formation of the infant's self-representations.

Stern also sees the caretaker's expressions and behavior as providing external symbolic representations for the child's inner experience, fulfilling this function long before language is available. He has identified a form of interaction, beginning when the infant is about 9 months old, which he terms "affect attunement," and which accounts for this process of representation. According to Stern (1985):

> An attunement is a recasting, a restatement of a subjective state. It treats the subjective state as the referent and the overt behavior as one of several possible manifestations or expressions of the referent. For example, a level and quality of exuberance can be expressed as a unique vocalization, as a unique gesture, or as a unique facial display. (p. 161)

The process of affect attunement may be seen as the first stage in the referential process, as this applies to the verbalization of emotion. The caretaker's response serves as a representation and extension of the infant's feeling state, not simply an imitation of external behavior, as in the following example:

A nine-month-old girl becomes very excited about a toy and reaches for it. As she grabs it, she lets out an exuberant "aaaah!" and looks at her mother. Her mother looks back, scrunches up her shoulders, and performs a terrific shimmy with her upper body, like a go-go dancer. The shimmy lasts only about as long as her daughter's "aaaah!" but is equally excited, joyful, and intense. (Stern, 1985, p. 140)

The mother's bodily action is isomorphic with the infant's vocalization but not identical to it, expressing the same inner experience but in a different modality. The mother's shimmy may be characterized as a nonverbal, *cross-modal,* and also *cross-subjective* symbol referring to the child's intense inner state of excitement and joy. It symbolizes the inner experience in an expression that may be jointly observed and also communicates to the infant that there is another being with similar inner experience, an answering "emotional intelligence" outside of herself. Direct imitation of the vocalization alone would not provide evidence for a separate, responsive subjectivity in this sense.

In his empirical research, Stern has identified three basic features of behavior—intensity, timing, and shape—for which matches without actual imitation, including cross-modal matches, are possible, and which thus form the basis for attunement. For each of these features, specific categories of matches were identified, and matching criteria were established. Ten mothers with infants 8 to 12 months of age were observed in a controlled play setting. Stern found that attunements, most frequently cross-modal, were the most common responses to infant expressions of affect, accounting for about half of all maternal responses. In some cases, mothers also carried out purposeful misattunements, which Stern refers to as "tuning," and whose purpose appeared to be to change, either to increase or decrease the infant's level of activity or affect. Mothers were largely unaware of their attunement or "tuning" behaviors. Even where there was some awareness of the interaction, mothers were generally focused on the desired consequences of what they were doing rather than on properties of the behavior itself.

The new forms provided through attunement and its subtle variants develop the interpersonal meaning for the infant's inner representations. All of this is generated on the largely subsymbolic level that best represents the emotions, and that the child is equipped to understand from the beginning of life. The basic interpersonal aspect of the development of the referential process may be seen precisely here. The infant, in the normal course of development, finds that the actions and expression of another person are related to his own inner state and his own expressions, and provide a new meaning for these. He also learns that a range of expressions of others or of one's self may be functionally equivalent in representing a feeling state, thus forming an emotional class in this sense.

Development of Verbal Emotional Meanings: An Extension of Vygotsky's Concept

The expression of emotion in verbal form requires a new integration, beyond the expression in vocalization and action that is intrinsic to the emotion schemas. While no model exists as yet to account for this development, we can begin to provide such an account on the basis of Vygotsky's formulation of the development of word meanings. Partially paralleling Vygotsky's formulation, as discussed in Chapter 9, and adding to it, we can make the following statements concerning the development of verbal emotional meanings in the early life of the child.

1. In their ontogenetic development, emotion and speech have different roots. The first emotion structures are constructed without linguistic mediation, in the first interpersonal contexts of life. Emotion differs from other forms of thought in that it is also expressed directly in vocal form. This begins with crying at birth and continues to develop, with moans, squeaks, screams, gasps, whines, guffaws, giggles, hisses, and many other forms throughout life.

2. We can identify a nonemotional stage in the speech development of the child, in which the child actively experiments with phonemes, which will develop into language. We can also identify a nonlinguistic stage in his emotional expression, in which he is unable to say how or what he feels but expresses emotion in the natural vocal and other expressive forms—crying, screaming, laughing, kicking—of which he has full command. The relationship of the vocalization of emotion to other types of early vocalizations remains to be studied.

3. The development of emotion and speech follow different lines, independent of each other.

4. At a certain point, these lines can meet, whereupon emotion can be verbalized, and speech attains the power of containing and expressing emotion. The verbal emotional meanings have the form first of describing specific images and events that figure in the schemas. The child who is upset or excited learns first to describe "what happened" and later, perhaps, becomes able to characterize or name the feelings. The process depends on the caretaker's acceptance and acknowledgment of the feelings that are evoked, so that the child is not overwhelmed by them.

The joining of the lines of emotion and language requires an adequate interpersonal context. Vygotsky assumed that the social context required for the development of word meanings would be universally available for all children who are raised in human society. This is not the case for emotional expression; there is great variability in the degree to which the interpersonal context needed for development of verbal-emotional meanings is present in the early life of a child. This variability will be reflected in the integration—or dissociation—of the emotion schemas and the individual's capacity for adaptive emotional development throughout life.

THE REFERENTIAL CYCLE AND
THE DISCOVERY PROCESS

The development and verbal expression of emotional meaning, as this occurs in psychoanalytic treatment, is not a function of either subsymbolic or symbolic processing only but requires working back and forth flexibly between systems. This is a process of building new categories and dimensions, which may then be used to direct further search, rather than classifying experience on the basis of categories that have already been constructed. This interactive function is the core of the referential process; new classes of functionally equivalent experiences emerge in the subsymbolic systems, while identification of these new clusters occurs in symbolic modes. Optimally, the process operates recursively in a continuously deepening progression as the new symbolic systems serve to open new connections in nonsymbolic ones. Thus, in its most adaptive expression, the referential process would be characterized as *spiral* rather than cyclical in form.

The referential cycle, or spiral, is central in the discovery of new meanings and their communication, as this occurs throughout life, in emotional and cognitive domains. The stages of the referential cycle that I have identified in the organization and verbalization of emotion have illuminating parallels in both creative scientific work and in the arts. Here I will take a brief manifest detour to look at the operation of the referential cycle in scientific and artistic exploration as a basis for understanding its application in the discovery process of psychoanalysis.

In his studies of creative thought, based on extensive reports by leading scientists and mathematicians, the mathematician Hadamard (1949) has identified four stages in the process of discovery, which he terms Preparation, Incubation, Illumination, and Verification. He illustrates this process from the introspections of mathematicians and scientists, including those of the great French mathematician Poincaré.

Preparation

There is first a phase of preparation for the creative work. On a general level, in science and mathematics, the preparation is the ongoing, lifelong acquisition of knowledge that makes one an expert in a field. The specific preparation for a particular problem is the translation of the problem from its verbal formulation into a domain in which the subsymbolic processing can operate. This preparation depends on a "back-translation" movement from verbal-symbolic to subsymbolic forms. The mathematician hears about or raises a problem verbally; then starts to formulate this in a mathematical or scientific mode, which may have geometric or topological form. The person works actively for a while, then may experience the effort as futile and frustrating; he feels he is working without direction, "in the dark." This is what it feels like to work in the subsymbolic systems—to search without clear direction and without categories and dimensions having been defined.

Incubation

The subsymbolic search occurs to a large extent outside of awareness and without intentional control. The person may turn attention away from the problem, to other questions or other pursuits, but the subsymbolic processor, once prepared and activated, continues to work, following its own connections, which may not be available in the symbolic mode. In Poincaré's descriptions, we see that each of his major mathematical insights was prefaced by some such version of *turning away*—a trip to the seaside, entering his military service, a geological excursion—and each of his insights concerned relationships among questions that had seemed entirely unrelated at first. In these subsymbolic operations, new categories and dimensions are delicately and gradually built. At each stage, an interactive exploration of the implication of the categorization is carried out, which may occur within or outside of awareness. From today's perspective, it is precisely creative work of this nature that is not accounted for by classical symbolic information-processing models. Symbolic systems, which include the von Neumann class of computers, require that categories be explicitly defined and rules of operation be specified; they cannot make selections among possible combinations based on implicit rules.

Illumination

In the Illumination phase, the connection that has been sought appears, as if coming from outside:

Just at this time I left Caen, where I was then living, to go on a geologic excursion under the auspices of the school of mines. The changes of travel made me forget my mathematical work. Having reached Coutances, we entered an omnibus to go some place or other. At the moment when I put my foot on the step, the idea came to me, without anything in my former thoughts seeming to have paved the way for it, that the transformations I had used to define the Fuchsian functions were identical with those of non-Euclidean geometry. (Poincaré, quoted in Hadamard, 1949, p. 13)

As the poet Paul Valéry has described it, the state or process known as poetic inspiration is essentially similar to the process of creative scientific work:

The man whose business is writing experiences a kind of flash—for this intellectual life, anything but passive, is really made of fragments; . . . elements very brief, yet felt to be very rich in possibilities, which do not illuminate the whole mind, which indicate to the mind, rather, that there are forms completely new which it is sure to be able to possess after a certain amount of work. Sometimes I have observed this moment when a sensation arrives in the mind; it is as a gleam of light, not so much illuminating as dazzling. This arrival calls attention, points, rather than illuminates, and in fine, is itself an enigma which carries with it the assurance that it can be postponed. You say, "I see, and then tomorrow I shall see more." (quoted in Hadamard, 1949, p. 17)

This illumination may be experienced as deriving from some external source—a gleam of light, the voice of God, the muse—"without anything in my former thoughts seeming to have paved the way for it" as Poincaré said. However, it is also the case that the muse visits only those who have worked for years to find new questions, new answers, and new forms, to furnish the mind with the components of the "good combinations" to which Poincaré refers. The new forms or new categories do arrive from outside, that is, from outside the symbolic system. The work of the subsymbolic processor in the Preparation and Incubation phases, going on outside of awareness as if outside of oneself, has prepared the ground for the Illumination. This is the referential phase of the discovery process, in which subsymbolic experience is connected to symbolic form.

Reflection and Verification

The next phase is the process of reflection and interpretation, which includes making the results precise and their continuation and utilization. This occurs primarily within awareness in the verbal processing mode; for the mathematician, this may include explicit numeric or geometric processing. Poincaré feels a "perfect certainty" about the truth of the result that appeared to him in Coutances but later verifies it for his "conscience's sake."

Recursion of the Cycle

The process of discovery is cyclical or recursive, as the mathematician extends and makes further use of—works through—the results. Following the result of Coutances, Poincaré then turns his "attention to the study of some arithmetical questions apparently without much success and without a suspicion of any connection with my preceding researches," and becomes frustrated in this search:

> Disgusted with my failure, I went to spend a few days at the seaside, and thought of something else. One morning, walking on the bluff, the idea came to me, with just the same characteristics of brevity, suddenness and immediate certainty, that the arithmetic transformations of indeterminate ternary quadratic forms were identical with those of non-Euclidean geometry. (quoted in Hadamard, 1949, pp. 13–14)

Following this illumination, he reflects on his results and explores their implications. In this recursive process, the new connections open a new set of questions, which he addresses with conscious effort:

> Returned to Caen, I meditated on this result and deduced the consequences. The example of quadratic forms showed me that there were Fuchsian groups other than those corresponding to the hypergeometric series; I saw that I could apply to them the theory of theta-Fuchsian series and that consequently there existed Fuchsian functions other than those from the hypergeometric series, the ones I then knew. Naturally I set myself to form all these functions. I made a systematic attack upon them and carried all the outworks, one after another. There was one, however, that still held out, whose fall would involve that of the whole place. But all my efforts only served at first the better to show me the difficulty, which indeed was something. All this work was perfectly conscious. (Poincaré, 1956, p. 2045)

The new difficulty is dealt with, as the previous problems have been, while his attention is turned away:

> Thereupon I left for Mont-Valérian, where I was to go through my military service; so I was very differently occupied. One day, going along

the street, the solution of the difficulty which had stopped me suddenly appeared to me. I did not try to go deep into it immediately, and only after my service did I again take up the question. I had all the elements and had only to arrange them and put them together. So I wrote out my final memoir at a single stroke and without difficulty. (Poincaré, 1956, p. 2045)

Hadamard's (or Poincaré's) phase of Incubation corresponds to the phase of subsymbolic activation in the referential cycle. The Illumination incorporates the two phases of construction of prototypic imagery and its connection to narrative forms. In Hadamard's formulation, further connections within the formal verbal system are made in the Reflection and Verification phase; this corresponds to the reflection phase, in the expression of emotional experience, through which the emotion may be categorized and named, and the power of the verbal system, including the shared logic code and information concerning the perspectives of other people, may be brought to bear.

I would suggest that the descriptions of their processes of nonverbal thought, by Poincaré and other scientists, mathematicians, and artists, should put to rest the conventional categorization of nonverbal forms as regressive—in the service of *ego* or any other agency. The point is made most emphatically by Einstein:

The words of the language, as they are written or spoken, do not seem to play any role in my mechanism of thought. The psychical entities which seem to serve as elements in thought are certain signs and more or less clear images which can be "voluntarily" reproduced and combined. . . .

There is, of course, a certain connection between those elements and relevant logical concepts. It is also clear that the desire to arrive finally at logically connected concepts is the emotional basis of this rather vague play with the above mentioned elements. But taken from a psychological viewpoint, this combinatory play seems to be the essential feature in productive thought—before there is any connection with logical construction in words or other kinds of signs which can be communicated to others. . . .

The above mentioned elements are, in my case, of visual and some of muscular type. Conventional words or other signs have to be sought for laboriously only in a secondary stage, when the mentioned associative play is sufficiently established and can be reproduced at will. (quoted in Hadamard, 1949, pp. 142-143)

I may note that the use of verbal reports such as those of Einstein and Poincaré has become an increasingly important technique for studying human mental functions within the cognitive science field (Simon &

Kaplan, 1989). This does not mean necessarily accepting these reports at face value, any more than we accept the reports of analytic patients concerning their inner representations as such; in both cases, the reports are used as a basis for systematic inference as to the meanings that are expressed and the processes that are described. It is clear that such self-reports provide a rich source of data on complex subsymbolic mental functions, as the self-reports of analytic patients do concerning their emotional functions. In all cases, the challenge of research is to develop reliable and valid techniques for extracting the meanings that are expressed. I will demonstrate this approach, as applied to the processes of emotional exploration of psychoanalysis, in Chapter 17. The same processes of exploration and discovery may be traced in many areas where new perspectives and new knowledge are sought.

THE PROCESS OF DISCOVERY IN DETECTIVE FICTION

Detective Chief Superintendent Wycliffe, the Cornish detective created by W. J. Burley, does not see himself as a logical thinker and generally deprecates his cognitive abilities. Yet, his methods seem to work, and he has achieved considerable fame for his success in solving difficult cases. Wycliffe knows he does not think in the accepted way; he himself doesn't quite understand what his methods are.

> Wycliffe closed the file and put it away. He was thoughtful, but he suffered from an inherent difficulty in putting his thoughts into words, or indeed, into a strictly logical sequence. His mind lacked precision; vague pictures, words and phrases, recollected sights, sounds and smells seemed to drift in and out of his consciousness as a substitute for true "thought." The same images turned up again and again in different associations, forming ever-changing patterns. He was rarely conscious of selecting one pattern rather than another but somehow, given time, a particular one would command his attention and then he would act. (Burley, 1975, p. 133)

Wycliffe (or Burley) might or might not be interested to know that his methods can be accounted for by our model of the referential process— subsymbolic activation, repetitions of associated patterns; emergence of a particular prototypic image—leading, usually, in Wycliffe's case, to action, and then to the explanation and verification that the reader awaits.

CHAPTER 14

The Referential Cycle in Free Association

And this is how it is: if only you do not try to utter what is unutterable then nothing gets lost. But the unutterable will be—unutterably—contained in what has been uttered!
—LUDWIG WITTGENSTEIN (from a letter to
Paul Engelmann; quoted in Monk, 1990, p. 151)

The analytic patient, like the scientist or detective, is in search of new discoveries and new understanding, and there are many parallels (as well as differences) among their pursuits. Whereas Poincaré was motivated to further the shared knowledge of his field, psychoanalysis is undertaken to alleviate pathology and pain, and the explorations of psychoanalysis focus internally, on one's self and one's life. At the same time, the discovery process in psychoanalysis is intrinsically a collaborative effort, in contrast to the creative explorations of other fields, which are carried out to a large extent alone (although influenced by work that has gone before). The explorations of psychoanalysis are thus both more inwardly focused and more intrinsically collaborative than those of science or the arts. This is not paradoxical—although it may appear so—if we see the analytic patient as focused on an internalized, interpersonal world.

The process of symbolizing, as this occurs in emotional development and in treatment, is intrinsically dependent on the presence of another person. The presence of the other has many roles in reality and in fantasy: the stimulus activating an emotion schema; the listener who understands, supports, and accepts, or who brings a new perspective to bear on the material that has been brought forth.

The referential process in the special interpersonal context of the treatment provides the basic model for the transformation of private emotional experience, with its dominant subsymbolic components, to the verbal code in which experience may be shared. The cycle operates in different ways for patients for whom representations of objects were in place to varying degrees in the individual's early life, and for whom dissociations of varying levels of severity between nonverbal subsymbolic and symbolic processes have occurred. The explorations that occur in free association, like the cycles of scientific or mathematical discovery, follow the general phases of the referential process. The phases of the cycle may be described as follows.

SUBSYMBOLIC ACTIVATION: PREPARATION AND INCUBATION

The work of the analytic patient depends on the capacity to access and use subsymbolic experience. Part of the treatment must be to develop this capacity: to give oneself up to such experience while maintaining direction and control. To connect to such material in the treatment, one must be willing to talk without knowing what one is talking about, to turn away from a conscious direction, or a conscious goal, and let the subsymbolic processes direct the search. We can see that the method of free association is uniquely suited for such turning away; it seems, in a sense, to have been invented, intuitively (subsymbolically) for that purpose. The patient cannot take a trip to Coutances, to the seashore, or to military service, but the method of free association enables the patient to turn away from direct focus on the problem while remaining present and in communication with another person.

In treatment, the connection to subsymbolic experience proceeds interactively with the development of the relationship, the connection to the new symbolic object, the analyst. The availability of both types of connection depends on the structure of the emotion schemas with which the patient enters treatment, as well as on the availability of connections to symbolic objects in the patient's early life, as I have discussed.

In addition to the general preparation for the analytic work, specific preparation for each session may occur outside of the treatment in the days intervening between sessions, during the trip to the analyst's office, in the waiting room, and in the beginning of the session itself. The preparation may include a focus that is intentionally problem directed, in which the patient sets a problem verbally for himself, as the mathematician or scientist may do. However, in psychoanalysis, as in science, the most productive preparation is often "thinking about nothing" in a special way, letting contents of the previous session, or fantasy and dream material drift in and out of view. The nature of the preparation phase is likely to change markedly, with more productive "thinking about nothing" as treatment continues. In the recursion of the process, each playing out of a cycle also serves as preparation for the one to follow.

In the session itself, as the patient turns inward, new components of a dominant, problematic emotion schema gradually come into focus. The dominant schema is determined by the events of the patient's life, including the events of the treatment. The schema is likely to be operating in dissociated form; the activation is likely to involve subsymbolic, including sensory and somatic components, coming into focus without connection to specific objects, or with objects that have been displaced. The affective core itself remains unspeakable, *unutterable*, because it is painful, and also because it is inherently unutterable in its subsymbolic form.

The schema may at first be expressed nonverbally by facial expression, gesture, emotive vocalization, and action, or may be represented in general verbal terms: "I feel tired"; "I feel angry"; "It's hot in here"; "It smells funny"; "You look weird today." The patient may avoid the symbolic elements of the schema, if he recognizes them as such, as he lets the subsymbolic components operate. However, the basic rule constrains him to go on, to continue verbalizing and symbolizing whatever he can—bodily feelings, vague images, whatever comes to mind.

SYMBOLIZING AND ILLUMINATION: IMAGES AND WORDS

This phase is the process of connecting subsymbolic components of the emotion schemas, which may operate in dissociated form, to images and then to words.

Construction of Prototypic Imagery

The conversion of the subsymbolic to the symbolic format operates first within the nonverbal system. The continuous stimulus variation of the subsymbolic flow is chunked into patterns or classes of representation that lead to the production of prototypic images. The patient thinks of an event, an image, a memory, a dream that may seem trivial or irrelevant. He does not know why it comes to mind or what its connection to his current experience might be. This material may include memories of the past and also events in the relationship in the here and now. It represents the emotion schema or aspects of this, often peripheral aspects whose relation to the schema is unrecognized. The symbolic material is more likely to be permitted into awareness, to the extent that its connection to the painful affect is distant.

Narrating Images and Events

While the patient does not as yet recognize the emotional meaning of the discrete images and episodes that begin to surface, she has contracted to continue speaking and so goes on to describe these representations in words. The narratives reveal the patient's emotion schema as it exists now, or a peripheral piece of this, as it has been retrieved from memory or played out in the context of the current situation.

The telling of the narrative is where the possibility of breaking the vicious circle is found, and the reorganization of the schema can begin. This brings in the central "illumination" phase of creative psychoanalytic work. The old story in a new, interpersonal context is potentially a new story, not just a retelling. The construction of a new schema in the treatment parallels in some respects the initial construction of emotion schemas in early development. However, the patient has the cognitive powers of an adult, her life situation is different, and the new relationship is different from the old. The somatic elements of the activated schema occur in the session in titrated or trace form; the event is represented in a code that is shared. The person of the analyst and the therapeutic context constitute prototypic imagery in the here and now, which may be entered newly into the dissociated schemas. The new relationship potentially enables internalization of a more benign object and development of new schemas of self-care and self-regulation. The new imagery and new schemas enable new interactions to occur within the treatment and outside it; these work to modulate the earlier malevolent expectations, permit new information to be taken in, and old memories to be retrieved.

The analyst listens, processes the patient's communication (including all paralinguistic as well as verbal components) within his own emotion schemas, and responds, providing new emotional experiences, and in some instances new categories through interpretation. In some cases, the analyst follows the direction of the patient's associations. In other cases, the analyst's vision will lead him to redirect the patient where a useful direction seems available that the patient can take, but has not yet. If the process is successful, the patient is able to use the new ideas, information, and experience—including what she herself produces and what the analyst provides—to develop new categories and new dimensions, and to symbolize aspects of the emotion schemas that have been dissociated.

REFLECTION AND VERIFICATION

The patient, with the analyst, reflects upon the images and stories that have been told. The analyst may take the lead at this stage. The tools of logical differentiation and generalization are intentionally invoked. The connection of the displaced object to the activated memory schema may be recognized; the differences in the situation in which the activation occurs may be recognized as well. As in Hadamard's phase of verification, the results are made more precise and their implications further explored. The interactions and interpretations lead to new perspectives on old expectations, which enable reconstruction of the schemas to occur.

If the schema is altered, we would expect that the next narrative that emerges from this schema would be altered in form, deepening the recursive progression. The reconstruction of the schema will characteristically proceed from the periphery. As one bit is reconstructed, a connection to another component may be revealed, just as the resolution of one question led Poincaré to another in his recursive discovery process.

THE REFERENTIAL CYCLE IN THE "GOOD HOUR"

Kris's (1956) formulation of "the good analytic hour" takes the essential form of the referential cycle, as outlined here. As Kris says, "Many a time, the 'good hour' does not start propitiously. It may come gradually into its own, say after the first ten or fifteen minutes" (p. 446). I suggest that this first 10 or 15 minutes is not fallow or empty; it is the necessary phase of preparation and incubation, while subsymbolic work is under way. Much is happening inside the patient but not much that can be talked about or shared. The patient, adhering to the basic rule, brings in whatever elements of the schemas emerge; however, the emotional meaning of this material is not yet apparent.

Eventually, the second phase of the cycle, the symbolizing or illumination phase, will occur. As Kris says, "Then a dream may come, and associations, and all begins to make sense. In particularly fortunate instances a memory from the near or distant past, or, suddenly, one from the dark days may present itself with varying degrees of affective charge" (p. 446). The dream or memory, and the associations, symbolize the schema and develop its emotional meaning.

The possibility of intervention to facilitate a change in the schema may occur here. But it need not always be a formal interpretation, as Kris also notes: "And when the analyst interprets, sometimes all he needs to say can be put into a question. The patient may well do the summing up by himself, and himself arrive at conclusions" (p. 446). The interpretation or questioning by the analyst and the summing up, by patient or analyst, constitute the third phase of the cycle, dominated by reflection and reworking of the new material that has been brought forth. Optimally, this is a process of emotional insight in which some reorganization of the schema may occur. New connections may be made within the verbal system, which then feed back to activate other nonverbal aspects of the schema. A new cycle, at a deeper level, may then begin.

The various forms of spurious insight to which Kris refers may be accounted for as failure of one or more aspects of the referential cycle. For example, emotion schemas may be activated in the treatment but not represented in symbolic form; or symbolic, verbal expressions may occur without being connected to subsymbolic somatic and sensory elements of the affective core.

THE REFERENTIAL CYCLE IN A "BREAKTHROUGH SESSION"

A session discussed by Thomae and Kaechele (1992), which they specifically characterize as a "good hour" in Kris's sense, illustrates the playing out of a referential cycle and its recursive progression. This was the 115th session in the treatment of Arthur Y., who had suffered from obsessive thoughts since his youth, including a thought that he had to murder his own children. According to the authors, this was a "breakthrough session" in which the patient underwent a spectacular, positive change.

Subsymbolic Activation

In the beginning of the session, Arthur Y. talked about a surgeon who had removed his tonsils under a local anesthetic. The doctor had barked at him to keep his mouth open; Arthur talks now about wanting to swallow and fearing suffocation. The analyst responds to Arthur's bodily feelings and elaborates them; he says it is "as if you were up to your neck in water, or rather blood." The focus in this phase is on somatic and sensory events. Arthur's symptoms were experienced in this session as an aid in the formation of productive ideas, as Thomae and Kaechele explicitly state. The symptoms are appropriately construed as steps toward symbolizing, not as resistance. Arthur Y.'s analyst used the patient's experience of his symptoms "to emotionally revive his recollection of situations of suppression."

Symbolizing: The Illumination

The symptoms that were verbalized were connected to the activated emotion schemas. The emotional meaning of the activated schema, the desires and expectations involving other people, then begin to surface. The patient reports a fantasy about attacking the surgeon with a scalpel: "If I were a 9-year-old boy and simply took the next object and shoved it through his face, then as a child I would expect him to finish me off." The analyst expands on this:

> **A:** Yes, and with the scalpel you're the powerful surgeon, SS officer, Hitler, etc., God the Almighty with the knife, and in the small children you yourself are a child; you're a victim. . . . But you don't mean your children, of course. You mean the immense power, but it's so terrible that nobody can point the scalpel at you, and this has implications for more distant, seemingly harmless things, such as you're not permitted to criticize the therapist, me. (p. 473)

As the session proceeds, Arthur Y. experiences the wish to destroy and the fear of being destroyed in the new context of the analytic relationship, as well as in the context of his adult values and adult powers. He sees that his anxieties aren't about his children, but about an enemy that he doesn't dare to defend himself against. He sees that he has the same feelings toward the analyst, who has talked about increasing his fee.

Reflection and Verification

After the somatic and sensory material, and the emergence of images and episodes, Arthur Y. can then go on to examine his identification with both victim and perpetrator in reflective ways. He can now differentiate his wish to destroy his children or himself from his wish to destroy his tormentors. Both schemas have elements of the same affective core, while the objects have been displaced. The reflection occurs in the joint discourse, and the theme also incorporates the analyst.

As we can see, Thomae and Kaechele's analysis of this "good hour" is compatible with the theory of the referential cycle. The patient, in this symbolizing progression, has moved from the in-body experiences of swallowing and suffocation to the fantasy of shoving the scalpel in the surgeon's face, then being destroyed by him, then to some exploration and elaboration of the emotional meaning of these images and fantasies. As the authors point out, this session contrasts with the previous one (114), which the analyst had characterized as a "bad" hour. The work had broken down, according to the authors, because the symptoms were contained verbally rather than being experienced in the session and allowed to develop further in a symbolic transformation. Turning too quickly to verbal analogies in Session 114, before the playing out of the symbolizing process within the nonverbal system, foreclosed the operation of the referential cycle there. The experiences of Session 115 allowed the development of emotional meaning to proceed.

Recursion of the Cycle

In this productive hour, Arthur Y. goes on to an outpouring—even a flood—of narratives involving issues of revenge and powerlessness, in which a sequence of displaced objects, including the analyst, appear:

> Although he had just been submissive in his attitude that he was a victim, he suddenly began, in dramatic monologues, to settle old scores with his various oppressors: his father, who had not attempted to understand him, but instead had punished him after a boyish prank and then gone away to war—never to return—without even saying goodbye; the patient would most of all have liked to attack him with a weapon. He would have liked to have his way with his sadistic teacher. He was mad at his mother for cheating him out of his childhood. Finally he attacked me, the analyst, because I had forced him to confess. He compared this compulsion, grinning, with the image of a dog that you have to carry to the hunt, i.e., he felt forced to do something that he actually instinctively wanted to do. (p. 474)

The old schema activated in the session becomes changed in form. He accuses the analyst of provoking feelings of revenge in him that he could not satisfy. "He made this accusation part of an impressive image of a man who could not even release his excitement by masturbating because he did not have any hands" (p. 474). A new component of the schema, a theme of sexual excitement that cannot be released, associated with the theme of revenge, begins to emerge:

> P: Yes, and here come all of these figures and become alive, and I get terribly mad about all of these years—who should I pay it off to? There's nobody there [mumbling]. I had the following thought.

What's the use of getting horny somewhere if I don't, well if I don't have a woman or even two hands to satisfy myself? (p. 474)

The progression of objects and narratives about them that emerges in this session constitutes part of the process of working through. Gedo (1995) and Goldberger (1995) have discussed working through in relation to the referential process in these terms. In this flood of narratives, the referential cycle, with its central symbolizing function, is occurring repeatedly in highly intense, concentrated form.

Arthur Y.'s new insight—following on the narratives and interacting with them—was emotional insight: neither cognitive insight only, nor a corrective emotional experience, but the emergence of new connections within the emotion schemas. The affective core of the schema was first experienced somatically in an interpersonal context; this led to expression of narrative imagery, which was then reflected upon. As Thomae and Kaechele say, Arthur Y. "not only complained intellectually about having been denied his elementary rights as a child, but experienced this as an existential loss, and reacted to it by becoming enraged" (1992, p. 475).

The case of Arthur Y. provides an illustration of the processes of pathology and its cure in treatment, as outlined in the previous chapter. In the dissociation of the emotion schemas, which produced Arthur Y.'s neurosis, the somatic and sensory components were split off from their initial objects, the various oppressors of his life. When these subsymbolic components were activated in different contexts later in life, Arthur connected them to new symbolic objects, in this case, his children. However, this attempt at repair of the schema, to provide symbolic meaning of some sort for it, was destructive in itself. In the treatment, it was necessary to separate off the displaced object of the children, so that a more veridical and adaptive version of the schema could be developed, one that incorporated Arthur Y. as both victim and perpetrator, and reflected more accurately what he might expect of others and of himself now. As part of the process of reorganization, the person of the analyst became a new symbolic object, and symbolic objects arose as well from memories of the past.

THE REFERENTIAL CYCLE IN THE LISTENING PROCESS

I have focused here on the process of translating nonverbal, including subsymbolic somatic and emotional information, into the verbal code. As we have seen, the referential process is necessarily bidirectional, and this needs to be emphasized as well. The referential process is involved as listeners (or readers) translate the words of others back into their own subsymbolic and emotional representational systems. The back-translation process is also involved in a continuous and iterative way as the individual uses language to direct and regulate himself.

The special skill of the psychoanalyst, to listen to verbal material with the "third ear," to find the underlying thread among the elements of the emotion structures, depends on the engagement of the bidirectional referential function in the listening process. Arlow's (1979) account of the listening process, in his paper "The Genesis of Interpretation," follows essentially the progression of the referential cycle:

1. The analyst begins by suspending critical judgment, listening passively and indiscriminately to what the patient is reporting. Modes of behavior, including facial expressions, body posture, gestures, voice timbre, and speech rate all transmit information concerning the patient's emotional concerns. Information is provided as well from changes that the analyst experiences in his own affective and physiological state. We may note that Arlow is giving a rather exact description of subsymbolic processing here. The analyst is accepting, connecting to the patient's currently activated emotion schema with its subsymbolic affective core, without imposing emotional categories as yet.

2. At a certain point, mental representations from the analyst's own memory and experience enter into his consciousness and cause a shift from what he terms a passive–dependent—what we call "subsymbolic"—stance. These representations generally come, as Arlow says, in "the shape of some random thought, the memory of a patient with a similar problem, a line of poetry, the words of a song, some joke he heard, some witty comment of his own, perhaps a paper he read the night before, or a presentation at the local society meeting some weeks back" (p. 200). The connection of the new representation to what the patient has been saying may not be apparent at first. This is the symbolizing or illumination phase of the analyst's listening process, which may come in the form of imagery or as verbal thoughts.

3. The association of the analyst's representations to the patient's emotional concerns is made either immediately or shortly thereafter. The analyst makes these associations for himself; then must decide, on the basis of his clinical judgment, what aspects to communicate to the patient and how. The response "has to be made consonant with the patient's material according to disciplined, cognitive criteria before being formulated into an interpretation" (p. 205). This is the third, reflective phase of the listening process by which interpretations are generated.

It is important to see that the representations on which the analyst's response is based are the symbolizing of his own schema of what the patient has been communicating to him. It is the analyst's emotional meaning of the patient's material that is being developed here, regardless of how fully the patient may now be represented in the patient's mind. The analyst's understanding must be affected by his own emotion schemas, including schemas that may not be fully known to him. In his comments on the session, Arthur Y.'s analyst says he thought of his allusion to water, because the patient had once been in a very dangerous situation and almost drowned. The tonsillectomy also reminded the analyst of a tooth extraction he himself had had as an adult, in which so much blood collected in his pharynx that he felt as if "I were up to my throat in water." The meaning of the analyst's associations to the patient's expressions may seem self-evident to the analyst, and to the reader of a case report, but remains to be validated.

In principle, we should be able to determine from the patient's response and the subsequent course of the treatment to what extent the analyst's schema of the patient represents the patient's concerns. Some of the problems of this determination within the treatment context have been discussed in Chapter 2. The application of empirical research procedures to address such issues of veridicality will be discussed in Chapters 18 and 19.

PSYCHOANALYSIS AS EXPLORATION
AND DISCOVERY: TURNING AWAY

In the patient's process of working through and in the work of the analyst in listening and responding—as in the poet's, mathematician's, or scientist's work of invention and discovery—the symbolizing function is central. In all cases, the individual is exploring in the realm of subsymbolic representations and processes, and is connecting these to symbols, which may be images or words.

We can intentionally control and direct our symbolic processing to a considerable degree, and can generally do this even better for language than for imagery. However, we cannot directly tell a subsymbolic processor what to do. We can only develop our questions and work as best we can to answer them, and then wait for the subsymbolic processor to do its work. We load the system with information the subsymbolic processor might need, even if we cannot say exactly what this information is or how it will be used.

When Lieutenant Joe Leaphorn of the Navajo Tribal Police is asked by Kennedy, the local FBI officer, to look for a killer's tracks on a sagebrush flat, he walks in widening circles and crisscrosses the terrain:

> "What were you looking for?" Kennedy asked. "Besides tracks."
> "Nothing in particular," Leaphorn said. "You're not really looking for anything in particular. If you do that, you don't see things you're not looking for." (Hillerman, 1989, p. 23)

The scientist, the detective, the analytic patient, and the analyst as well, all learn when to pursue the solution actively, even when the work appears futile, and they feel that they are working in the dark; and also when to stop and wait, with patience and openness, for the system to operate on its own and some clarity to emerge. The subsymbolic system, once adequately primed, carries out its content-determined processing on the dimensions and in the directions of its own problem space. If it achieves a solution that can be symbolized, this may then appear to us as if from outside. This processing in subsymbolic modules is the essential core of creative work, the basis for the mysterious and longed for visit of the "muse," and the basis for the illumination, the "surprise," that we hope for in analytic work.

Turning attention away from direct attack on a problem to look without knowing what one is looking for is crucial for the discovery process of psychoanalysis, as for the sciences and the arts. However, turning away also plays a particular role for the mental contents being addressed in psychoanalysis. Beyond the general function of subsymbolic processing in any creative search, there is an intrinsic need for such processing when the things one is looking for are representations that were initially developed early in life in subsymbolic form and have never been explicitly stated. Such experience can only be expected to emerge when the subsymbolic system is given the freedom to do its work.

The need to let the subsymbolic processor operate is still more crucial when the information that is sought is not only unstateable in words, in a cognitive sense, but unspeakable, in an emotional one—associated with dreaded thoughts too horrible to say (or know). The integrative processes of the symbolic mode cannot work with such unbearable images and conflicting goals. In the symbolic domain, we cannot discover and avoid the same images and thoughts. Here, the special powers of the subsymbolic modes, operating in a multiple processing system, come into play. The independent, subsymbolic processors operate in their own modalities and their own formats, without being directed—or blocked—by the organizational processes of the symbolic modes. In this way, subsymbolic processing can facilitate connection to the unutterable before the integrative processes of the symbol system take over to forestall this and to direct the movement away. In retrieving an experience and then telling a story that is connected somehow to the emotion schema, but whose relation to the schema is not recognized, the patient shares information before its emotional meaning is known to her. One cannot directly utter the unutterable, but it will necessarily be present in what one does utter, if one is able to turn attention away.

If the representation of a dreaded emotion schema emerges in the context of the new, interpersonal setting of the transference, material that has been previously unbearable may begin to take a new—and less unspeakable—meaning. As his own aggression *and* his own victimization are both experienced in the treatment, in relation to the analyst, Arthur Y.'s fear of destroying his children takes a new meaning for him.

We may note a special danger of exploration in the psychoanalytic situation, not present in the explorations of science. The turning attention away that is permitted in the free association and essential in any creative venture may itself operate in the service of an attempt to avoid, and may be driven or supported in part by this. Rather than activating the connections between subsymbolic and symbolic processing modes, turning away in this sense may operate to shut the connections down. To be productive in the service of emotional discovery, the patient needs to develop a kind of "emotional vision," which is comparable to the vision of the creative mathematician, and also needs the courage to follow this vision—to distinguish the useful directions from circles and dead ends. In the beginning, the work depends crucially on the emotional vision of the analyst concerning the patient, to guide the patient's explorations in the direction set by the patient's own issues. Gradually, the patient may develop and use her own emotional vision as the guide for her associations. The development of emotional vision is a major component of successful analytic work that begins in treatment but then continues throughout life.

The patient's capacity to search freely and to symbolize depends initially not only on the analyst's vision but also on the power of the analyst's presence as directly affecting the computation of danger in the patient's interpersonal world. This occurs first in the transference. Through the reorganization of the emotion schemas, the patient's expectations of danger will gradually be recomputed in a more general way. We need to recognize, however, that the analyst, who has been incorporated as a new symbolic object in the patient's emotion schemas, will play a continuing role in her emotional life. The analyst may be internalized in a variety of forms in schemas that have played out in the relationship and have been reconstructed, and also may become a benign symbol in the construction of new schemas of soothing and self-regulation. The resolution of the transference, in this sense, can never be more than partial. There may also be cases where treatment fails, and the internalized representation of the analyst will lead to new dissociations. In either case, termination of treatment does not terminate the analyst's presence and power. The analyst as object-symbol remains an active agent in the patient's inner representational world.

CHAPTER 15

The Referential Cycle in Fantasies and Dreams

Freud saw the theory of dreams, with its central concepts of the primary and secondary processes, as his most original and significant contribution:

> This book, with the new contribution to psychology which surprised the world when it was published (1900), remains essentially unaltered. It contains, even according to my present-day judgement, the most valuable of all the discoveries it has been my good fortune to make. Insight such as this falls to one's lot but once in a lifetime. (1900, p. xxxii)

FREUD'S THEORY OF DREAMS

Dream interpretation has remained of central importance through all the shifts that have occurred in psychoanalytic theory and technique. While the psychoanalytic theory of dreams has evolved and changed, as have other aspects of the theory, the major phases of dream construction, as postulated by Freud, may be outlined in general terms as follows:

1. *Activation.* The energies of the repressed wishes, which remain active during sleep, press for discharge, threatening to awaken the sleeper. The muscular apparatus, however, is decathected, thus inactivated.
2. *Latent dream thoughts.* The unconscious wish attempts to advance toward the preconscious and from there to consciousness. However, an unconscious idea, as such, is incapable of entering the preconscious and

can only exercise an effect there "by establishing a connection with an idea which already belongs to the preconscious" (1900, p. 601), by virtue of its connection to "the mnemic system of linguistic symbols" (1900, p. 613), thus binding the energy of the wish. The latent dream thoughts are complex, logical structures, with all the attributes of rational waking thought.

3. *Transformation to concrete form.* In an intermediate stage of the dreamwork, the complex and abstract latent dream thoughts are translated into more concrete verbal form—the kind of language that can more readily be illustrated pictorially. Freud relates this to a comparable phase in the process of replacing a political article by a series of illustrations. In both cases, one step in the process involves giving the abstract thoughts of the latent content "a different wording, which may perhaps sound less usual but which will contain more components that are concrete and capable of being represented" (1916–1917, p. 175).

4. *Pictorial representation.* The concrete, verbal expressions of the dream thoughts can then be represented in pictorial form. The representation of a verbal thought in pictorial form parallels the process by which normal thoughts are transformed into symptoms in the neuroses, and is the function of the censor, exercised against unacceptable unconscious wishes. This reflects "a retrogressive movement in the psychical apparatus from a complex ideational act back to the raw material of the memory-traces underlying it" (1900, p. 581).

5. *Verbal narrative.* The pictorial representation of the manifest content is then translated back to verbal form to produce the dream report. The process of secondary revision contributes to the construction of a coherent and communicable narrative.

6. *Association and interpretation.* In the associations to elements of the dream narrative, aided by interpretation, decoding of the dreamwork takes place. The dreamer may then begin to recover the repressed dream thoughts, the latent verbal contents of Stage 2, which constitute the statement of the unconscious wish, and which the dream conceals.

There are many problems with this formulation, including both the internal inconsistency of the model and its lack of support in current psychological and neurophysiological research. The processing sequence represented in Freud's theory of dream construction flips back and forth between nonverbal and verbal forms—from activation of an unconscious wish; to complex, abstract, latent dream thoughts; to concrete, verbal representations of these; to concrete imagery; then to verbal reports and associations to these. A schematic outline of this sequence is shown in Figure 15.1. The convoluted "zigzag" formulation is a direct function of Freud's implicit verbal mediation model, in which organized repre-

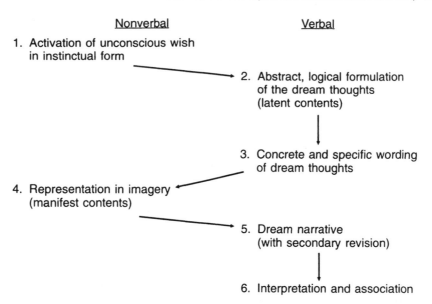

Nonverbal   Verbal

1. Activation of unconscious wish in instinctual form

2. Abstract, logical formulation of the dream thoughts (latent contents)

3. Concrete and specific wording of dream thoughts

4. Representation in imagery (manifest contents)

5. Dream narrative (with secondary revision)

6. Interpretation and association

FIGURE 15.1. Construction and interpretation of dreams: Freud's zigzag sequence.

sentation and transformation of meaning can only occur in a verbal mode. There is no evidence in current cognitive research for verbal mediation in this sense, as I have discussed.

The inconsistency of the theory is also seen in Freud's formulation of the operations of the dreamwork. There are two faces to this formulation that remain largely unreconciled. From one perspective, Freud viewed the pictorial representation of thought as the function of the censor, exercised against unacceptable unconscious wishes. The censor is seen as operating to disguise and distort the latent dream elements in a manner parallel to the operation of symptoms in pathological states (1900, p. 636). This "abnormal psychical treatment" is characteristic of regression or psychosis and other altered states. The parallel between dream symbols and pathological symptoms was central in Freud's view throughout his writings, as I have discussed.

On the other hand, Freud also characterized the dreamwork as a means of representation, the means by which the complex, abstract ideas of the dream thoughts can be expressed in pictorial form. He offers an extensive and original cataloguing of the systematic forms of representation provided by the dreamwork, by which abstract concepts may be translated into concrete imagery. The heart of the process of dream construction and the most original aspect of Freud's formulation lie in his concepts of the dreamwork, the varied mechanisms by which the images of the dream are generated.

In developing his theory, Freud is brought to question whether the dreamwork is indeed the function of the censor: "But although condensation makes dreams obscure, it does not give one the impression of being an effect of the dream-censorship. It seems traceable rather to some mechanical or economic factor" (Freud, 1916–1917, p. 173). Similarly, the process of visual representation of abstract ideas in the relation between a manifest dream image and the latent content "is not so much a distortion of the latter as a representation of it, a plastic, concrete portrayal of it, taking its start from the wording" (Freud, 1916–1917, p. 121). Symbolism is a means of expression, a process of representation based on perceptual and functional similarities.

While Freud recognized the function of the dreamwork to represent rather than disguise, the energy model has no mechanism enabling an account of imagery as a systematic and organized representational mode. The operations of the dreamwork are the modes of operation of the primary process, thus associated with unbound energy seeking immediate discharge in accordance with the pleasure principle. Energy is bound through the operation of the secondary process, which operates with verbal symbols. There is no basis in Freud's energy model for intrinsic organization in the nonverbal mode.

At some points in his writing, Freud attempted to reconcile the representational functions of the dreamwork with the notion of the primary process by emphasizing the archaic nature of the form of representation that was possible in dreams. Thus, writing in 1933, he characterized dreams as constituting a distinct mode of thought, phylogenetically antecedent to the verbal mode. The characteristics of dreams, based on pictorial rather than verbal language, are explained by Freud as manifestations of the phylogenetically more ancient modes of operation of the mental apparatus, which can come to the fore during regression in the sleeping state (reported in Thomae & Kaechele, 1987, p. 140). From Freud's perspective, such modes of thought would constitute a distinct form, phylogenetically ancient and regressive, but capable of attempting some kind of problem solving in rudimentary form. This speculation of Freud's is interesting in presaging the notion of systematic nonverbal processing, but still without recognizing the continuing significance of this function in mature mental life or identifying the mechanism of its operation.

The structural theory adds the view of psychic events, including dreams and fantasies, as multiply determined by id, ego, and superego tendencies, rather than necessarily or directly activated by instinctual impulses or unconscious forces (Arlow & Brenner, 1964). The structural theory also questions the necessary connection of linguistic symbols to the preconscious or conscious modes; thus, linguistic representations may occur in the unconscious as well. This carries us closer to a consistent account of dream construction. Nevertheless, within the structural theory, as in the topographic model, the concept of the primary process with its energic implications is retained, and there is no basic mechanism that can account for the expression of systematic, organized, complex meaning in nonverbal form in the sleep or waking state.

The inconsistency of the model has been recognized by many writers, from Arlow to Holt, and some solutions have been attempted, as discussed earlier in this volume. As Holt and others have finally conceded, the theory of the primary process remains in "sad disarray." Systematic information processing in dreams, like organized unconscious fantasies in waking life, "embarrass" the methodology of the classical psychoanalytic accounts (Arlow, 1969).

THE PERSPECTIVE OF CURRENT DREAM RESEARCH

The psychoanalytic dream theory has been generally rejected in the field of empirical sleep and dream research. The empirical study of dreams opened with the identification of periods of rapid eye movements (REM) that occur during sleep and appear to be associated with dreams involving visual imagery (Aserinsky & Kleitman, 1953). According to current views, the dreaming process depends on eye movement activation originating in the pontine brain stem (Hobson & McCarley, 1977). The brain-stem impulses are randomly initiated and are not influenced by higher order cognitive functions. The neural impulses reach the cortex in the form of pontine–lateral geniculate–occipital (PGO) spikes during REM periods, while afferent input is inhibited. The cortex then functions to bring some order into the representations activated by these spontaneous, random impulses, constructing a synthesis of the activating impulses with other ongoing representations. By this means, the dream acquires its specific contents, which the dreamer experiences, and some of which he can then remember when he awakes. According to this formulation, dreams have hallucinatory and delusional features, because the dreaming brain is cut off from the reality of sensory input. The distortions and bizarreness that are characteristic of dreams occur because the neural signals are randomly activated, and the cortex succeeds only partially in bringing order into these.

The activation–synthesis formulation has been interpreted by some as postulating that dreams reflect only random neurological firing, without psychological meaning. This is an oversimplified interpretation.

Hobson (1988), for example, does not deny the possibility that dreams have psychological meaning. The activation of dreams may be dependent on the randomly generated activity of the brain stem, rather than specific to repressed material; however, once REM sleep and dreaming have been physiologically triggered, wishes and other ideas may be expressed and shape dream plots. Hobson's critiques, and those of other dream researchers, have focused not so much on the possibility of dreams having psychological meaning as on several specific assumptions of the psychoanalytic theory: the assumption that the dream derives from the *energy of an unconscious wish*; the view that dreams have the purpose of *maintaining sleep*; the notion of a *censor* functioning to distort and disguise the latent contents; and, by implication, the assumption that the manifest contents function to *conceal* the actual meaning of the dream.

These and related assumptions derive from the energy theory, as we have seen; however, the core psychoanalytic insight—the special function of dreams to represent emotional meaning—does not entail these assumptions. The development of emotional meaning in dreams can be accounted for using the machinery of multiple coding, without being trapped by energic concepts and their inconsistent implications. The model to be proposed here is compatible with the basic psychoanalytic formulation and also with current dream research. Like all models, the elements of this theory need to be tested and supported or disconfirmed.

THE MULTIPLE CODE MODEL OF DREAMS

The operation of the referential process in dream construction parallels its operation in waking fantasies, free association, and other forms of thought and expression, with modifications arising from specific differences of afferent input and cortical activation in the sleep and waking states. The stages of the referential process, as these operate in the construction and interpretation of dreams, may be characterized as follows.

Subsymbolic Activation: The Latent Contents

The dreamer is concerned with events and problems of the day, although he may not be aware of their emotional meaning. As in waking life, the individual's focus on particular questions or problems serves to activate an emotion schema, with its subsymbolic processing systems. Subsymbolic processes are more accessible in REM sleep than in any other state. The activation of subsymbolic elements—including visceral and kinesthetic, as well as other sensory experience—is facilitated by the absence of external visual input, along with the high cerebral activation that is characteristic of REM periods (Hobson & McCarley, 1977; Hobson, Lydic, & Bagh-doyan, 1986; Antrobus, 1991).

The activated emotion schema constitutes the latent content of the dream. The contents of a dream may be as varied as the schemas that make up the individual's emotional world. The activated emotion schemas may include an unconscious wish seeking fulfillment, but may equally well be some other emotion structure—a fear, worry, or conflict, or a problem the individual is trying to solve. In some cases, absorbing cognitive problems may also continue to be processed during sleep and emerge in dreams. In the initial activation of an emotion schema, the subsymbolic processes are likely to be dominant; this is particularly the case for emotion schemas that are dissociated.

The Symbolizing Phase: Manifest Content and the Dream Narrative

The symbolizing process in the dream construction includes two sub-stages: (1) representation by images in the manifest content, and (2) representations by words in the dream narrative.

Dream Imagery

A range of visual activation occurs spontaneously in the REM state, as dream researchers have shown; however, the images to which the dreamer attends, and the associations to these, will be determined by the emotion schemas that have been aroused. In REM sleep, visual activation is stimulated, and somatic and sensory experience from inside the body are also relatively accessible, while afferent input and motor activation are greatly reduced. The activated images in all modalities are available to be connected to the dissociated schemas that have been aroused. They provide objects to replace the original objects that have been warded off and *thus provide symbolic meaning for schemas whose meaning has been lost.* The manifest imagery may be dominated by the visual, but may include somatic and other sensory components as well. The images serve as objective correlatives of the feeling states, precisely as images do in creative art forms.

The processes of the dreamwork are standard mechanisms of the nonverbal system that apply to many types of experience in waking life as in sleep. For condensation and symbolic representation, the associations and connections that are made follow the general principles of organization of the nonverbal system. The choice of images to represent other ideas or entities might be based on perceptual and functional similarity, or on contiguity of occurrence in time and place. Thus, entities are associated that look or sound alike, or that occurred together in the same time or place. The symbolic objects that are newly entered in a schema often reflect recognizable associations that are culturally shared (purses, rings, towers, cigars, trains coming into stations). In such cases, a person who listens to a dream report may also be able (or thinks he is able) to enter into its explication. The profession of dream seer—and in some sense of analyst—is built on the power to explicate such shared symbolism. While Freud distinguished displacement as entirely the operation of the censor and as not having a representational function, we can see that the shifts in affect and emphasis that Freud characterized as displacement may be systematic as well. Here, however, the basis for the association may be found in the individual's internal life, so that the connections are often idiosyncratic and thus more difficult—sometimes impossible—to find.

Representation of the emotion schemas by such discrete, manifest imagery is the first stage in the symbolizing process. While the possible elements of the manifest contents range widely, their organization and transformation occur within the nonverbal system, without verbal mediation being required at any point. Verbal material may appear in the manifest contents in a variety of ways, usually as speech sounds or written words, or in word play, but verbal thoughts do not direct the construction of the dream.

The Dream Narrative

The discrete imagery of the manifest contents may then be verbalized. The symbolic images and episodes are the type of nonverbal representations that can most readily be connected to words. In the development of the narrative, the scenario as it emerges in the dream is also reworked to varying degrees by the organizing principles of the verbal system. This reworking (or "secondary revision") includes logical associations, imposition of syntactic structure, sequencing of episodes and images, and a variety of communicative and storytelling devices. Some of these may enhance, some interfere with, the representation of the emotion schema that has been retrieved.

Reflection: Association and Interpretation

The understanding of a dream then depends on explication of its new symbolic organization through new associations and interpretations of the images and memories. The verbalization has the power to facilitate elaboration of the meaning of the dream, as the explication of a metaphor may enrich the latent meaning of a poem. Eventually, the patient may be able to generate a verbal statement of some of the emotional meanings expressed in the latent contents of the dream. In treatment, the work of reflection and interpretation may be collaborative in this verbal mediation phase. The analyst helps the patient to acknowledge the new meanings and to contain and explore them.

We see that in the model of the referential process, as in Freud's model, the goal is to connect latent emotional material to verbal thought, and the means of the connection is via concrete, specific images and words referring to them. The difference is the direction of processing that is assumed. In the multiple code theory, subsymbolic representations and processes are connected to imagery and then to verbal narratives that describe these concrete images; more abstract reflection on the concrete and imagistic narratives may then occur. As described by Freud, the process is, in part, the reverse: Abstract dream thoughts are transformed into concrete verbal form and then to imagery. Here, the systematic organization and transformation of thought takes place within the verbal system. Once we recognize systematic information processing in the nonverbal system, however, we see that it is not necessary to shift the burden of transformation to the linguistic mode; the nonverbal system does its own organizational work. Thus, we can dispense with steps 2 and 3 of Freud's *imagery–language–imagery* zigzag model, and the two models can be seen to correspond. A schematic outline of the referential process as this operates in dream construction and interpretation is shown in Figure 15.2.

Parallel Processing in Fantasies and Dreams

The symbolizing process, as it operates in dreams, parallels the operation of the referential process as it occurs throughout waking life—in children and adults, in the information processing of everyday life, in scientific and literary work, and in free association as well. The continuity of processing in dreams and waking thought is compatible with current research. According to Hobson et al., "At the level of extracellular recording, there is no visible difference in the mechanisms of cortical activation observed during REM sleep and waking" (1986, p. 379).

Like Hobson and his colleagues, Antrobus (1991) views the processing of imagery and dreams as similar in many ways: "The overall picture is that the cortical structures that support associative cognitive processing

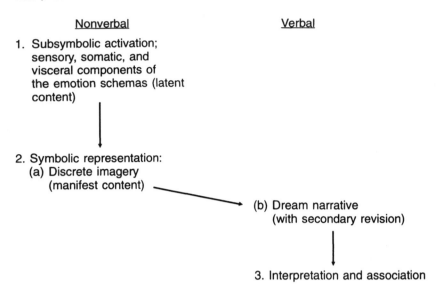

FIGURE 15.2. The multiple code theory of dream construction and interpretation: the referential process

are similarly activated in waking and in REM sleep, but markedly reduced in NonREM sleep" (p. 99). As he also points out:

> The imagery and thought of sleep occur periodically when, in Stage 1 REM, subcortical processes activate in a distributed manner a large portion of the cortical processes that, in the waking state, compute perceptual, cognitive and motor responses to external stimuli. Sleep imagery and thought, therefore, share many of the characteristics of waking responses to sensory stimuli. These responses include the creation of perceptual features that are predominantly visual but also include the auditory and haptic modalities. (p. 107)

There are also important differences between processing in REM and waking states, which account for the special features and special information-processing role of dreams. Dreams may in principle concern any types of contents. During waking life, however, afferent input is generally active and dominates the ongoing conceptual integration. In contrast, during REM, afferent input is inhibited, while internally generated visual images and bodily experience are dominant. The REM state is thus particularly well suited to facilitate the activation of the emotion schemas; the individual is looking inward, and subsymbolic experience and imagery dominate the field. In addition, because of the inhibition of external stimuli during sleep, there is no obstacle to interpreting dream images as veridical perceptions.

We can see that hypnosis and other altered states, and to a lesser extent, free association, particularly on the couch facing away from the analyst, operate as analogues to the sleep state in these respects: diminishing perceptual input, and permitting subsymbolic experience and imagery to be more prominent. The special features of mentation in the analytic situation, contrasting with the dream state, are the constraints of verbalization and the presence of another person to whom experience is reported. In essence, free association supports activation of subsymbolic functions in an interpersonal context that facilitates the symbolizing process and enables private images to be shared.

APPLICATIONS AND ILLUSTRATIONS

In this section, I provide several examples of how the theory of the referential cycle may be applied to account for the construction and interpretation of dreams. I first examine a session that shows the development of the emotional meaning of a dream in the context of the transference, then several types of dream material that raise specific problems for the standard psychoanalytic account. I then turn to Erikson's (1954) demonstration of the *expression* of meaning (rather than its disguise or distortion) in the manifest content of the Irma dream and show how the multiple code model provides a general psychological account for this.

Dreams and the Transference

In a research case discussed by Bucci (1993), the patient (a young unmarried man whom I will call Mr. A.) has been stood up by a woman on a first date the previous night.

Subsymbolic Activation

In the beginning of the session, before he talks about the previous night's events, and before telling his dream, Mr. A. talks of feeling cold and itchy. He feels the cold coming through the mattress of the couch. He felt calm and cool the previous night and did not get upset when the woman stood him up. He has a terrible itch on his penis. These sensory and somatic experiences are part of the arousal of the schema in the subsymbolic phase. As we have seen, the nature of a dissociated schema is precisely that it is dominated by somatic and motoric components without access to the objects of the emotion, which would enable connection to symbol systems to be made. In the construction of dreams in the sleeping state, this activation will occur in the bodily experience of the dreamer and then be integrated in the dream. In telling the dream, the bodily components of the emotion schema may be reexperienced in the session.

Symbolizing: Imagery and Narrative

Mr. A. then tells a dream in which he is riding a bicycle or unicycle with his male friends. He is in a village square with three movie theaters; he feels that the scene has appeared in his dreams before and describes the setting and his actions in elaborate detail. He feels some responsibility for his friends, which he has been unable to fulfill adequately, and feels blamed by his parents for his failure.

The scene of the dream shifts, and he is in an upstairs apartment with his male friends. He describes an image of a room, seen through a door, in which there is a couch and a chair; all his friends are in the room; he is having a great time talking to them. Then he sees five good-looking girls in the doorway, who intrude on this. He first says that the dream ended there, then remembers another part that was quite important. On his way upstairs, he got quite upset and had to go to the bathroom. For some reason, there was no toilet, and he ended up holding his feces in his hand—not just in his hand, but in paper, toilet paper in his hand. He had no place to put it. He went upstairs and couldn't find anything. Under a table, there was a wastepaper basket, so he dumped the whole thing in there and then covered it up. He was hoping that it wouldn't smell. He was sort of embarrassed; in telling his dream, his penis starts to itch again.

Reflection: Association and Interpretation

The dream imagery provides symbols for elements of the dissociated emotion schema. Eventually, through associating to the dream, and through communication of these associations in the shared discourse, Mr. A. begins to generate a verbal statement of some of its latent emotional meaning.

P: I'm afraid of women, I tell you, I am. They scare me. They're not compassionate and not reasonable like men, ah, (*pause*) ah, well, so I understand it and intellectualize. Still, the feelings, I don't know what the feelings were. Embarrassing with the feces, and annoyance with the women, frustration that I couldn't find the, ah, right movie. And I wasn't doing a good job. Ah, those were the feelings.

A: Suppose the bowel movement and the shit represented some kind of very violent feeling that is hidden behind that image. What would it be? If you suddenly blurted it out?

P: Rage.

A: Yes?

P: Rage. What right does that girl got to do to stand me up? That's it. I'm pretty important. I'm a pretty good guy. Rage, that would be the feeling.

He connects the experience of rage to feelings in the session, events of the previous night, and early memories or fantasies that may not have been formulated before, including a fantasy concerning a battle for control between his mother and himself.

P: I got the feeling ... my mother must have been sitting there with her hand out waiting for the goddamn thing, you know, and maybe I, ah, that would be a funny one, it's as though that it was a battle between me and my mother who'd get hold of my shit. She wanted it, and I wanted it. She wanted it; by getting it she had possession of me, or something. I don't know.

Mr. A. then moves on to additional connections and associations. This is the recursive and interactive operation of the cycle, as seen also in Poincaré's creative explorations.

In an apparent shift of focus, he recalls a memory associated with the loss of his father, which also represents his identification with him.

P: (*pause*) Another interesting thing, the feces were very small and I sort of questioned whether (*chuckles*) whether they were mine or not. Because in my present-sized body, my adult-sized body, this was definitely baby's feces. They were little, little ones. And that's something else, too.

Um, here's another one. When my father was dying at the house, on _____ Street, one day I guess I went to his john and he had, hadn't flushed the toilet, and there was his feces there. It was long and it was thin, and it was small like a baby's and, ah, it was sort of frightening. I guess he didn't eat much; his rectum was closing up or this or that. And I'm not sure if this reminds me of that. But if it did, man, I could see why I want to get rid of that stuff. This might be, this might be, ah, a curve I'm throwing, but that comes to mind.

In this phase of reflection and shared exploration, the analyst may take the lead at some points in elaborating the metaphoric meanings of the dream imagery:

A: Looks as though you retreated from sort of the excitement of the world [inaudible] and the anxiety to this upstairs room, with the couch and with the man, holding all this dirty, filthy stuff in your hand.

The wastebasket in the upstairs room (the analyst's office) was a repository for dirty things that had been concealed and carried around. Mr. A.'s feces incorporated many sensory features, including the special feature of their size. His associations and images, like any metaphoric representation, bring in meanings not recognized before, including a recognition of some of the emotional meanings of the analysis for him. In the selection of images from those activated during REM sleep, and in the interpretation of these, the process of dreaming, like the process of free association, gives the individual the chance to repair the dissociation, to connect the subsymbolic desires, yearnings, and terrors, to new objects that share some features with the original ones but are different as well.

The theory of the referential process accounts for the construction and interpretation of Mr. A.'s dream and the new meanings that emerge in the interpersonal context of the treatment. He begins with subsymbolic experience—feeling calm and cool the night before, feeling an itch now—leading to imagery and naming the emotion, and to new images and ideas not previously retrieved. (We may also note that many aspects of the dream imagery remain uninterpreted in this session.) There is no basis for assuming that a statement of the emotional themes of the dream had been generated prior to its construction, as Freud's formulation of the latent dream thoughts would require, or that the imagery of the dream was intended to conceal its underlying meaning. The imagery was a systematic vehicle for organization and communication of the emotional ideas of the dream, which have become accessible to him, in his sleep state and in the context of the transference. It is also possible that the new meanings, seen for the first time, may have led to changes in the emotion schema that was being expressed.

Symbolic Representations of Oral Issues

Freud's theory has general difficulty in accounting for organized unconscious fantasies, as we have seen, and particular difficulty in accounting for organized contents based on issues of preverbal times. Arlow (1955) discussed several examples of dreams in which latent contents of orality, including wishes to eat and to be eaten, are represented in symbolic form by fire, tools, and the fantasy of being crushed. In one case, a female patient dreamed of a "tremendous crematorium furnace," with "a huge oval-shaped opening into which the people had been thrust and two smaller round glass windows through which she could see the flames destroying the victims" (p. 65). According to Arlow:

> She connected the two round windows with her eyes and with her need to stare at the genitals of men. The huge aperture represented a devouring mouth. . . . During the session, the patient complained of excessive salivation, her stomach "growled," and she felt, as she put it, an intense "angry hunger." The fire in the furnace thus symbolized her consuming oral rage against her husband's castraters and her own. (p. 65)

The patient was concerned at this time with her identification with her father, including fantasies of revenge for a mutilating injury he had suffered. The issues were activated by her husband's recent failure in an important professional competition, which she had been raging about in her treatment. She attributed this failure to "Jewish competitiveness and favoritism," identified with her husband in his defeat, and saw the analyst in the victor's role.

The dream schema is dominated by visceral imagery of destruction. The patient's actual somatic experiences in the session, including salivating and stomach growling, represented the visceral, autonomic component of the emotion schema and also related to the consummatory act of devouring, as expressed in the dream. The central symbolism of fire directly represents the consummatory act. The subsymbolic visceral representations are also connected to concrete and specific images of objects, including the furnace with its two windows and huge oval-shaped aperture. The object of the rage and destruction is not represented in the dream. Through the occurrence of these experiences and the telling of the dream in the session, these elements of the dissociated experiences could be symbolized and also jointly experienced and observed.

In this dream, as in the previous example of Mr. A., we see the playing out of the dream in the context of the transference. The analyst, seen as the victor, became a symbolic object in the warded-off schema of oral rage and revenge, connecting to these subsymbolic, somatic components. We may also note that information known through reading and shared cultural experience—the crematoria of the Holocaust—were incorporated in the patient's overarching emotional organization and provided additional objective correlatives for the elements of the schema. The analyst may also have had some related feelings evoked by the images and the historical context, so that the subjective experience could be transmitted and shared.

In other representations of oral issues discussed by Arlow, pronged or wedge-shaped chopping tools represented teeth in emotion schemas of destruction or incorporation. Similarly, suicidal fantasies of being crushed were interpreted as representing a wish to be devoured and reincorporated, thus reunited with the mother, in sleep and death (Arlow, 1955). In general, the manifest contents of these dream and fantasies representing oral schemas are dominated by imagery of the consummatory act, the visceral imagery associated with it, and visual imagery of the agents of this act. As in the dream of Mr. A., there is no need to call on the assumption of a "censor" functioning to disguise the latent contents, or the assumption of the manifest contents as functioning to conceal meaning, to account for the representation of emotional meaning in this dream. The imagery directly represents the underlying schema in the medium available in the REM state.

Dissociation in Masturbation Fantasies

The process of defensive dissociation and its repair in dreams is supported in Arlow's discussion of masturbation dreams. Arlow (1953) has proposed that the processes of masturbation may be divided into two major components: the actual manipulation of a part of the body for the purpose of obtaining pleasure; and the fantasy that accompanies such physical manipulation.

The component of manipulation is represented separately, according to Arlow, in the following dream: "I see myself in the bathroom. I have stuffed too much paper into the toilet bowl. It overflows and I have to clean the mess up. I keep scrubbing and scrubbing; it seems as though I have been scrubbing all night. I awoke very tired" (1953, p. 52). The patient reports that she has just finished menstruation and has washed herself very carefully. The toilet bowl and toilet are equated with the vagina. The stuffing of paper into the toilet bowl reminded her of the way in which she used to masturbate—by bunching up a blanket between her thighs and rubbing her genitals vigorously with it. The cleaning was associated with actual cleaning that she had done that day. According to Arlow, the "vigorous scrubbing motions in the toilet, therefore, may be interpreted as representing a pictorial portrayal of the muscular activity of masturbation" (p. 53).

The separation of the two components of masturbation is an example of splitting or dissociation within the underlying emotion schema. The visceral and motoric representations associated with the consummatory act are split off from the object who would figure in the fantasy of desire. The dream represents such dissociation. It is precisely the object of desire that is missing from this dream. The emotion schema is symbolized primarily by representations of vigorous scrubbing movements. Actions, like somatic symptoms, can serve as new symbols in schemas in which objects have been dissociated, facilitating the organization of the schema and its connections to language. Actions or symptoms are less likely than visual images to enable wide-ranging associations involving other persons but can serve as early steps in the symbolizing process, before the transference objects or other objects can be incorporated.

The "Dream Screen"

An unusual type of dream phenomenon, described by Rycroft (1968) and Lewin (1946, 1948), perhaps carries dissociation and failure of symbolizing a schema to its logical extreme. These are dreams that have as their visual element what appears to be a blank, usually white background or screen, often with no discrete objects, actions, or even sensations to be named. According to Rycroft, such dreams are likely to occur in patients "with deep oral fixations, whose paramount wish is for union with the breast" (p. 2), when they are "attempting to re-establish emotional contact with the external world" (p. 11). Rado (1928) has suggested that the process of the dream screen "is the faithful intrapsychic repetition of that fusing with the mother that takes place during drinking at her breast" (quoted in Rycroft, 1968, p. 6).

Such dreams are formed essentially without representations of specific, discrete objects or events to serve as symbols. As in the masturbatory dreams described by Arlow, objects, particularly human objects, are not available as symbols. However, in contrast to the other examples, the dream screen contains no other types of symbols or images to represent the affective core. One might argue that such phenomena, with no apparent symbolism, and no dreamwork, are not actually dreams at all. On the other hand, we might speculate that these dreams represent powerful dominance of subsymbolic perceptual components, derived from very early emotional schemas related to oral needs and satisfactions, including representations of hunger, sucking, and bodily softness and warmth, as well as the associated visual experiences.

The unarticulated visual image of the white screen might indicate incomplete development of the visual system at the time the schema was laid down, or incomplete cognitive development with respect to representation of objects in memory. Alternatively, as Isakower (1938) suggests, the screen may represent the maternal breast, flattened out and taking up the whole field of vision, as the infant might perceive it while falling asleep. In a more general sense, the dream screen resembles the type of visual experience associated with trance states or the sense of nothingness, or "nirvana" of the type sought after through meditation. In these terms, the dream screen might also be understood as a subsymbolic visual representation of a highly gratifying emotion schema of merger or bliss. Such dream phenomena may also have different implications in REM or non-REM sleep.

A Final Illustration: The Irma Dream

As Erikson (1954) tells us, the dreamer of the "Irma" dream was a 39-year-old Jewish physician, a specialist in neurology in *fin de siècle* Vienna. Austria was a Catholic monarchy; Vienna was "swayed both by liberalism and increasing anti-Semitism." The dreamer's family was growing rapidly, and his wife was again pregnant. He was at that time attempting to achieve academic status but was meeting with difficulties, in part because he was a Jew, but also because of the radical nature of his ideas.

The narrative of Freud's "Irma" dream, the original dream "specimen," is well known. In brief, the dreamer and his wife are receiving guests in a great hall. He sees Irma and reproaches her for not having accepted the solution he proposed, telling her that if she still has pain, it is her own fault. She tells him about pains in her throat, stomach, and abdomen; she is choked by them. She looks pale and puffy. He takes her to the window to look into her throat. He finds a large white spot on the right and also sees extensive grayish-white scabs associated with the turbinal bones of the nose. He calls Dr. M., the leading figure of their circle, who confirms the examination. Dr. M. looks unlike his usual self; he is pale, he limps, and he is clean-shaven. The dreamer's colleague and friend Dr. Otto is standing beside Irma. Another colleague, Dr. Leopold, standing nearby, also examines her and draws attention to another sign of infection on her left shoulder, which the dreamer can feel. Dr. M. confirms the presence of the infection. They agree that the infection originated with an injection of trimethylamin given to her by Otto. Probably the syringe was not clean.

Erikson's analysis of the Irma dream focuses on the representational function of the dreamwork and its similarity to other types of symbolic productions. As Erikson has claimed, the representation of the latent dream thoughts in the manifest contents of the dream parallels other forms of imaginative representation, as in projective techniques and children's play. The manifest contents are a type of symbolic production that then need to be explicated in the context of the dreamer's current emotional and interpersonal concerns. Erikson has identified a set of features, or "manifest configurations" that characterize the dream contents and provide a frame of reference for dream analysis. His inventory of such configurations includes sensory, somatic, and affective contents, location in time and space, verbal elements, and a range of interpersonal relations. Using this inventory, the meaning of the dream thoughts may be explicated through a "configurational analysis" of the manifest dream in interplay with the analysis of the latent dream thoughts. We can see that Erikson's formulation is compatible with the notion of the emotion schemas that underlie the emotional meaning of dreams, and also compatible with our view of manifest imagery as representing and expressing this meaning.

Erikson explicates in great depth and detail the many and complex ways in which the underlying emotional issues of Freud's personal life, activated at the time of the dream—his professional predicament, his intimacy with Fliess, and the context of the larger culture of his time and place—can be traced in the symbols of the manifest dream. Freud was troubled by swellings in his nose and throat at that time and was also concerned with his wife's health. Irma's oral cavity is associated with a woman's sexual organs. The emphasis on mouth and nose in the dream is associated as well with Freud's relationship with Fliess, the otolaryngologist. The older colleague is temporarily castrated—beardless; the dreamer temporarily joins the group in power in ostracizing Dr. Otto, who is associated with Fliess, and also with early images from Freud's own life.

Each element of the manifest content has far-reaching associations that aid in illuminating the complex emotional meanings of the dream. We would say that there are many meanings generated in parallel in the subsymbolic processors that are brought together by the symbolic integration of the dreamwork. Freud did the work of tracing these meanings in the specimen dream, showing us how the dream elements work to represent emotional meanings in complex, metaphoric ways, although his own energy model does not provide a reasoned account of this systematic representational process. The dreamwork does not obfuscate; it provides a representation of multifaceted underlying meanings that are, however, difficult to grasp, because they are not yet known in the symbolic domain. The Irma dream was a part of Freud's complex process of knowing, acknowledging his emotion schemas, which were not yet symbolized, or symbolized only in part, not an act of concealing them. The dream, like the incubation and illumination phases in Poincaré's explorations (see Chapter 13), lays the foundation for the insight that followed. The subsequent stages of interpretation by which the meaning of the Irma dream was developed could not have been effective if the initial stage of representation by manifest imagery was not itself meaningful in its own representational medium.

Reconstruction of the Royal Road

The multiple code theory retains the central psychoanalytic view of the value of dreams in providing access to emotional meanings that have been dissociated, and also meets the major critiques of the dream researchers concerning the psychoanalytic theory of dreams. The function of emotional information processing in dreams is continuous with emotional information processing in waking life, with the special limitations and special powers of the sleep—particularly REM sleep—state. The sort of "psychical treatment" that occurs in dreams is not "abnormal" but pervasive in normal waking life. Dreams operate to represent experience, following the laws of operation of the nonverbal system, and are likely to be dominated by the subsymbolic formats that are most accessible in the sleep state. The particular dream thoughts that are dominant may be driven by any type of current concern, not wish fulfillment only, although emotional issues represented in subsymbolic format are likely to be relatively more central in the sleep state.

The role of interpretation and association in understanding the dream material is entirely compatible with Hobson's view concerning the function of interpretive processes applied to the activated imagery of the REM state. This formulation is also compatible with the view of Antrobus (1991) that dream processing includes both "top-down" higher level symbolic processes and "bottom-up" visual and other perceptual and kinesthetic processing, which may not be accessible to introspection, and which are modeled by connectionist or PDP systems.

Dreams do not function only to enable retrieval of schemas already formed. Through the action of the dreamwork, a dissociated emotion schema may be reconstituted as new elements, with their manifold associations, are entered into schemas whose objects have been warded off. Like all mental schemas, the emotion schemas represented in dreams are active and interactive, determining the perception and processing of new input, and determined and altered by this in turn. It is also the case that the verbal formulation of the meaning of a dream is likely to be constructed for the first time through its narration.

Dreams and fantasies do indeed correspond to symptoms, as Freud claimed. However, the implication is the converse of this. It is not that dreams or fantasies are symptoms in the sense of being regressive or pathological forms. Rather, somatic or psychic symptoms may carry out a progressive symbolizing function, in the same sense as dreams and fantasies, where other symbols are not available to be used. Symptoms, like dreams, are fundamentally attempts at symbolizing, healing in the psychic domain, although symptoms may then bring new problems of their own.

We may end by saying that Freud's formulation of the dreamwork constitutes a major contribution to our understanding of the mind, as he claimed, and as the psychoanalytic community and its observers generally agree. Dreams are indeed a "royal road"—not the only one but a major means of access—to the dominant emotion schemas of one's life, including subsymbolic components that have never been verbalized and symbolic components that have been dissociated. It is possible that certain early issues, dating to preverbal times, could not be retrieved without emerging in a dream or fantasy, or being played out in the transference, or both. As Freud showed, as Erikson has explicated, and as the dream research has also shown in its way, dreams, like metaphors, serve fundamentally to represent concepts in their complexity and depth, rather than to conceal and distort. We have also seen that dreams serve to generate new meanings, not primarily to represent meanings that have already been formed.

CHAPTER 16

The Multiple Code Theory and the Metapsychology

Rather than trying to match Freud's concepts, I have tried to produce a coherent model of emotional information processing and emotional exploration that may be applied to the discovery process of psychoanalysis, and that may also have general application as a theory of psychological organization. Multiple coding is derived from current work in cognitive science but differs from most information-processing models in focusing on *emotional* information processing, and in addressing the central question of how disparate representational systems are connected in an integrated, goal-directed self, functioning in an interpersonal world. It is a general model of information processing that is applicable in normal life, as in pathology; some may see this as similar to Freud's enterprise, others as distinguishing the multiple code theory approach.

Some of the major features distinguishing the multiple code theory from Freud's model of the psychical apparatus include (1) psychological organization as a tripartite (at least) rather than a bipartite system; (2) the concepts of emotion schemas and emotional information processing in contrast to the concepts of energy and drive; (3) a broader understanding of symptoms as symbols; (4) the continued operation of multiple information-processing formats throughout conscious, rational, mature mental life; and (5) a different view of the goals of treatment. In this chapter, I will present a brief overview of these points and their implications, and will then provide an informal glossary of some psychoanalytic concepts that have been newly defined in this theoretical framework.

PSYCHOLOGICAL ORGANIZATION AS
A TRIPARTITE SYSTEM

The operation of modes of thought outside the conscious, verbal domain is central to a psychoanalytic theory. Freud's formulations of the primary process and its component functions constitute viable and original hypotheses, well ahead of their time, concerning the forms and processes of nonverbal or unattended thought. However, Freud's bipartite theory incorporates many assumptions, which can now be seen as untenable, concerning the concepts of the primary and secondary processes and their postulated properties.

The primary process, the domain of unbound energy, is defined as including unconscious, nonverbal, regressed, infantile, and pathological forms of thought, dominated by contents of wish fulfillment. In the secondary process, energy is bound; thought is conscious, verbal, mature, rational, and oriented to reality. As we have seen in the review of the architectures and functions of mind, however, the set of dimensions that Freud associated theoretically with the two basic modes of thought do not, in actuality, coincide. The organization of thought and memory is far more complex than was assumed in Freud's characterizations. In modern terms, we would say that the construct validity of the primary and secondary processes, as derived from the hypothetical dimension of mobility of cathexis, has not been supported. Implicit or unconscious thought may be either verbal or nonverbal; it may be symbolic or subsymbolic. The contents of implicit or nonverbal or subsymbolic thought may include complex, abstract scientific and mathematical concepts, and many other types of ideas, other than wish fulfillment in the psychoanalytic sense. Implicit and nonverbal forms of thought occur throughout normal, adult mental life and in waking states as in sleep. Explicit or conscious or verbal thought has a similarly varied range of functions, properties, and contents.

The structural theory (Freud, 1923; Arlow & Brenner, 1964) acknowledges some of these failures of correspondence. Freud came to recognize that the distinction between the qualities of mind did not necessarily coincide with the dimension of verbalization, or with the presence or absence of wish-fulfillment ideation, but did not carry out the implications of these observations for his model of the psychical apparatus.

As the review of the cognitive literature has shown, a bipartite system is not sufficient to account for the distinctions in modes of information processing that have been observed. In place of the duality of the primary and secondary processes, identified by Freud, the multiple code theory incorporates three major types of information-processing systems: *subsymbolic nonverbal* processing and *symbolic* systems that are both *nonverbal* and *verbal,* with multiple variations within each of these. The distinction between subsymbolic nonverbal processes and symbolic imagery is not recognized in Freud's system. Both subsymbolic processes and symbolic imagery are incorporated in the primary process, as defined by Freud, whereas the secondary process is associated with verbal forms. However, the distinction between subsymbolic and symbolic nonverbal forms is crucial to understanding psychological organization and communication. The subsymbolic mode accounts for the types of intuitive and implicit processing involving sensory and bodily functions that are central to the analytic understanding of the primary process, and that have eluded classical information-processing models. Symbolic imagery is the pivot of the emotional information-processing system, enabling organization of the nonverbal system independent of verbalization, and also enabling its connection to words.

I have not built a component of *subsymbolic verbal* processes into the outline of the multiple code theory that has been presented in this book; this does not deny the possible role of such processing in psychological organization and in the symbolizing of emotional experience. The paralinguistic features of speech, such as tonal variation, loudness, pitch, and pausing are aspects of vocalization that are processed on subsymbolic levels. Vocalization, the sound of speech, would be most appropriately included, along with facial expressions and body movements, in the nonverbal, subsymbolic mode. However, processes with subsymbolic features also play a role in semantic information processing in ways that are not yet well understood. PDP modeling has been applied to aspects of language development and to processes of word finding and language construction in adults as well as children. The role of a subsymbolic linguistic component in information processing, in emotional information processing, and in the production of communicative speech needs to be clarified and either integrated into an overall theory or reclassified and redefined. This is one of many ways in which future work on the multiple code theory and the emotion schemas can proceed.

EMOTION SCHEMAS AND MOTIVATION

In Freud's metapsychology, the functions of activation and regulation have been reified under the concept of drive. This descriptive approach has not enabled systematic identification of the factors—internal and external—affecting these functions. The organization and activation of human behavior cannot be accounted for adequately by a closed system of energy transformation, as many writers have noted. In place of Freud's energic construct, with all its contradictions and limitations, multiple coding incorporates constructs of emotion schemas and emotional information processing that account for the arousal and regulation of human behavior as well as its organization. The notion of the emotion schemas is a hypothetical construct, as is the notion of drive, but differs in its coherence within a general psychological model, which is amenable to empirical investigation. We base our theory on a modern view of emotions as particular types of information-processing schemas that enable evaluation of the meaning of events for an individual's well-being and provide the basis for directing action (Lang, 1994; Scherer, 1984). Motivational components, understood as programs of readiness and intent, are included, along with components of cognitive evaluation, physiological activation, and motoric action, as elements of emotion schemas. Subjective feeling states are also associated with emotion schemas; these will usually come into awareness when a schema is aroused but may be inaccessible in schemas where dissociation has occurred. Like all schemas, emotion schemas are active and dynamic, processing new information in an interactive way—determining our perception of new experience and continuously changing with new input.

SYMPTOMS AS SYMBOLS

A corollary of the emotional information-processing approach concerns the role of symptoms such as somatization and acting out in the symbolizing process. The notion of substitute discharge as such is meaningful only in an energy model. We have proposed that the emergence of symptoms indicates dissociation of the emotion schemas, and that, in certain pathologies, a dissociated schema may be organized around a symptom rather than around a representation of a person. In this context, symptoms and behaviors themselves function as discrete symbolic entities; they may be steps on the way to more adequate symbolizing, not regression or resistance. The pain, the acting out, the obsessive preoccupations may be the only discrete entities available to be experienced and jointly examined in early phases of treatment of patients with severe psychopathology, as discussed in Chapter 12. The symptoms and actions enable some connection to a dissociated schema to be made before new interpersonal objects can be accepted and more integrated schemas built.

The theory thus returns by a different conceptual path to the notion of symptoms as carrying systematic emotional meaning, which had initially been claimed by Freud. Ultimately, the reorganization of the schema requires construction or reconstruction of connections to other persons. However, the symbolic meaning of symptoms may need to be traced before further symbolizing in an interpersonal world can occur.

OPERATION OF MULTIPLE SYSTEMS
THROUGHOUT LIFE

Another major difference between the multiple code theory and the metapsychology concerns the operation of intuitive, implicit, and nonverbal processing throughout normal, mature waking life. The subsymbolic and symbolic nonverbal systems may be "primary" in their origins, both phylogenetically and in an individual's life, but they need not be archaic or infantile in their functioning in adults. Both subsymbolic and symbolic processing modes play a role in the construction of all types of meanings, including emotional meanings, throughout life. Mentation with the formal structure of subsymbolic processing, as we have identified this, is not necessarily rooted in primitive desires or libidinal or aggressive drives, is not necessarily focused on the self rather than external reality, and does not necessarily involve alien, mysterious, or perverse contents. Subsymbolic processing may apply to all such subject matter, but also applies far more broadly to a wide range of other content domains, as I have discussed; it may be focused on external reality, as in scientific and mathematical discovery, and may operate in the conscious mode. There are fine distinctions and complex patterns within nonverbal systems that cannot be captured in the general categorical medium of words but must be represented by modeling in their own particular subsymbolic media. Anyone who has observed a Casals or Balanchine master class does not need to be convinced of the complexity of the nonverbal, including the subsymbolic domain, and of its capacity for activation and communication in a mature, conscious mode.

INTEGRATION OF SYSTEMS
IN PSYCHOANALYTIC TREATMENT

The restructuring of the theory of the psychical apparatus also leads to a reformulation of the objectives of psychoanalytic treatment. The goal of psychoanalytic treatment has generally been understood as the dominance, or replacement, of one system or agency by another—*to make the unconscious conscious, to have ego where id has been.* We now see that multiple systems, with their own functions, contents, and organizing principles, continue to operate throughout normal, mature, waking life. The goal of treatment is defined within the multiple code formulation *as facilitating integration of systems and enabling reconstruction of emotion schemas that have been dissociated,* rather than replacing one function with another. This requires repairing disconnections and building new connections—between subsymbolic and symbolic elements within the nonverbal system, and between symbolic nonverbal representations and words.

NEW DEFINITIONS OF PSYCHOANALYTIC CONCEPTS

In building a new psychoanalytic psychology, with the features noted earlier, some familiar concepts will be retained, some revised and redefined, some given up. The goal is to develop a nomological network within which each of the concepts that are used by clinicians may be consistently defined in relation to other concepts and to observable events, and within which refinement of concepts and definitions, and verification of propositions may proceed. I have provided a few examples in previous chapters of the type of definitions that have been generated within the theoretical framework of multiple coding and will outline some of them here in very general terms. The examples are given to illustrate the potential application of this approach in generating working definitions. As the nomological network is developed, and as inconsistencies and gaps emerge, the definitions will be continuously elaborated and refined.

Defense is a broad and varied category that includes both dissociation of referential connections and dysfunctional attempts at resymbolizing; the latter involve entering new objects in schemas that have been dissociated, as in displacement. A componential model of the defenses may be developed, distinguishing those that are primarily dissociative and destructive of symbolic meaning from those that carry symbolic meaning of their own.

Repression, defined as dissociation of referential connections, may occur (1) among subsymbolic processes, (2) between subsymbolic process and images, and (3) between images and words. I would suggest that the concept of repression be reserved for blocking or destruction of connections that have previously been in place. Dissociations occurring because of connections never having been formed might be characterized as *dissociation* without repression and may be the more general case.

What I have called *uncovering* really refers to construction of referential connections among nonverbal, including subsymbolic and symbolic representations and processes, as well as between images and words. This may involve reconnecting systems through reconstructing referential connections, or may require building new connections; again, the latter may be the more general case.

In *transference,* the emotion schemas laid down through repeated interactions with central figures in the individual's past now come to incorporate the analyst; they are transferred to this new symbolic object.

The emotion schema then plays out in the treatment but—one hopes—as a reconstruction rather than a repetition.

Free association is *free* of conventional conversational or organizational constraints, so that the associative flow is available to be guided or determined by the underlying emotion schema that has been aroused. The patient reports as best he can the flow of sensory and somatic experience and the images, memories, and events that emerge. The assumption that Freud made implicitly, and that I make explicitly, is that the apparently trivial and irrelevant scraps of feelings, images, and ideas that come to mind are elements of the currently dominant and problematic emotion schema. The associative process activates retrieval of the peripheral elements of a warded-off schema, without immediate awareness of their connection to the dread wishes or expectations that are central to the search. In the new context of the treatment, this potentially facilitates further entry into the schema, so that its meaning can be explored. As I have noted, these basic premises that underlie the psychoanalytic method cannot be simply assumed but need to be tested as well.

Working through may be defined as the recursive process through which the telling of a narrative and reflection on this leads to accessing new components of an emotion schema; thus, additional images are developed, memories are retrieved in more complete sensory and bodily form, and new connections in the verbal system can also be made. Perhaps most fundamentally, working through involves incorporating the visceral and somatic information of the affective core in one's representation of an event.

I am not providing definitions of the concepts of interpretation or insight here, but the concept of working through does begin to provide an answer to Edelson's (1983) question as to why veridical insight, as generally understood, is not enough: "An additional task facing psychoanalysis is to specify not only what properties in addition to truth an interpretation must have for veridical insight to result, but what in addition to the acquisition of veridical insight is necessary for these desired objectives to be achieved" (p. 100). The best answer to Edelson's question, and the best definition that I have found of the concept of working through, is provided by Rilke (1982) in his semiautobiographical novel *The Notebooks of Malte Laurids Brigge*. I will excerpt briefly here from a long, beautiful, and relevant passage:

> I think I should begin to do some work, now that I am learning to see. . . . You ought to wait and gather sense and sweetness for a whole lifetime, and a long one if possible, and then, at the very end, you might perhaps be able to write ten good lines. . . . And it is not yet enough to have memories. You must be able to forget them when they are many,

and you must have the immense patience to wait until they return. For the memories themselves are not very important. Only when they have changed into our very blood, into glance and gesture, and are nameless, no longer to be distinguished from ourselves—only then can it happen that in some very rare hour the first word of a poem arises in their midst and goes forth from them. (pp. 19–20)

Working through is the process of changing a veridical insight into "blood, into glance and gesture." It is facilitated by the retrieval of specific memories, and by specific events, but not completed until one goes beyond the images and words.

Structural change is defined as change in emotion schemas; it occurs gradually as the product of the working through. Structural change may involve building new referential connections, entering new objects in schemas that have been dissociated, or replacing objects in schemas where displacement has occurred. The new symbolic organization that is developed in the schema has the power to affect the operation of its affective core. The individual comes to see things differently, feels differently, has new expectations and beliefs about how others will act toward him. The implication of this formulation of structural change, as in the concept of working through, is that it incorporates change in the somatic and sensory components of the emotion schemas, not in the verbal and symbolic components only. That is the unique goal of psychoanalysis. A major implication of this formulation is to demonstrate that the deeper goals of psychoanalysis, and the processes by which such goals may be achieved, may be stated meaningfully and are within the reach of empirical research.

While adaptive change in emotion schemas is the goal of psychoanalytic treatment, changes in the emotion schemas also occur in adaptive or maladaptive ways in the ongoing events and relationships of life; that is how we are all formed, and how we develop and change. The various means of effecting change, including insight or internalization, which occur in development and in different ways in the treatment, need to be systematically defined in terms of the types of symbolic or subsymbolic processes that are involved.

Conflicts occur in many different, complex ways in the repeated interactions of life and in the internalized representations of these interactions in the emotion schemas. In line with the position of Brenner (1992), as discussed earlier, I would not account for conflict in structural terms, as between ego, superego, and id, but instead see conflict as occurring pervasively, in relation to many types of wishes and many tendencies to respond. In some cases, the individual may be able to resolve these oppositions through reflection or action. In other cases, however, the meanings and consequences of the components of the opposition may be experienced as threatening or catastrophic for well-being or even survival, and incapable of being resolved within one's life situation—as a young child's feeling of rage and a wish to attack may exist alongside of and involve the same objects as a wish to be cared for and terror of being abandoned. Such conflicts figure as key factors in the formation of maladaptive emotion schemas. Defensive dissociation and displacement of objects are ways of trying to reduce such unbearable opposition.

The power of free association may be seen in a specific way as enabling access to conflictual desires and expectations that have been dissociated. The executive function of the symbolic processing system will, in general, not permit simultaneous registration of representations of entities and their negation, and will also operate to divert attention from painful and threatening images, as from external threats. Representation in the subsymbolic processor is more versatile and flexible; it is less controlling and less controlled. The conflictual elements can emerge into awareness, to some extent, prior to being recognized as such, as part of the flow of peripheral elements of the emotion schema, and can make their way into the shared discourse in this way.

The concept of *resistance* needs to be redefined within the new multiple code framework. The referential process is inherently partial and limited. The subsymbolic components of the emotion schemas, which are global, analogic, continuous, and parallel in their operation, cannot be connected directly to the discrete symbols, operating in single-channel sequential format, of the verbal code. To term all difficulties of communicating emotional experience as "resistance" represents a failure to recognize the essential diversity of representational codes and appears to assume, incorrectly, that code-to-code translation would be automatic and transparent if the motivation to avoid some ideas were not present. It is also the case, of course, that the intrinsic difficulties of the referential process may be increased by the dissociation involved in defense, and may interact with this. Motivated resistance, or resistance as a dynamic concept, is a special case in which communication of experience is blocked by conscious or unconscious defensive operations. The distinction between the inherent difficulty of the referential process and a conscious or unconscious avoidance of communication may not always be clear; the role of the former should always be considered when a patient is having difficulty "saying what he means."

Given the premise of multiple, diverse systems operating throughout normal adult life, the psychoanalytic notion of *regression* also needs to be revised. While Kris (1936) recognized complex nonverbal processing as a function of *regression in the service of the ego*, I would argue that it is misleading to characterize these processes as regressive in any sense.

Organized nonverbal processes, including imagery and subsymbolic representations, operate throughout normal waking life at all levels of functioning, including the highest level of creative scientific work, as illustrated in Chapter 13. Such complex, nonverbal functions are seen as "regressive" only if one assumes superiority of verbal processing over other processing forms. I suggest that the notion of regression might be restricted to reduction of capacity for particular functions, rather than applied to a shift from verbal to nonverbal modes. A loss or giving up of language functions might be seen as regressive; a loss of imagery functions might be regressive in the same sense.

A number of psychoanalytic concepts and distinctions have not been incorporated as such in the multiple code formulation. In turning from Freud's bipartite model to a multiple code structure, I have not retained the distinction between the *primary and secondary processes* as such; the construct validity of these concepts has not been supported, as discussed earlier. Imagery has features of both the primary and secondary processes; it is nonverbal but may also be organized, accessible to consciousness, and oriented to reality. Conversely, language may be processed outside of awareness; may be associated with regressed, infantile, and pathological forms of thought; and may be dominated by contents of wish fulfillment—all features associated with the primary process mode. The tripartite model that I have proposed provides a better fit for the reality of mental functions as we understand them today.

The concepts of *id, ego,* and *superego* have not been used within the multiple code framework as presented here. The concepts of emotion schemas and structural change have been defined from a different and more general theoretical perspective. There is, however, an interesting relationship to be seen between subsymbolic processes, as defined here, and aspects of Freud's concept of *das Es,* translated literally as "the it" rather than "the id," and distinguished from *das Ich,* translated as "the self." It seems possible that Freud may have been focusing, at least in part, on the domain of processes that are experienced as outside of oneself, in the designation of "the it." The subsymbolic system, as I have defined it, incorporates the same sense of experience as outside of oneself and also includes representations associated with biological functions. However, subsymbolic processing also includes a wide range of other processes as well, and thus is far broader and more systematic than the notion of the id, with its accrued meanings and metaphors of "chaos" and "seething excitation" (Freud, 1933).

Similarly, the concept of *ego,* as defined within the structural model, lacks construct validity in modern terms and would need to be comprehensively revised. The functions of the psychical apparatus that have been associated with the organizing functions of the ego may be seen from a current perspective as referring to the fundamental operations of psychological organization, broadly defined. Freud opened the search for such a general model of psychological organization, which would account for adaptive as well as maladaptive functioning but was limited in its development by the scientific context of his times. We can take a further step, in the context of modern cognitive psychology, although this scientific context has limitations as well, and can then hope that further steps will be taken as the field expands.

The objective of this work has been to propose a theoretical framework that may serve to stimulate debate and revision, and to provide a basis for empirical research. The objective has precisely not been to offer one completed and closed theoretical system to replace another. There may be many different views of what constitute the intrinsic and central concepts of psychoanalysis; there may also be alternative general theories that would serve as explanatory models of psychological organization. The architecture and modes of information processing that have been formulated need to be elaborated and refined. It is likely that there are multiple levels within each of the three major architectures and a far more elaborate series of stages that can be identified in the operation of the referential cycle. Each definition that has been proposed here may be continuously revised; the implications of each revision then need to be threaded through the entire system and other concepts revised as well. This is the corollary in theory development of the process of working through. Psychoanalysis needs to enter the arena of scientific work in the field of psychology, using its own special, controlled, naturalistic research context, to examine and test new ideas in the light of shared knowledge, to facilitate such working through, and to bring about the structural change of its own theory.

CHAPTER 17

Empirical Studies of the Analytic Process

Empirical research on the treatment process is essentially the psychoanalytic method in modern, scientific dress. Such research focuses directly on the discourse and the relationship in the treatment context itself, which cannot be reproduced in a laboratory setting. However, scientific study also requires shared observations. The fundamental difference between the methods of modern psychoanalytic research and the psychoanalytic method as formulated by Freud is the requirement that the processes of treatment be accessible to observers other than the participants themselves.

Much of the research on psychoanalytic treatment that has been carried out thus far, including the work that will be reported in this chapter, has relied on transcripts of tape recordings. These provide objective records not only unfiltered by the analyst's view of what is relevant, but also excluding whatever evidence may be produced in paralinguistic, facial, or bodily channels. A few studies have used additional procedures such as video recordings, ongoing measurement of the patient's physiological state during the session, or examination of the patient by researchers and clinicians other than the treating analyst (Horowitz et al., 1993; Eisenstein, Levy, & Marmor, 1994). For all of these approaches, one must balance the gains of increased information against the potential effects of the measurement procedures in changing what is observed.

In this chapter, I introduce empirical research on the treatment process, which has relied primarily on linguistic and clinical measures applied to verbatim transcripts of tape-recorded therapy sessions. General issues concerning the use of process research methods, including procedures based on sources other than audio recordings, will be discussed in Chapter 18.

In the accepted procedure for recorded treatments, as carried out in the research treatment to be discussed in this chapter, the analyst contracts with the patient regarding the recording procedures and the use of the treatment for research, and guarantees of confidentiality are established. Optimally, the taping is done for every session, with the expectation that it will become a part of the background context of the treatment. If only selected sessions are recorded, they cannot be seen as representative of the treatment as a whole. The taped record of the entire treatment provides the basis for a wide range of longitudinal studies. The selection of sessions for transcribing and further analysis is then made for purposes of particular study designs.

Verbatim transcripts are produced following standardized rules (Dahl, 1978; Mergenthaler & Stinson, 1992). The transcribing rules are designed to minimize ambiguity and distortion in the written record, and to permit representation of the verbal material in texts that are as close as possible to the natural spoken form. For current research purposes, the transcribed text must also be prepared so as to be amenable to computer analysis. Confidentiality is maintained by replacing names of all persons and places referred to by the patient in the transcripts, and masking them as well in the tape recordings themselves.

MEASUREMENT OF THE REFERENTIAL CYCLE

In our process research studies, the flow of the patient–analyst interaction and the operation of the referential cycle are examined using a wide range of clinical and linguistic measures whose meaning is established in the theoretical context of the multiple code theory. The cycle was initially defined on the basis of referential activity (RA) scales scored by raters, including scales assessing the concreteness, specificity, clarity, and imagery level of speech (Bucci, 1988, 1993; Bucci et al., 1992) and related linguistic measures. The scales and related measures are relatively easy to score, and high interjudge reliability has been achieved, as discussed in Chapter 11. However, like any measure scored by raters, they are limited in their application to long-term treatments. New computerized procedures have now been developed that permit application of this approach in studies of long-term treatments and multicase designs.

As discussed in Chapter 11, computer-measured referential activity (CRA), developed by Mergenthaler and Bucci (1993), parallels the RA scales in reflecting the phases of the cycle. Mergenthaler (1992, 1996) has also developed computerized measures of emotion-abstraction patterns (EAPs) that provide additional indicators of the phases of the cycle. The measurement of EAPs is based on two computer dictionaries, Emotional Tone (ET) and Abstraction (AB). The ET word list consists of items that demonstrate an emotional or affective state of the speaker and are likely to cause emotion in the listener. The AB dictionary consists of complex, abstract nouns that are understood as signs of reflection and evaluation.

To arrive at the CRA, ET, and AB scores for a particular text, the word lists are matched to the lexical items of a text. Counts of matched words and proportion of matched words to total word count of a text are computed using the Text Analysis System (TAS) developed by Mergenthaler (1985). Counts are based on tokens (total frequency of occurrence of a word) rather than types (each different word counted only once). Details on these computerized procedures are given in Bucci (1995), Mergenthaler (1996), and Mergenthaler and Bucci (1993).

Each of these measures, and combinations of them, represents a *particular clinical state associated with a phase of the cycle.* The computer-assisted measures provide a kind of linguistic CT scan of therapeutic transactions in a session, revealing the underlying structure of the process in a way that reading or listening alone cannot. The measures point to periods in the session at which the patient is working with emotional experience or moving away from this and also provide a way to assess the effects of particular interventions on the playing out of the symbolizing process. Content measures may then be applied to enable clinical characterization of the underlying themes that are being expressed, and to examine changes in these.

The use of computerized procedures eliminates the problem of interjudge reliability. The computer program segments and scores the text automatically, and no judgment procedures are required. The crucial psychometric question is that of validity. The construct validity of the linguistic measures, including the judge-rated and computerized procedures, as measuring phases of the cycle, has been developed through examining their convergent and discriminant validity in relation to other research procedures in the nomological network of multiple coding. The construct validity of all these measures, as representing the phases of the referential cycle, continues to be developed as the measures are used, and the nomological net is elaborated.

Phase One: The Subsymbolic Phase

In the subsymbolic phase, the patient is dominated by sensory and somatic concerns. Using judge-scored procedures, I have characterized this phase by relatively low levels of RA and by low clarity and specificity relative to the other scales. Using computerized procedures, we identify this phase as showing high levels of the ET measure and low levels of CRA and AB.

Of the three phases of the cycle, however, the phase of subsymbolic processing is probably the least amenable to measurement using linguistic techniques. The affective core of the emotions, including sensory, visceral, and motoric experience, is likely to be represented directly in facial expression and body movement, which themselves constitute components of emotion expression, whereas language is associated with these states only later and by indirect means. Videotape recordings could be used to score facial or bodily activity; however, we must be concerned with the intrusion of such procedures and their likelihood of affecting the treatment in significant ways. Vocalization, such as laughing, crying, and sighing; and paralinguistic indicators, such as pausing, pitch, and intonation patterns, assessed by listening to tape recordings rather than relying on transcripts, could add important information concerning the processes of the subsymbolic phase, without requiring additional recording procedures. Such studies are now under way in our work and in work by others. We are also developing a somatization word list, consisting of references to visceral and other bodily experiences that are central in our conception of the subsymbolic phase but are not represented in the ET measure.

The qualities and contents of language associated with the initial subsymbolic phase have also been captured in part, on a verbal level, in the Gendlin Experiencing Scale (Klein, Mathieu, Gendlin, & Kiesler, 1970). The Experiencing scale assesses subjective, phenomenological feeling states rather than the specific, concrete, sensory details of imagery and events that are valued in scoring RA. In several studies, we have found that levels of Experiencing scores do not vary with RA, and that Experiencing is likely to be high in the subsymbolic phase, when RA is relatively low (Bucci, 1993; Fretter, Bucci, Broitman, Silberschatz, & Curtis, 1994).

Phase Two: The Symbolizing Phase

The symbolizing phase is identified as the CRA peak; using the RA scales, we expect to see all four scales converging at high levels. As we have shown, prototypic narratives of activated emotion schemas, including objects, actions, and visceral feelings that figure in the schema, are most likely to be found in the specific memories, dreams, and episodes that are told in the RA (or CRA) peaks. The use of RA or CRA as an indicator of narrative speech has been verified in several studies, using widely different populations, speech samples, and narrative measures. Working from a psycholinguistic perspective, Moore (1992) examined the relationship between narratives identified according to discourse analysis criteria, and RA measured by the RA scales. In a series of interviews with a sample of nonclinical adult subjects, and in verbatim transcripts of recorded psychoanalytic sessions, Moore found that narrative passages were consistently marked by RA peak scores. In a study of several specimen hours, I (Bucci, 1988, 1993, in press) found that narratives expressing central relationship patterns were concentrated primarily in the RA or CRA peaks. These patterns included the relationship episodes (REs) on which the core conflictual relationship theme (CCRT; Luborsky & Crits-Cristoph, 1988) is based, other indicators of relationship patterns such as the frame structures as defined by Teller and Dahl (1986), and central transference themes as defined by Hoffman and Gill (1988). Kalmykova et al. (1997) have found significantly higher levels of CRA in passages defined as REs than in non-RE passages in verbatim transcripts of psychodynamic psychotherapies.

All of these studies provide validation for the RA or CRA peaks as identifying the points in the session at which central emotional themes are being expressed in narrative form, and where measures of thematic content may most usefully be applied. In addition to measures of relationship patterns scored by judges, we are also developing computerized content measures that will capture central clinical themes. The computerized language style and content measures serve as scanning devices to locate the points in a session where particular thematic content is being expressed, which may then be subjected to further, more intensive clinical investigation.

Phase Three: Reflection and Verification

In the third phase of the cycle, the individual reflects on the significance of the narratives that have been told; new connections are made within the verbal system, and the discourse is more likely to be shared; the analyst may take the lead to some extent. This phase is generally associated with some decline in CRA; using the RA scales, we might see relatively low levels of concreteness and imagery. We may also see increases in ET, accompanied by rising AB. The patient "names" the emotional experience that has been played out in the narratives ("I guess I was really angry at her"), then brings the powers of the verbal system to bear in examining the meanings of the narratives that have been told ("I guess I was so angry because . . . "). This phase would also be reflected in other insight measures (Bucci, 1993).

Computerized Version of the Referential Cycle

The basic referential cycle, as measured by our computerized text-analysis procedures, would thus include high ET, indicating verbalization of emotional experience; followed by high CRA, the narrative, which may describe a dream or memory or recent event; followed then by concomitant increases in ET and AB, indicating that emotions are active and connected to verbal reflection. This phase might be characterized as emotional insight. Optimally, AB then begins to decline and ET to rise, indicating new connections to emotional material, and a new cycle begins.

Variants of the cycle might occur; for example, the patient might begin with expression of emotion or somatic concerns in movement or facial expression, without corresponding verbal report. Thus, the language measures would show the cycle as beginning with a CRA peak without preceding ET. The cycle might be interrupted defensively in various ways, often indicated by a period of high AB following the CRA peak, as the patient defends against the contents that have been opened up; she then may (or may not) resume and reach the third phase of emotional reflection, the concomitant ET and AB. I will illustrate various types of completed and interrupted cycles, as well as material in which no cycle is identified, in the empirical study to be reported next.

STUDIES OF A PSYCHOANALYTIC TREATMENT

In this illustration of empirical measurement of the referential cycle, I will present the three computerized measures—ET, CRA, and AB—applied to verbatim transcripts of a tape-recorded psychoanalysis. I will provide overall scores for sessions as a whole to assess the course of the treatment over time and also examine the process within three individual sessions representing different phases of the treatment.

The patient, Mrs. C., was a young married woman who was experiencing severe sexual difficulties in her marriage and also reported general feelings of anxiety and dissatisfaction at work and in her personal relationships.[1] The analysis lasted 6 years, with five sessions a week, for a

---

[1]The discussion of the case of Mrs. C. includes revision and elaboration of some material presented in Bucci (1997), as well as new session material.

total of 1,114 sessions. All of the sessions were audio-recorded for research purposes, and some have been transcribed. Aspects of the treatment have been studied by several researchers, including Jones and Windholz (1990), Weiss et al. (1986), Dahl, Kaechele, and Thomae (1988), and Spence, Dahl, and Jones (1993), in addition to our own work.

Figure 17.1 shows the application of our three computerized measures to a sample of 105 sessions representing different phases of the treatment. For this application, ET, CRA, and AB scores were computed for sessions as a whole. The TAS program (Mergenthaler, 1985), matches each instance of the dictionary items to the transcribed patient or therapist speech for the session as a whole, and computes the proportion of words matched in each dictionary to total word count. In Figures 17.1 and 17.2, ET scores are shown as black bars, AB as grey bars, and CRA as grey dots connected by a dashed line. The convention of the dashed line is used to indicate that the sessions selected here include nonadjacent blocks; thus, no inference can be made to scores of sessions intervening between such blocks. All scores are presented as standardized scores, fluctuating around their means, with units of one standard deviation from the mean. In Figure 17.1, the mean is computed from patient speech only for sessions as a whole, for the 105 sessions included here. Thus, we see the three computerized measures for each session as deviating above or below their averages for the 105 sessions covered here.

The patient's ET is highest for the beginning of the treatment, in the sample of 22 sessions from the first 100 hours. CRA is also generally high at this time; AB is low. The pattern changes dramatically as the treatment continues. By the second year of treatment, the patient's use of emotional speech reflected in ET declines and never recovers consistently; CRA also shows general decline, with occasional peaks.

One can see the same patterns of patient speech reflected in Figure 17.2 for a subset of these sessions and can compare this to the analyst scores. Here we see summary scores for seven sets of 10 sessions, spaced throughout the treatment, which were used in the Jones and Windholz (1990) study. Scores are presented as standardized scores fluctuating around the means for the 70 sessions represented here, for patient and analyst separately. The patient never again reaches the CRA level that she showed in the first 10 sessions; she shows some increase, but still to a lower level, in the 10 sessions from the fifth year of treatment (Sessions 765–774) in which Jones and Windholz see her as struggling with feelings of aggression and guilt. In contrast to the patient's pattern, the analyst shows an overall increase in CRA across the treatment, with a local peak in the third year (Sessions 429–438). We may note that this is a special, not a representative, time in this treatment; these are the patient's

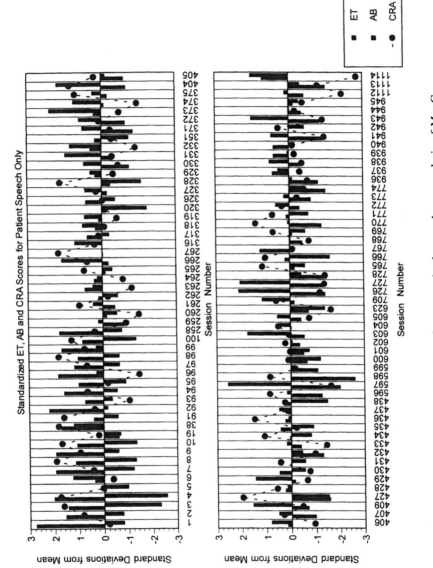

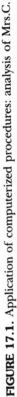

FIGURE 17.1. Application of computerized procedures: analysis of Mrs.C.

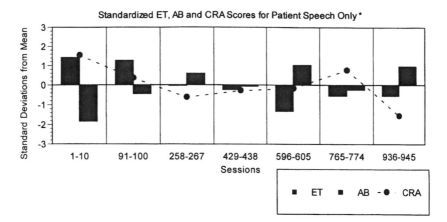

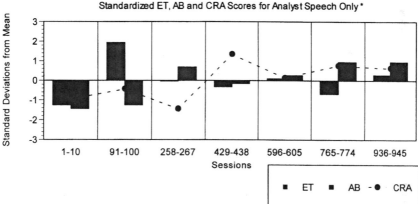

FIGURE 17.2. Application of computerized procedures: seven sets of 10 sessions studied by Jones and Windholz (1990). *Scores are averages of 10 consecutive sessions selected from seven distinct phases of the treatment.

immediate predelivery and postparturition sessions. It is noteworthy that the analyst's speech shows a CRA increase, while the patient's CRA remains low. We have discussed the issues of the transference and countertransference in this phase (Friedman, Udoff, & Bucci, 1994) and are considering these issues further in our current work.

The implications of our linguistic overview are at variance with some of the conclusions of Jones and Windholz (1990) concerning this case. In their study, the selected sessions were rated in random order by clinical judges using the Psychotherapy Process Q-Set (PQS) technique developed by Jones. The PQS was designed to provide a basic language for the description and classification of patient and analyst actions and attitudes, and their interaction. On the basis of these ratings, Jones and Windholz found: "Over the years the patient's discourse was less intellectualized and dominated by rationalization, and increasingly reflected greater access to her emotional life and a developing capacity for free association" (Jones, 1995, p. 100). In contrast, our linguistic overview indicates that Mrs. C. shows a general decline in expression of emotional experience across the 6 years of her treatment, as reflected in declines in both CRA and ET, and that her language style in treatment becomes more intellectualized and abstract, as indicated by the increase in AB. In effect, we reach essentially opposite conclusions from those of Jones and Windholz, using the same set of 70 sessions. I will return to these findings in the analysis of several individual sessions from this case, to be reported later.

Weiss, Sampson, and their colleagues (1986), using a set of process research methods based on assessment of the patient's unconscious plan, studied the first (1–100) and last 100 hours (1,015–1,114) of this case. According to Weiss (1993), the patient's plan, as inferred from the first 100 sessions, was still guiding her behavior during the final 100:

> Throughout her analysis, Mrs. C. was unconsciously worried about the analyst for whom she felt omnipotently responsible. During the first 100 sessions she tested her belief in her responsibility for the analyst by attempting to demonstrate to herself that she could not push him around. During the last 100 sessions she tested this same belief by attempting to demonstrate to herself that she would not hurt the analyst if she made clear to him her wish to terminate. (p. 25)

Weiss discusses this consistency of Mrs. C.'s unconscious plans and goals as a demonstration of the psychometric stability and reliability of their plan formulation measure. I would raise the question, however, as to whether one would expect pathogenic belief systems to remain unchanged across a successful analysis, and what it means if they do. From one perspective, the stability that is observed in this case raises questions about the interpretation of the Weiss et al. plan construct; from another perspective, which is central to the discussion here, this must lead us also to question the effectiveness of Mrs. C.'s treatment in addressing her pathogenic beliefs. Presumably, if an analyst repeatedly passes the patient's "tests," in the terms of the Weiss et al. approach, one would expect the patient's pathogenic belief system to change rather than remaining stable.

CHANGING PATTERNS OF INTERACTION:
A STUDY OF THREE SESSIONS

We can see that these formulations raise questions concerning the nature of change in the interpersonal discourse and in the patient in this treatment, and also the reasons for these changes. We can begin to explore these questions by looking at the process within sessions at different phases of the treatment, using our computer-assisted procedures, combined with examination of some of the clinical material that is identified as salient by these measures.

In the examples that follow, I will examine three sessions from three different phases of this analysis. The first session, number 38, is from the first year of the treatment, when ET and CRA levels are at their highest. The second session, number 326, is from late in the second year of the treatment, after the general linguistic pattern of the treatment had changed, and is the Monday of the week in which she decided to have a pregnancy test. The third example, number 726, is from the fourth year.

The Early Phase: A Partial Cycle

Session 38 is the session from the sample shown in Figure 17.1 that had the highest combined score on all three language measures—ET, AB, and CRA—in our sample of 105 sessions. The high levels of our measures might or might not indicate productive work, depending on the patterning of the discourse, but was our best bet, using our measures as a screening device, to find a session in which all aspects of the cycle are likely to be found.

Figure 17.3 shows the three dictionaries—ET as black bars, AB as grey bars, and CRA as a continuous line—applied to Session 38 of Mrs. C. For this and the subsequent two figures (17.4 and 17.5), the transcript of the session is divided into 150-word blocks[2] and the scores, proportions of words matched, are computed for each measure for each word block, then converted to standard scores. The computerized procedures, which incorporate the TAS techniques described earlier (Mergenthaler, 1985), take

---

[2]The minimum word block size that is required to produce reliable results is determined by the expected coverage—average proportion of words matched—of the dictionaries to be applied. ET and AB require at least 150-word blocks on average to produce reliable results. While CRA matches a larger proportion of words and can produce reliable scores with smaller word blocks, 150-word blocks are used here for correspondence with the other measures (Mergenthaler & Bucci, 1993).

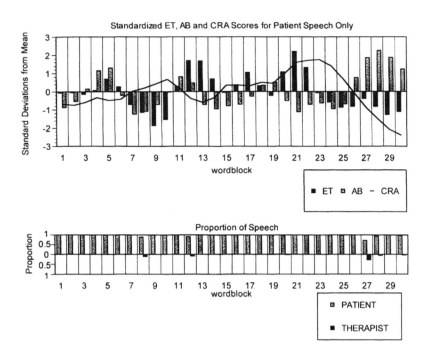

FIGURE 17.3. Application of computerized procedures: Mrs. C., Session 38.

take the verbatim transcript, which has been prepared according to specified transcribing rules (Mergenthaler & Stinson, 1992), and carry out all phases of the segmentation and scoring automatically, dividing the speech into 150-word blocks, scoring each block, and generating the graphs. The upper graph shows the computerized content analysis for patient speech only; the lower graph shows proportion of each 150-word block accounted for by patient speech (height of bar above the midline) and analyst speech (below the midline). As we can see, the analyst speaks very little in this session, only in Word Blocks 8 and 12, very briefly in 20, and then again in 27 and 28. This is somewhat, but not substantially, below the average for his interventions throughout this classical treatment.

Hour 38 opens like an example of the good hour as described by Kris (1956). The hour does not start propitiously; little happens in the first 10 or 15 minutes, according to our measures. The patient tells of her feelings of rejection by her mother; she says that she is afraid she will not be able to control her anger at her mother. In Word Block 12, the analyst asks:

A: What would you like to do?

The patient responds with a vivid answer, reflected in high ET:

P: Shout something awful at her, or throw something, break something, generally create a disturbance . . . I want to attack her, hurt her back in some way.

She follows this description of feeling and action with a series of narratives, lasting approximately from Word Blocks 15 to 25: first, an incident concerning a man whom, she says, she had been petrified about dancing with, but then she danced with him and enjoyed it, because "he was wild enough and strong enough as a leader so it made me do things that I might not have dared to do otherwise." It is not a big inferential leap to see a reference to the analytic relationship in this; this inference is validated by the subsequent associations. She reports a dream—still following Kris's model of the "good hour," and also following the pattern of the referential cycle. She was at a gathering of people, connected with the dance. The analyst was there; he told her that he knew what she was doing, and that she had better stop. This leads to a description of a movie she recently saw, about a girl who wanted to be a free spirit, then to other associations and narratives, ending with her telling about her fears of being left alone and rejected. Dreams are, of course, characteristic contents of the RA peaks. For this patient, it is also quite characteristic to use narratives drawn from movies or books as vehicles for expression of her own emotional themes.

Following the RA peak, the analyst intervenes with a clarifying question in Word Block 27:

A: You said that, um, in the dream I said to you, in effect, "You know what you're doing and stop it." Right? What was it?

P: What you said?

A: What was it that was being referred to? Do you recall?

P: I think I was actually sort of, um, gradually hunching up more and more and putting my face in my hands and just kind of hiding my face.

A: Ah, that's what I was referring to.

The patient then goes on to considerable summing up on her own for the remainder of the session. She says that she feels understood, cared for, comforted. However, her language becomes increasingly abstract. She attempts to probe the meaning of the analyst's being in her dream, and her feelings about it; she is uncomfortable about his being in the dream, of having him "take an importance with me that was just fantasy." At the same time, she has a feeling of freedom that she can say what she thinks. She has this feeling more when she thinks about being in the session than when she is actually there. She talks about fooling herself; she distrusts everything that she says.

In this session, we see the opening of a cycle, with emotional arousal indicated by high ET, leading to narratives of an incident, a dream, and a description of a movie, constituting a CRA peak. The analyst's brief question in Word Block 12 may have contributed to the unfolding of these narratives. Optimally, according to our model of the referential cycle, the sequence of narratives of the CRA peak would then have been followed by concomitant increases in ET and AB, indicating emotional insight. Here, it is followed by high AB alone, while ET is low, indicating reflection without emotional connection. She becomes locked into ruminative doubting of the feelings that have been opened up, rather than moving forward with them. She is moving away from her connection to emotional experience and also withdrawing from the analyst; she recognizes this withdrawal herself, at least to some degree.

The Pregnancy and the Session Time: An Interrupted Cycle

In the next session to be presented here, Session 326, a Monday from the second year of treatment, Mrs. C. reports her decision, made over the weekend, to have a pregnancy test. As can be seen in Figure 17.1, the language measures for the session as a whole are generally in the midrange. ET has a local peak on that day, AB is relatively low, CRA is at the midpoint. The CRA score will peak several days later, in Session 328, the day she is expecting to receive her test results, and will decline sharply immediately thereafter, when she learns she is pregnant and reports this to the analyst.

A graphic representation of the computer-coded process analysis of Session 326 is shown in Figure 17.4, in the same format as for Session 38. In discussing this and the subsequent session, we will rely on our technique of using the contents of the CRA peaks as indicators of the major themes, including transference themes, being expressed in the session. We will also take a step further in identifying the nature of the theme (or themes) using the measure of CCRT developed by Luborsky (Luborsky & Crits-Cristoph, 1988, 1990). We will then provide an evaluation of the analytic intervention in terms of its effects in facilitating the

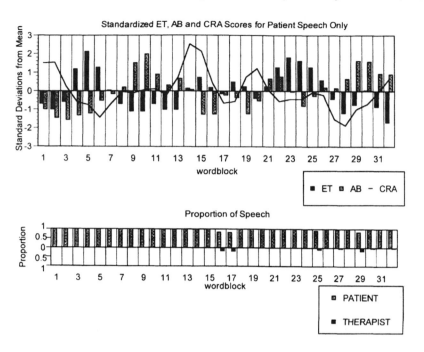

FIGURE 17.4. Application of computerized procedures: Mrs. C., Session 326.

patient's access to emotional experience, as indicated by the effect on development of the cycle.

In Session 326, we can identify three points at which the CRA rises more than one standard deviation above the mean as well as one brief increase to almost that level at the end of the session. The session begins with a CRA peak, in Word Blocks 1 and 2. Mrs. C. tells about an incident in which she tried to collaborate with a colleague on a project. She felt less competitive than she usually does, but the colleague acted in an unpleasant and rivalrous way, and Mrs. C. felt angry and tense.

Following this story, her expression of emotion is relatively high, indicated by the high ET levels. This leads to her introduction of the fact that she has gone today for a pregnancy test; she then brings up the possibility of changing her session times. ET declines, CRA is low, AB begins to rise. The following passage is from Word Block 7:

P: In any case I wanted to definitely do something about finding out whether or not I was pregnant, and it's the first time I've felt I really wanted to know. Before when I've thought about wanting to know I've thought, "Well, do it as soon as school's out," or something like that.

And something else that just makes me think of it, too, saying when school's out, but also it was on my mind today, and again, I've mentioned it here before, that I'd thought of it, but I don't know, today it was on my mind in a different way. I really wanted to now ask you about being . . . ; if it would be possible to change the time once school is out.

She has difficulty in making this request and goes on to speak in an abstract way, indicated by the continuing increase in AB.

The second CRA peak, lasting from about Word Blocks 13 to 15, is the major central narrative of the session. She reports a childhood memory of an injury, presumably accidental, by her older sister, who was always antagonistic to her. She was age 5 or younger, and she and her sister were playing hide and seek. She was hiding behind a door, her sister moved the door, and it crashed into her and cut her face. In the same CRA peak, she goes on to tell another story about her sister teasing and frightening her, talks about her feelings of rivalry with her sister for their mother's love and care, and then, in Word Block 16, returns to the thoughts of nursing and her mother's always being very much on schedule, with no sense of relaxing:

P: And all I can do is imagine how I think my mother would have been, and I can't imagine her being anything but very much on schedule, and that the schedule said at this time she nursed me for so many minutes, and that I better be on schedule. No sense of relaxing and just enjoying it, which may be very untrue.

The analyst's first intervention of the session follows immediately:

A: But it may explain why it's important to you to find out whether I'm going to hold you to your schedule.

P: You mean because I do have that feeling about my mother.

A: Well, you say you imagine how important that may be and that that's the way she was, and earlier you were wondering, how am I?

This intervention is followed by the third, smaller increase in CRA, in Word Blocks 19 and 20, concerning another incident at the school where she works. She feels angry and annoyed toward her colleagues, but in contrast to the narrative that opened the session, she sees herself here as in the wrong, selfish and unfriendly. She connects this to some conflicted feelings about her husband. Her expression of these feelings is marked by increases in ET and AB, which we see as characterizing emotional insight, in Word Blocks 21 and 22, leading then to an increase in emotional expression. She had rejected her husband's bid for intercourse, as she often did, using events in the analysis as an excuse; she reflects on his response and her own:

P: And he got mad at that, too—and I can—I mean it meant I was taking absolutely no responsibility for our relationship. I was expecting him to foot it all and putting up with me in any way I wanted to be while I go through this and—so I felt badly afterwards, when I thought about it I guess, because I realized—I don't know what I realized, but I just suddenly felt I don't want to be so alone and I want to be with [husband] and so I asked him to make love to me, really. I mean—I didn't say it in so many words, but I did something that—I don't know why it's so hard for me to say this, but I was starting to make love to him, and I find it very hard to say that.

She goes on to talk further about ambivalent feelings toward her husband. The analyst comments, in Word Block 25:

A: You don't say what you did when you started to make love.

She says she doesn't want to talk about that. She doesn't want to remember what she did; she just wanted to be close to him, and to kiss him, and to put her arms around him; that's what she did, and she doesn't want to remember that. She speaks briefly about one of her cats, who was wanting more attention than she usually does, and then clawed up a chair. Mrs. C. tried to discipline her by hitting a paper against her hand. She connects this to herself, asking the analyst for a change in session time:

P: She [the cat] acted like she thought it was a game today, but in any case, I had an angry feeling toward her for a minute, and then I thought again of the fact that I want to ask you to change the time. And I don't know whether I connect it with angry feelings, that I think you'll be angry, or if I'm getting ready to be angry with you if you don't.

In the fourth brief CRA increase, at the end of the session, she talks about her feelings of competitiveness and anger toward men, and about the birth of her brother, when she was about age 6. She saw him as the favored child; he was the fourth, after three girls. She talks about wanting to be a male, and also wanting to be a female, and also about "feeling the way my mother feels."

The Core Conflictual Relationship
Theme for Session 326

According to our model of the treatment process, the narratives in the CRA (or RA) peaks represent the central emotional theme of the patient in this session; we expect that this theme will be found in the transference as well. Measures of central themes such as the CCRT may then be applied to these narratives. In the standard procedure for scoring the CCRT, judges read the transcript and identify the REs, narratives about self–other relationships from which the CCRT is then extracted. An important contribution of the computer procedure is to enable us to bypass the step of requiring judges to identify REs by using the CRA measurement as a scanning device. Evidence for the use of RA or CRA elevation as an indicator of narrative speech and as a basis for locating REs has been presented earlier in this chapter.

Once the REs have been identified, three components of each episode are then scored: (1) the *wish* being expressed in relation to the other person; (2) the *response of the other,* actual or expected (RO); and (3) the *response of the self* (RS). Both positive and negative components may be identified. The components that have been identified are categorized and summed across all REs in a session; the CCRT of the session is then identified on the basis of the most frequently appearing components. Ten REs are generally used for reliable identification of a CCRT; for purposes of this illustration, however, we have identified a summary CCRT based on the REs that occurred in the four points of CRA elevation in this session:

> *Wishes*: (Positive) To collaborate with the other, to feel close.
>   (Negative) To compete; to control.
> *Response of Other (RO)*: Be angry and rejecting.
> *Response of Self (RS)*: Feel angry and hurt.

We see this central theme in various forms and contexts throughout the session, with changes as to the objects in the various roles and the identifications that are expressed. In the beginning, in the episode about her colleagues in the work setting, and in her childhood memory with her sister, she sees herself as trying to collaborate and as being rebuffed. In the next narrative about her colleagues, she sees herself as in the wrong, deserving of the anger. Later, it is she who takes the role of the angry or powerful person, and she disciplines her cat. Finally, related to this role, she talks of her competition with her brother and identification with her mother.

The CCRT is understood by Luborsky et al. (1993) as "a significant central relationship pattern that is related to the concept that clinicians call the transference pattern" (p. 328). The patient recognizes both roles in the treatment relationship; she is not sure if it is she who is angry at the analyst or he who is angry at her. The analyst's first intervention of the session, in Word Blocks 16 and 17, does address the theme that has been identified in the CCRT, relating her feelings about her mother's rigidity in scheduling her nursing to her anxiety about asking him to change session times. He focuses on her wish for control and her expectation that she will feel angry. As he says in his final intervention, in Word Block 29:

A: Well, it seems to me the central thing is that the very idea that I wouldn't do what you want makes you mad.

The study of Friedman et al. (1994) provides a perspective on the patient's themes, which is different from the analyst's view, but is also compatible with components of the basic CCRT. Friedman et al. have argued that unconscious themes of affiliation, nurturance, receptivity, and bodily concerns are dominant for the patient at this time, in the early phase of her pregnancy. According to these authors, these and related themes are incorporated in an emotional schema of "maternalism," a central aspect of female sexuality that is biologically as well as psychologically determined. The emotional themes of maternalism are present for all women, to varying degrees, at different times in their lives, but are biologically, hormonally, dominant in pregnancy. We know, although Mrs. C. and her analyst were as yet uncertain, that she was indeed pregnant at this time, so that the biological factors were in play. The psychological factors are also particularly likely to have been aroused for her on this day, when she finally faces the possibility that she is pregnant and decides to submit to a pregnancy test.

The manner in which the themes of maternalism play out for each individual woman will depend on her own emotion schemas and conflicts within them, and will particularly reflect the manner in which these themes are negotiated in her early relationship with her own mother. For Mrs. C., we see the themes of maternalism as expressed in the positive wish component of the CCRT of this session, to feel close to another. In the major phase of emotional insight following the CRA peak, she talks specifically about not wanting to be alone. Based on her relationship to a cold and rejecting mother, this leads to the expected negative RO; the other will be angry and rejecting. We may also see that her request for a time change follows immediately after her reference to the possibility that she is pregnant, and seems to be related to this. Rather than indicating only her wish to control the analyst, it is possible that this may represent her wish for him to recognize the special nature of this time in her life, her feeling that she needs him to care for her.

In this ministudy, we thus see two versions of the same central theme: one focusing on wishes associated with rivalry and control, and expectations of anger in others and herself; the other, on a wish for closeness, attachment, being cared for, an expectation of rejection, and feelings of anxiety and abandonment. Given Mrs. C.'s pregnancy and its psychobiological implications as we understand them today, we would suggest that the latter may have been dominant, although not recognized as such.

Evaluation of Interventions

Our measures enable us to evaluate and compare differences in clinical views by examining the effects of interventions derived from them. We do not look for the patient's direct agreement or disagreement, whose meaning is intrinsically ambiguous, but for indirect indicators in the patient's language style that the interventions serve to facilitate or block access to emotional experience and the fuller playing out of the referential cycle (Bucci, 1989).

The sequence from Word Blocks 4 to 22 is an example of a cyclical pattern that is interrupted but then resumed and carried through. The emotional expression reflected in the high ET in Word Blocks 4–6 is temporarily warded off by an intervening period of abstract speech; the patient breaks through this again with the long central narrative. The analyst intervenes, in Word Blocks 16 and 17, with a transference interpretation related to the time change, which picks up an aspect of the CCRT theme. The patient then completes the cycle with the period of emotional insight, as we have seen. At this point, AB declines again; her language becomes more emotional, indicated by an increase in her ET scores, in Word Blocks 22 to about 25; she also pauses frequently during these segments. The increase in ET would mark this as an example of the iterative cyclical (or spiral) process, a point of opportunity in the treatment process, in which emotion schemas may potentially be deepened and new connections made.

The analyst then intervenes briefly, in Word Block 25, to comment on her not saying what she did when she started to make love. This leads to a decline in CRA and ET, and a subsequent increase in AB. The intervention in Word Block 29, referring to her demands and her anger, also leads to a decline in ET and continued high AB.

Our results indicate that the transference intervention in Word Blocks 16 and 17, in which the analyst addresses Mrs. C.'s feelings concerning her mother's rigidity and connects them to her expectations of him, was effective, serving to facilitate the cycle. The latter interventions, in which he focuses on themes of erotic sexuality, and on her anger, lead to an increase in the patient's defensive stance. The measures suggest that the period following Mrs. C.'s description of starting to make love to her husband, with its indicators of emotional insight and subsequent emotional activation, represent a lost opportunity in the treatment, in which the patient's explicit statement of not wanting to be alone and wanting to be with her husband (and perhaps with the analyst) might have been, but was not, addressed. We do not know what might have happened had the analyst responded to the affiliative or attachment themes and explored other possible implications of her request for a time change, or her feeling of closeness to her husband, or the emotional meaning of her decision to have the pregnancy test that day. We do have some preliminary indications of what happened—a decrease in CRA and ET, and increase in AB—when he continues to focus on the themes of aggression and sexuality that seem central to him.

We may also note that the shift in her role in the session CCRT—from herself as the one who is unfairly rebuffed, to herself as deserving of the anger, and as identified with the angry and powerful person—provides evidence for the theme of omnipotent responsibility emphasized by Weiss et al. (1986). The patient sees herself as powerful, and as responsible for the other's anger and for her own. The nature of Mrs. C.'s issues of control, as well as the interplay of attachment and aggression themes in her pregnancy, and in her overall emotion structures, are being explored in our current intensive studies of this case.

The Tape-Recording: Linking in Stalemate

The last example, Session 726, occurred in the fifth year of the treatment, just prior to the phase characterized by Jones and Windholz (1990) as the period of transference neurosis and resistance. In the intervening years, Mrs. C. had delivered a healthy baby girl. Session 726 is the first of a series of three sessions that occurred in the week prior to the analyst's vacation and were characterized by low CRA and ET, and high AB, as we can see in Figure 17.1. The measures mark these sessions as a generally unproductive period in which emotional connections were not made, and intellectualization was dominant. The graphic representation of Session 726, constructed as described earlier for Sessions 38 and 326, is shown in Figure 17.5.

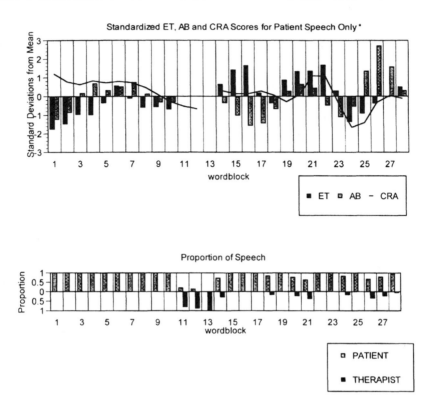

FIGURE 17.5. Application of computerized procedures: Mrs. C., Session 726. Because of the extensive analyst interventions, patient speech for Word Blocks 11–13 was insufficient to permit reliable computation of ET and AB for those units; CRA only was computed for Word Blocks 11 and 12. Word Block 13 was entirely taken up by analyst speech.

The session begins with an extended silence of approximately 3 minutes, typical for Mrs. C. at the opening of a session. (Silences are not indicated on this graph, which is based on word count rather than time.) Her first utterances are relatively high in CRA. When she came into the room, she noticed an odor that made her think of cat urine. She has the fantasy that somehow cats had gotten in and urinated on the couch— although she knows that must be impossible— and then she had to lie in it. The other thing she was thinking, which seemed more likely, was that the material on the couch had somehow gotten damp; it had that kind of a smell. She says that perhaps she started thinking about cats having urinated on the couch to avoid thinking about someone having been on the couch just before her and what they might have done. She had the idea of that person sweating profusely, so that it would make the material damp.

An idea comes into her mind that she was not aware of when she was first talking about this smell; sometimes her husband will sweat a lot when they are making love. She doesn't want to get to that kind of thinking, but now she feels stuck. She talks about a general feeling of panic that had overtaken her yesterday and today, related to the analyst's impending vacation at the end of this week. She feels that her understanding of what they have talked about is vague and out of reach; she needs to come to treatment in order not to lose it. She needs something to happen before the end of the week; otherwise, it will be too late.

She falls silent for 2 minutes, around the end of Word Block 5; she changes the topic to a room she is redecorating, then begins to ruminate in a vague and dissociated way. She knows that she is getting blocked; her perception is validated in declines in all three language measures, from Word Block 8 to Word Blocks 11 and 12.

P: And then somehow I think I stopped that feeling of, of, that was the initial one of sharing. And, I don't know, somehow it seems like that, um, well I suppose it can't be really separate, but it was a different thing from my, um, forgetting what I'd remembered and using it in the way I did. (*Pause*) Well, I, I kee—I think I wonder because I think maybe I was wondering this yesterday, too, if, if I'm trying to separate the two because, um, there, there might be something if I don't, that I don't want to see. I mean, somehow I guess it seems—I don't, I don't—um, maybe I'm, I'm getting too tangled up in this . . . [Word Block 10]

The analyst intervenes for the first time in Word Blocks 11–14, while the patient is in this tangled, ruminative phase. His intervention here is far longer than his usual utterances, taking up almost the entire word count for these segments, as shown in the bottom portion of Figure 17.5.[3] He first refers to her fantasy about the cats; he suggests that she was saying that his place stinks. He then refers to her fantasies about provoking a male to attack her, which he has previously noted with respect to her husband and himself.

A: So you keep, in one way or another, by your behavior, inviting me to, as you say, break through, to rape you, to attack you; then you'll have an occasion to fight back and kick me in the groin and destroy me. And it's this kind of a fantasy behind all the things that you're doing,

I think. And now you're saying, you haven't got much more time. "I, if I'm going to do it, I've got to do it this week." Ah, in a way this is very similar to the way you've behaved toward [husband] for years. [Word Block 13]

In response to this intervention, Mrs. C. speaks with some emotion, as reflected in higher ET in Word Blocks 14–16. Her CRA is around the midpoint for the session. She disagrees, in part, with what the analyst has said. What she actually wants is to be overcome, not to fight back. Perhaps she wants to fight some with her husband, but she wants him to be stronger.

The analyst responds, in Word Block 18, that he is struck with how nonspecific the things she is thinking are. She responds directly to this; she asks herself, "What am I not thinking by not being specific?" She seems to comply with the analyst's interpretation; she goes on to describe a situation in which she passively resists her husband's wishes and gets him to become angry at her. She sits around on a Sunday, reading the newspaper, doing nothing, not getting dressed; she doesn't feel good, but she does it anyway. Her husband doesn't like her doing that; she waits for him to nag her. Then, she would get dressed "and it would be, the end result would be something that, even though we'd fought to get there, was one I really kind of wanted." This is part of the CRA peak of Word Blocks 21 and 22. She thinks that maybe what she does could be interpreted two ways—as setting up the fighting to make her husband control her, or as related to her wish to destroy her husband and attempting to control that wish. This brings her back to her wish, discussed in previous sessions, to have tape recordings of the session to listen to during the vacation. Her CRA is declining steeply at this point.

P: Well, the thing I'm thinking now, I, um, I can see it could be interpreted two ways. And I'm not sure, um, (*sighs*) but something led me to, um, think back to what you had said that got, got us started on thinking about these things, or me started, um, in the way that I am right now. And, I don't know, it's as if I'm, what I'm trying to do is replay exactly what you said and then everything that's been said since then, um, as if it's a recording in my mind so that when I leave here I'll have it. And if I can't do that then I won't have it when I leave here. [Word Blocks 23–24]

All language measures are declining at this time. The analyst interprets her wish for the recording, as he has done previously, as further evidence of her wish to have what he has and by implication, to destroy him:

A: Well, the recording for you is equivalent to—it's my penis. I have it and you don't and you want it. And that's what the fight is about. That's what you want to get revenge for. That's why you're trying to defeat me, frustrate me. That's what you want to do to the guy in the movie, it's what you'd like to do to [husband]. That's why you're thinking this. [Word Block 26]

Mrs. C. resists this interpretation, as she has done in previous sessions, and returns to what she sees as her own reasons for wanting the recordings, her feelings about the forthcoming separation. The analyst does not acknowledge the possibility of alternate interpretations, and the issue remains unresolved.

Comparison of Patient and Analyst Themes

As discussed earlier, we view the narratives of the RA or CRA peaks as derivative expressions of the patient's dominant emotion themes. The difficulties that occur in this session may be examined by comparing the patient's themes in her CRA peaks with the analyst's interpretations. In terms of the CCRT, her theme in the first peak may be seen as incorporating an explicit wish component only: She has not taken in enough to keep her going while he is away; she thinks about what happens when she is not there; her *wish* is *for him to do something to her, to give her something to take with her while they are separated.* She leaves the expected responses from self and other as implicit; she may be setting up the situation so that he will fill them in for her—which he does.

The analyst does not respond at first, leaving her to her rumination and withdrawal. His intervention, when it comes, does not reflect her theme but continues one that he has been pursuing in previous sessions. In terms of the CCRT structure, he identifies a different *wish*: *to provoke him;* and explicit *expected responses* from the other and herself: *he forces her to do something or is angry with her; so that she is then free to fight back and destroy him.*

The contents of the patient's CRA peak in Word Blocks 21 and 22, a narrative about her husband, in some respects appear to support the analyst's preceding interpretation, with a different perspective. She acknowledges that she tries to provoke her husband. Perhaps she does have destructive wishes toward him; however, she also provokes him (her husband—or her analyst) as a way to control herself or to activate him to restrain and overcome her. She continues to resist the connection of wanting a tape recording to wanting his penis, and as representing envy and destructiveness. Thus, she identifies a *wish* that is similar to the one the analyst has previously attributed to her: *to provoke him;* but with a different agenda as to *expected responses* from him and from herself: *he restrains and overcomes her; she feels relieved.* The analyst's interpretation following this peak reiterates the theme of his earlier intervention in essentially unmodified form.

Effects of the Interventions

As in Session 326, one way to evaluate the validity of the analyst's view of the case is to examine the patient's responses to his interventions using our language measures. The lengthy series of interventions in Word Blocks 11–14, pursuing his theme of envy and destructiveness, is followed by an increase in ET and a decline in AB. As the measures indicate, the patient has been emotionally aroused by the interventions, but she does not bring in new associations; she responds to what the analyst says, and struggles to get across her opposing view.

The analyst's intervention in Word Block 18, which refers to the nonspecific nature of her thoughts, may be seen as having its intended effect. She experiences this as exhorting her to be more specific. His comments appear to empower her to express her hostile wishes, reducing her censorship of them. This leads to a series of narratives that are indeed more specific than the material that has gone before, reflected in the CRA increase in Word Blocks 21 and 22.

The analyst's interventions in Word Blocks 20 and 21 continue his earlier theme. The *contents* of the patient's subsequent material appear to provide partial confirmation for the analyst's interventions. She acknowledges her feelings of anger and her wish to provoke him. Her language *style*, however, tells a different story, with steep declines in CRA and declines in the other language measures as well. The patient's language here, even more clearly than in her response to the first, very long intervention, indicates that the analyst's view, as expressed in his interpretation, did not succeed in opening connections to her emotion schemas; she remains disconnected and defended. All language measures show some increase in the remainder in the session; however, this phase is dominated by high levels of abstraction, as the patient struggles to defend her views. Her language at the close of the session reflects her anger and frustration, conflicting with her wish to comply with the analyst, and the disorganizing effects of these feelings:

P: Well, I don't know. I mean, maybe I'm doing just what we were talking about in, in wanting to set it up so that then I could fight you, but I'm feeling, I guess, very resistant to, um, not everything that you just said but, but the, um, the fa– connecting my wanting a recording or, or trying to, to get what seems to me is like a mental recording of what was just said here. Um, and connecting that with why—my wanting your penis. And, um, I mean I know I did, too, in that I, if I thought you have the recording and I don't, then it did occur to me immediately, well, you have a penis and I don't. But I still feel very resistant to thinking I've made an equivalent of your penis and the recording. Because it just seems ridiculous. I mean, there doesn't seem to be any possible comparison that, in that the recording isn't anything. And, of course, then, then it, I, I think, well, maybe what's happening is, um, once you've exposed that I've made a substitute right just this minute, um, for what I really want, then it clearly is not what I really want. I mean the substitute—(*Pause*)

A: Well, our time is up.

We may also note that her difficulty in connecting to emotional experience continues in the next two sessions following this one, Sessions 727 and 728, as indicated by continued low levels of CRA and ET, shown in the overall analysis of Figure 17.1. Based on these measures, the analyst's view, as reflected in his interpretations at this phase of the treatment, is not validated in the patient's response.

From today's perspective (about a quarter of a century after this analysis was completed), it seems apparent that for Mrs. C., as a woman (and now the mother of a small child), there can be important meanings for having the analyst's tape recording other than taking away his treasures and destroying him, just as her pregnancy can have emotional meaning other than that assumed in the classical theory. The theme of having the analyst's baby emerged during the pregnancy, but her fantasies concerning the infant were interpreted classically there as attempted reparation for her lack of a penis. We now see affiliative, nurturant, and dependent themes as primary in her maternal strivings, perhaps operating alongside of, and in interaction with, sexual and aggressive motivations, but not secondary to them. Along these lines, we can see that the patient's wish to have something of the analyst to take with her does not necessarily mean that she is envious or has destructive wishes toward him. A property of objects such as tape recordings (and babies), in contrast to bodily parts, is that they can be propagated, can be jointly held, and can even increase in value, substance, and meaning in various senses when they are shared. In the instance of the pregnancy, the infant is something that she has created with a man; the analyst as father of her child figured centrally in her fantasies around her pregnancy. In the instance of the tape recording, this is also something they have made together. If such images and motivations were present for Mrs. C. at this time of impending separation, and were not understood, they would account quite directly for her anger and hurt.

On the basis of these results, it appears likely that Mrs. C.'s anger and wish to provoke the analyst, as expressed in her second CCRT, is at least multiply determined by the interaction in the session, rather than stemming only from primary motives of envy and revenge, as the analyst assumes. Our analysis of this session suggests alternate explanations (as the patient herself does). Her anger may be a response to his initial rejection, to his preceding interpretation, or to his unwillingness to see alternative interpretations. It may also, ironically, be an indirect compliance with his formulation (which is characteristic of this patient); she indeed becomes angry, as he claims she has been.

Recursion of the Emotion Schemas

In the first session discussed here, Session 38, which occurred early in the treatment, we see a pattern of opening up and expressing feelings more freely at first, then defending against them. She reports a dream that incorporates her emerging feelings of freedom, and that incorporates the analyst, then describes a movie about a girl who wanted to be a free spirit. She is threatened by the new possibilities, however, and withdraws from her open position, as indicated by the decline in emotion-related speech and the increase in abstraction at the end of the session. A similar pattern is seen in the treatment as a whole, with high levels of ET and CRA in the first 100 hours of the treatment, and their subsequent decline, along with an increase in abstract speech, reflected in high AB. We may suggest that the discourse pattern that is seen in this early session signals the structure of the discourse as it will unfold throughout the treatment. The possibilities for emerging emotional freedom exist but are not realized; the patient remains defended in the end. As Weiss et al. (1986) have argued with respect to their application of the concept of the unconscious plan, this stability may be seen as a demonstration of the reliability of our measures and our portrayal of Mrs. C.'s emotion schemas. On the other hand, as I have also pointed out, one might argue that in a successful treatment, this pattern, like an unconscious plan, might have been expected to change.

We may also suggest that the difficulties that are seen in the third session described here, Session 726 (and to a lesser extent also in Session 326), may be seen as related to the difficulties in the treatment as a whole. In Session 326, she begins with a feeling that others are angry at her, talks about her wishes not to be alone, and ends with herself as identified with the angry and powerful person. In Session 726, the patient begins with fantasies of what happens in the office when she is not there; she is anxious about the impending separation; she wants to have something of the analyst, or the treatment, to take with her. He persists in his interpretation based on themes of envy and destructiveness; she disagrees but offers a compromise; he retains his position; she feels angry. In both sessions, we see anxiety over separation and feelings of anger intertwined with it; in both sessions, she moves toward identification with an angry and powerful person.

In our examination of the pregnancy phase of this treatment, we have seen Mrs. C.'s relationship to a cold and rejecting mother as salient (Friedman et al., 1994; Udoff, 1996). We have also seen that this structure is pervasive for Mrs. C., not restricted to the pregnancy period. We have identified a central emotion schema of desire for closeness and attachment, with expectation of rejection and consequent feelings of anger toward the object, leading to fear of further rejection. She turns away from her desire for closeness to the object and identifies instead with the powerful, angry person. This pattern characterizes her position from the start, is reenacted in the latter two sessions we have studied, and characterizes the outcome of the treatment as a whole. Her acceptance of the interpretations of hostility and destructiveness may be seen as overdetermined; her version of compliance as well as identification is an expression of her affiliative theme.

We should note that Mrs. C.'s second theme in Session 726 is very close to the statement of her unconscious plan, as formulated by Weiss et al. (1986): She feels responsible for the other (the analyst, her husband); she tests her pathogenic belief (and presumably attempts to disconfirm it) by trying to demonstrate that she cannot push him around or hurt him. The analyst's rejection of her request for the tape recording may be seen, in that respect, as passing her test (although the analyst would presumably not be likely to formulate an unconscious plan in this way.) On the other hand, his focus on her wish to destroy him (and other males) implicitly supports her belief in her power and her responsibility in this regard; *she is dangerous, as she fears, and can feel safe from doing damage only if the male is stronger and able to restrain her.* In Weiss et al.'s terms, the patient's unconscious plan for cure is not fulfilled; her belief in her responsibility for the analyst's feelings and her own is repeatedly confirmed.

The Blind Man and the Elephant: Complexity of the Emotion Schemas

Each of the researchers and clinicians who studied this case has seen it through a different lens. The analyst focused on Mrs. C.'s structures of envy and aggression, stemming from the birth of a favored younger brother. From his perspective, her problems and complaints, like those of the two patients in their first analyses, discussed by Grossman and Stewart (1976; see Chapter 2, this volume), seemed to be best accounted for in terms of the classical psychoanalytic concept of penis envy. Weiss et al. (1986) emphasized feelings of unconscious guilt, based on unconscious feelings of superiority, and saw her envy and belittling of herself as secondary. We have emphasized themes of affiliation and anticipated rejection, with anxiety and anger consequent on this. Our language analysis provides some support for our position and that of Weiss et al., and also some indication that the analyst's interventions may not be connecting to Mrs. C.'s emotion schemas as the treatment proceeds.

From today's perspective, the main conclusion we may derive from this descriptive study is that a variety of emotion schemas representing a range of clinical views were present and operative in this patient to different degrees and at different times. We expect that such complexity will generally be the case as a patient's emotion structures unfold in psychoanalytic treatment. As Grossman and Stewart (1976) demonstrated, the issues seen in one light in the patients' first treatments took a different form in the second. The challenge in understanding a patient's emotional organization is to move away from fixed doctrine and identify which of many operative schemas are salient, conflictual, and contributing to the individual's maladaptive functioning at a given time.

The greater complexity of this approach makes the role of research more obvious and central—and this must include research on basic psychological organization as well as on the therapeutic process. In place of the clear guidance of a received theoretical doctrine—penis envy, control mastery, issues of attachment—we are now talking about a broad domain of emotional information processing in which conflict and maladaptive functioning may occur. We need a general psychological model to encompass the complexity of emotional organization, and reliable and valid methods to evaluate hypotheses concerning particular views of a case—to distinguish which of many possible schemas, many possible emotional meanings, are being expressed at particular points of a patient's associations and interactions. I have shown a first step in this direction in the single-case study that has been presented here. In the next chapter, I will discuss additional aspects of the interface of our research with clinical work, and will also outline some of the general challenges that we face in building a psychoanalytic research program.

CHAPTER 18

Notes Concerning the Psychoanalytic Research Agenda

I have presented these examples from a single case to demonstrate the methodological power of this research approach to raise clinical questions and provide means of addressing them. The measures point to the location of central themes and enable evaluation of the work of the treatment, including the analyst's interventions in facilitating the patient's explorations. Using these measures, differences in theoretical views and in technique may be evaluated as these affect the access to emotional experience and the changes in emotional meanings that are the fundamental objective of analytic treatment. The psychoanalytic session provides a unique research setting for evaluation of specific clinical hypotheses that may contribute as well to evaluation of more general propositions concerning emotional and cognitive functioning within the context of a basic theory of psychological organization.

The material presented in Chapter 17 may be seen as an outline—or promise—for a process research project rather than a completed study. In this chapter, I discuss some of the major components of the psychoanalytic research agenda and the challenges that need to be met, so that such promises can be fulfilled. I will first discuss some specific clinical implications of the research, to show how our findings may potentially be of direct value for the clinician. I then return to the question of the role of theory as a framework for empirical psychoanalytic research, then turn to several of the major methodological issues confronting the psychoanalytic research field.

IMPLICATIONS FOR CLINICAL WORK: THE CRITICAL PERIODS HYPOTHESIS

A particular clinical implication of the formulation of the referential cycle is that the different phases of the cycle call, intrinsically, for different types of therapeutic response. This provides a general framework for timing of interventions, which would, of course, need to be adapted for different cases and different phases of a treatment. I will focus here on the telling of a narrative and the period immediately following this as one type of critical period in the symbolizing process and in the relationship. The computer-measured referential activity (CRA) peaks in all three sessions identify points in the patient's associations where the underlying emotion schemas, activated in the here and now of the relationship, are being "told" in narrative form. Changes in these narratives serve as indicators of underlying structural change. I have provided validation for these claims in the research that has been discussed. The peak indicates that referential connections have been activated. The access to emotion schemas, with their subsymbolic components, has been opened and is being expressed; the emotional wound has been opened sufficiently for treatment to be effective.

The direction of the treatment is significantly affected by the manner in which analyst and patient negotiate this critical phase. The *back-translation* process, in which priming and preparation in the symbolic, verbal system activate the subsymbolic processors, is most likely to be successful following CRA peaks. This back-translation may occur in the form of the patient's own reflection on the meaning of the story that has been told, and may also come in the analyst's verbal communication and in shared reflection by analyst and patient. Substantive interventions, including interpretations, are most likely to have impact at such times, when the patient is moving from inner exploration to a communicative, reflective mode, and has access to both. Other things being equal, interventions are less likely to be effective, may not be understood, or may even impede the patient's flow of associations and reflections at other points in the cycle.

There are several directions that the patient may take following a CRA peak. One story may lead her to another; if left alone, she may be able to follow the path of her emotional connections to deeper levels and to new illuminations, as Freud's patient Elizabeth R. (who is said to have invented free association) wished to do. Patients sometimes decline from an initial CRA peak and move on to another, as Mrs. C. seems to have done in Session 326. Alternatively, the patient may move out of the narrative phase and turn back to reflect on the stories and images that have been retrieved and told with useful results. On the other hand, if she now glimpses emotional meaning that she does not wish to see, she is likely to mobilize defenses of various types, and further exploration may be closed down.

Patients frequently pause following a referential activity (RA) or CRA peak, as Mrs. C. did in many sessions, including those discussed here. (Pausing is not reflected in the graphs, which are based on word count only). Such pausing would be interpreted as a call for turn-switching in normal conversational discourse (Jaffe & Feldstein, 1970). It is likely that both analyst and patient are aware, at least intuitively, that an intervention is expected following a high RA narrative, particularly when it is followed by a pause. The analyst then makes a decision as to whether to intervene or remain silent. He computes (within his own subsymbolic as well as symbolic systems) the direction and momentum of the patient's associations, then determines whether the patient may need support or even a bit of navigation in her further search for what she is trying *not to find,* or if she might better be left alone.

In our empirical work covering several different treatments, we have provided evidence that analysts show increased tendencies to intervene as the patient's CRA declines following such peaks (Baerson, 1993; Dove & Bucci, 1997). Given the regularities of the intervention process that have been observed, the absence of an intervention, when one is expected, is as much an action as an intervention would be. Baerson (1993) has characterized the nonoccurrence of an intervention at times when one is "expected" as a "silence intervention," with particular meaning of its own. Silence may have the effect of turning some patients away from their current direction to search for material that will engage the analyst. In other contexts, silence may encourage autonomous exploration. Silences— or "silence interventions"—may be used to send a message to the patient that certain unconscious manipulations will not succeed and may operate as passing a test, in the terms of Weiss et al. (1986). Silence may also indicate to the patient that others are indeed not responsive to her, as she may have learned in the early—dysfunctional—interactions of her life. The emotional effects of silence must be interpreted individually for each patient and each patient–analyst dyad, and for different periods of the treatment as well.

It is possible that part of the analyst's computation in deciding whether to intervene is based on his own view of what the direction of the patient's associations *ought to be,* rather than what they are. It is obvious that issues of countertransference need to be addressed at this point. Either decision by the analyst following a CRA peak—to remain silent or to intervene—will be experienced by the patient as significant and meaningful, and will enter into her computations of what to say next. The effects of interventions, or failures to intervene, must be seen as particularly powerful in a classical treatment in which each intervention is a noteworthy event. Thus, we can examine the effects of timing, as well as the effects of contents of interventions, and the interaction of these. We have seen variations of these effects in the three sessions studied in the preceding chapter.

In Session 38 of the analysis of Mrs. C., the analyst intervened for the first time in Word Block 8, while the patient was involved in her narrative, indicated by RA rising above the mean; the intervention was a simple clarification question that appeared to facilitate the associative flow. The other substantive interventions in this session occurred at the critical period I have described, following instances of decline from the CRA peaks. The intervention in Word Block 12, a question addressing her feelings, was followed by an increase in emotional tone (ET) and a substantial CRA peak. The next intervention, in Word Block 27, followed the large peak and referred to the analyst's role in her dream. This was not so effective, leading only to increased abstraction (AB) within the brief time left in this session. The timing of the intervention, in terms of our critical period hypothesis, was appropriate; the contents, or the occurrence so near to the end of the session, may have interfered with the potential effect.

In Session 326, the analyst does not respond following the CRA peak and decline that open the session. The patient shows a temporary defensive decline in ET and increase in AB, which constitute a retreat from emotional connections; however, she then seems to recover her connection to emotional experience on her own, moving into the central CRA peak. The analyst's silence may be seen as effective here in that sense. His first interventions, in Word Blocks 16 and 17, follow the second CRA peak and lead to further, moderate CRA increases and to emotional insight.

Subsequent interventions, however, are not so successful, as we have seen. The intervention in Word Block 25 comes at a time when, as our model would suggest, substantive interventions are less likely to be effective and may even be disruptive. The patient has completed a period of emotional insight, has shown an increase in direct emotional expression, indicated by the increase in ET, and is now moving to an increase in CRA. This pattern is indicative of the deepening of access to an emotion schema and the possible beginning of a new cycle. This is a critical period in a different sense, a point at which the patient is turning inward, searching within her own inner experience, perhaps experiencing arousal of subsymbolic somatic and sensory experience, and might better be left alone to continue her search. CRA and ET both decline following this intervention, suggesting that it may have impeded her exploration and, at the least, did not facilitate it.

In Session 726, as in 326, the patient shows a decline from her initial RA level, accompanied by declines in ET and AB and by long pauses, which are not indicated on the graph. The pattern indicates an expectation of a response; her language becomes increasingly tangled, as I have shown. The analyst eventually intervenes at length, in what seems to be an attempt to rescue the patient from her morass, but the interventions are of limited effectiveness, as discussed earlier. The interventions in Word Blocks 20 and 21 do have an effect in activating emotion schemas, although with problematic implications, as I have discussed. The interventions at the close of treatment appear to push her back into an abstract mode.

This discussion has suggested hypotheses concerning points in the treatment where interventions are more or less likely to occur and to be effective in reaching the patient. Interpretations have more connecting power at certain times—for good or ill. The hypotheses are amenable to empirical study; such studies, including investigation of the interaction of content and timing of interventions, and their effects, are part of the research agenda now under way.

INTERPRETATION OF MEASURES: CONSTRUCT VALIDATION AND THE NOMOLOGICAL NETWORK

To analyze the process in a treatment and in a session, including evaluation of the effects of interventions, a wide range of different measures assessing clinical contents, as well as measures of discourse characteristics, need to be applied. The language style measures tell us *where* in the session significant events are occurring. Other content measures, as well as clinical analyses keyed to the linguistic analyses, can then be applied to tell us *what* is happening and help us understand why and how. In the preliminary study reported in Chapter 17, clinical evaluation and a general core conflictual relationship theme (CCRT) formulation, applied to the CRA peaks, were used as indicators of underlying themes. In a systematic process study, the CCRT, in either its tailor-made or standardized versions (Luborsky & Crits-Cristoph, 1990), could be applied to all sessions, with reliability computed among several judges. The new version of the fundamental repetitive and maladaptive emotion structures (FRAMES) measure currently under development by Dahl, based on his emotion theory (Dahl, 1978), might also be applied as an indicator of underlying themes. Measures of the patient's defenses and changes in these in the course of treatment, developed by Perry (1993) and his colleagues, add further clinical information to our understanding of the patient's issues. Content dictionaries, including measures of maternalism and affiliation (Udoff, 1995), and measures of aggression and hostility, have also been developed for evaluation of clinical themes. My colleagues and I are currently carrying out studies applying multiple measures of these types to the case of Mrs. C. and other recorded psychoanalytic treatments, and using statistical means of evaluating intervention effects.

The measures have been developed as operational indicators of internal events such as underlying themes, transference, structural change, and defenses of various types. The central point of the research strategy, which needs to be emphasized here, is that all such events are conceptualized as psychological constructs defined in terms of one another and inferred from observable events within a theoretical context or nomological network. Without a general theoretical framework, the meanings of the operational indicators remain vague and unresolved, and the inferences from these measures are likely to differ in unclear ways from study to study, leading to the ambiguity of findings that has been and remains a major obstacle to research in this field.

The study outlined in Chapter 17 was based on the theoretical framework of multiple coding and the referential cycle. The measures that have been applied to the case of Mrs. C. are interpreted in this context. This does not mean accepting the theory as veridical, but it does mean using it as a set of principles and propositions that may then be supported or disconfirmed. Specific clinical theories may also be developed and built in to the nomological network, and studies carried out to evaluate these.

While the multiple code theory is one such theoretical framework, within which our measures have been interpreted, alternative theories of psychological organization might also be developed by others. The important point is that we need to have a theoretical framework, to use the framework to define the measures, and to use the observations to support or disconfirm the theory.

SAMPLE SELECTION AND ISSUES OF REPLICATION

In Chapter 17, I reported on discourse patterns for a large sample of sessions selected to represent different phases of the treatment of Mrs. C. Using the computer-measured language analysis as a screening device, three sessions representing different discourse patterns and different phases of treatment were selected for more intensive analysis. The computerized procedures enable us to select sessions systematically in this way, rather than relying on the usual methods of selecting generally defined periods of the treatment (such as early, middle, late) and choosing sessions randomly within those phases.

The use of large samples of sessions, selected systematically and studied with reliable and valid techniques, takes us well beyond the level of the clinical case report, and also beyond the single-session or small-sample treatment studies that have previously been the state of the art in the process research field. The excellent research volume edited by Dahl, Kaechele, and Thomae (1988), for example, is based on convergent studies of a single hour of the case of Mrs. C. Similarly, a special issue of *Psychotherapy Research* (1994), edited by Luborsky, Popp, Barber, and Shapiro, covered seven transference-related measures applied to a single interview. The studies by Weiss et al. (1986) and by Jones and Windholz (1990), cited earlier, used large samples of sessions from the case of Mrs. C. but did not look at process within sessions or compare her treatments to others.

Ultimately, systematic process research requires large-sample and multiple-patient designs. To reach conclusions about the case of Mrs. C. and the factors affecting the treatment course, a large number of sessions, beyond the 105 sessions used here, would be required for the overall treatment study, and the intensive process component would need to be considerably increased. The *maternalism* study of Friedman et al. (1994), now under way, covers all sessions during the entire period of Mrs. C.'s pregnancy, from the gestation point (known by inference) to the several postpartum months. Another project will examine the dramatic shift, manifest in a steep decline in ET and general increase in AB that took place early in this treatment and was never reversed.

The study of large samples of sessions is feasible only through use of computerized procedures. In addition to the language style measures illustrated in Chapter 17, computerized content measures are also being developed; these enable automatized evaluation of the expression of particular themes. Computerized measures of the construct of maternalism, reflecting affiliative and nurturant themes, have been developed (Friedman et al., 1994; Udoff, 1995); construction of a measure covering aggression themes is also under way.

No matter how large the selection of sessions from a single case, however, we also need to move on to multiple-case designs, to answer the type of questions with which clinicians and theorists are concerned. For example, following our studies of the pregnancy of Mrs. C., we expect to understand her individual, intrapsychic issues, including her conflictual identification with her mother, and how these issues play out in her pregnancy, expectations of motherhood, and current relationship with her husband, and in the analytic relationship as well. We also expect to examine issues of countertransference in general, and those surrounding the pregnancy in particular, in this dyad. We will, however, not know to what extent the patterns that are identified for this patient and this analyst are specific to them, or generalizable to others, until we find other, parallel cases of pregnancy in analysis that may be studied in a comparable way. The same question arises with respect to any clinical issue. We need to develop a cohort of fully recorded treatments, to screen them using automatized procedures, to select samples of sessions for more intensive study, and to develop the type of replicated single-case designs that are most appropriate for providing the answers we require. An excellent survey of the types of replicated single-case methods that are needed, including quasi-experimental and patient-series designs, has been provided by Fonagy and Moran (1993).

METHODS OF RECORDING:
THE UNCERTAINTY PRINCIPLE

Another major issue that needs to be faced in developing a viable psychoanalytic research agenda is the nature of the recording method itself. A few projects have employed multiple channels of data collection, including video recordings and measurement of physiological indicators such as blood pressure, heart rate, and galvanic skin response, as well as interviews and testing by researchers and clinicians other than the treating analyst (Eisenstein et al., 1994; Horowitz et al., 1993). At the other extreme, clinical case studies have generally relied solely on the analyst's memory, or his session or process notes. The studies of Mrs. C., by ourselves and other researchers, like most psychoanalytic research studies, have used transcripts of audio-recorded sessions. In selecting a recording method, we must make a scientific choice that balances gain or loss of information, on the one hand, against the interpersonal effects of various types of data recording on the other, and we must consider pragmatic issues of feasibility and expense as well.

The use of audio recording, as described in Chapter 17, is now generally accepted in our research. It is nevertheless the case that in all methods of objective recording, that is, all methods other than note taking by the analyst, the problem of intrusion of another observer into the psychoanalytic process must arise. This has been an issue of considerable concern to clinicians and an obstacle to their participation in research. Even those clinicians who support the process research effort are often unwilling to tape-record their own work. Parenthetically, one might perhaps question why recording for research purposes is experienced as intrusive or otherwise unacceptable by many clinicians, while recording for presentation in supervision is generally accepted as standard clinical practice. It seems likely that the supervisory relationship affects the treatment relationship in ways that go well beyond that of a potential research presence. The impact of this powerful clinical interaction *à trois* may not always be considered—even by the same clinicians who are so aware of the potential impact of the research presence.

I think we do need to face the question, from a scientific as well as a professional perspective, of the possible effect of a third participant represented by a recording device, an outside interviewer administering research instruments—or a clinical supervisor—on the interpersonal relationship that is being studied. The researcher, as well as the clinician, does, I believe, need to be concerned as to whether the research treatments that we study are representative of treatments as they are practiced. We know that any psychological measurement has the potential of changing the entity that is being measured to some degree. Analysis is a uniquely sensitive interpersonal domain in which all trivial actions—changing appointments, taking a phone call, being a few minutes late—have emotional meaning that is potentially significant and needs to be explored. In such a setting, we particularly need to know the impact of our measurement procedures; this applies for both participants, not the patient only.

The reliance on audio-recorded and transcribed session material also introduces other types of bias from an opposite perspective. While we generally rely on audio recording as the minimally intrusive (as well as least expensive and most easily managed) research approach, the question then arises as to the extent to which the rich array of human expression can be meaningfully studied when it is reduced to a stream of words. In most cases, our research relies on transcripts rather than the recordings themselves, and thus uses only words printed on a page, even lacking the paralinguistic cues, such as pausing, intonation patterns, and emotive vocalization, that are available when listening to speech. Modern transcribing techniques have incorporated conventions for representing some of these paralinguistic indicators; however, the transcribing can include only a small proportion of the rich overtones and melodies of speech transmission outside of the lexical items themselves.

While considerable emotional information may be lost, there are nevertheless several justifications for studying the words of psychotherapy in isolation from other expressive and interactive cues. The first arises from the characterization of psychoanalysis as the "talking cure." Psychoanalytic theory and practice have given a privileged place to the power of words, the information that is carried in words, and the role of language in the organization of experience. In emphasizing the more general function of *symbolizing*, which goes beyond verbal encoding, and in recognizing mature and complex forms of nonverbal thought that continue to operate and develop throughout life, the multiple code theory raises questions concerning the basic psychoanalytic emphasis on verbalization. Nevertheless, it remains true in the multiple code approach, as in psychoanalytic treatment in general, that language is the primary medium for sharing information. The bidirectional operation of the referential process—connecting inner emotional experience with the shared language code—is the multiple code formulation of the talking cure. From this theoretical perspective, we can study many aspects of the process of expressing emotional experience by studying the characteristics of language, while recognizing that some aspects of emotional expression are likely to be lost. A related justification for reliance on the verbal record is that in the analytic situation, particularly for the patient on the couch, the importance of the transmission of information by facial expression or body movement is considerably reduced.

This brings us to what is perhaps the most commonly cited justification for relying on the verbal record: an assumption concerning the redundancy of human emotional expression. We assume that the meanings that are communicated in facial expression and movement are also expressed, perhaps implicitly or indirectly, in verbal channels. Such redundancy may indeed operate for the majority of cases. There may, however, also be cases in which the emotional information that is communicated in the alternate modalities is different and even contradictory, and the convergence or divergence of information carries a message of its own. We do not, in fact, really know to what extent the general redundancy that is assumed is actually present. Studies need to be done to compare the communication of emotional experience as carried in words and in accompanying paralinguistic indicators, and also in body movement and gesture.

Clinicians may not have been sufficiently concerned about the potential biases that affect the notes they take during or after the session. On the other hand, researchers also need to become more fully aware of the potential biases associated with their recording techniques. The adequacy of verbal transcription as representing the patient's expression and the interactions that occur in a session cannot be assumed but should be investigated. The effects of intrusion of a research presence, even in as minimal a form as a tape recorder, also needs to be assessed. Studies can be done to screen transcribed material for derivatives of the recording process and possible changes in these derivatives as the treatment proceeds; we might also look for derivatives in the analyst's, as in the patient's, speech. Studies can also be done comparing a variety of measures scored by judges for session material gathered under different recording circumstances. In a study by Samstag (reported in Bucci & Miller, 1993), different groups of judges scored the same session material for RA by reading transcripts, listening to audiotapes, or viewing videotapes; systematic differences in RA were found as a function of recording method. Every audio-recorded research treatment now being used as a source of transcribed material could be used as a data source for such comparative studies.

The degree and nature of potential bias in transcripts, as compared to process notes, might also be addressed empirically in studies in which the analyst keeps such notes and audio (or even video) recordings are also made. We could learn to what extent or in what ways the overlooking of some material in session notes is motivated. We might also find that the analyst's notes contain information as to nonverbal behavior—including the style of entering and leaving the office, the nature of movement on the couch, or facial expression and gesture where these can be observed—that colors the material of the session in crucial ways. Studies of all available indicators, including information from the analyst's notes, as well as paralinguistic cues from recordings, in addition to the verbal text, have the potential of building the construct validity of our measures and increasing our understanding of the analytic process.

The conclusion to be drawn is that the choice of recording medium is far from simple. We need to be aware of the effect of measurement on the individuals being observed—analyst as well as patient—and the relationship between them. It was the impression of the analyst observers of a recorded treatment carried out by Franz Alexander (Eisenstein et al., 1994) that the patient, following an initial period of discomfort, appeared to be essentially unaffected by the research setting and to function in a manner comparable to other patients in traditional treatments. The therapist, however, appeared to remain aware of being observed. The judges argued that the therapist's awareness of "performing" was not a significant factor but, if anything, had the effect of increasing his efforts to function effectively. It seems clear that the apparent enhancement of the therapist's performance was, in itself, an indicator of the impact of recording, although apparently with positive rather than negative consequences in their view. We also need to design innovative empirical approaches for evaluation and comparison of recording methods, including investigation of the different types of bias associated with different recording techniques, and the different types of information available with each. The examination of these issues emerges as particularly important in the context of the multiple code theory, with its assumptions concerning the richness and diversity of information in different processing channels.

TREATMENT PROCESS AND TREATMENT OUTCOME

The final issue to be considered here, in the development of a psycho-analytic research agenda, concerns the evaluation of treatment effects. Psychoanalysis, like other therapies, has the goal of alleviating human distress. The special agenda of psychoanalytic treatment is that we do not treat the symptoms but attempt to address the underlying source of distress, to bring about change in the way an individual experiences and structures her interpersonal world. The techniques of treatment need to be evaluated specifically in terms of such psychoanalytic goals. The concepts of the referential cycle, the emotion schemas, and changes in these schemas, all concern inner events. Our process research focuses on development and application of operational indicators of such inner events. Using these empirical tools, we are investigating the basic questions of when and how change occurs in the psychoanalytic process and whether specific curative factors can be identified. We should note that measurement of process, in analytic terms, is intrinsically linked to measurement of outcome. On the one hand, there are mini-outcomes that may be addressed in each phase of the treatment, and even in each session; on the other hand, the process of analytic change is expected to continue well beyond termination, potentially throughout life.

While analysis has its own special treatment goals, ultimately, as practitioners, analysts must also be concerned with standard indicators of treatment effects. The assumption of psychoanalysis is that analytic change will improve one's capacities for adaptive functioning, and will be reflected in improvement in standard measures of well-being, including reduction in symptoms and behavioral change. That expectation cannot be assumed but needs to be tested as well. A full psychoanalytic research agenda needs to show that internal changes are indeed related to changes in health, social adjustment, and quality of life. We would also claim—and need to demonstrate—that the kinds of measurable change that are brought about through psychoanalysis are different from those produced in other treatments—more generalizable, more pervasive, more capable of withstanding life crises, and more likely to persist and develop further after the close of treatment.

Ideally, there should be a general outcome component in every process study, including indicators of external symptomatic and behavioral change, as well as internal structural change. We need to look at the relationship between analytic and symptomatic change, and to look at process factors contributing to good and poor outcomes measured on both levels. In collecting new research treatments, assessment of change should be derived from assessment of the patient, on both levels, at the beginning and end of treatment, including evaluation by clinical judges other than the treating analyst, and also including long-term follow-up of the patient's mental state and life events following termination.

In ongoing work, Luborsky and his colleagues (1996) are developing methods of assessing changes in health–sickness, social adjustment, and related dimensions in archival treatments where change measures are not available, using the contents of early and late sessions. This would potentially allow us to incorporate an outcome component in the process studies of archival treatments, so as to enhance the research potential of these valuable resources.

Small Particles and Large Black Holes

In studying changes in emotion structures and the effects of these, the research agenda of psychoanalysis resembles the agenda confronting theoretical physicists who must find ways of studying very small particles, and also the tasks of astronomers who study very large black holes and related phenomena. The research goals may be somewhat more difficult to achieve in our field than in those but seem realistic nonetheless. Through a collaborative and theory-driven approach applied to the material of the psychoanalytic situation, we can potentially derive data about a human psyche in interaction with others that are available in no other way.

LAST WORDS

1. *The Tower of Babel*

Psychoanalysis is the "talking cure"; our theory retains the psychoanalytic view of the fundamental role of language in the therapeutic process. However, the human information processor is an imperfect device; the new and powerful representational system of language has been overlaid on a set of other representational systems that were previously in place, but without adequate mechanisms for integration of the systems having been developed. From the viewpoint of communicating subjective experience, including emotion, it seems somewhat premature, even misguided, in the grand, evolutionary scheme of things, to have inserted a powerful new system such as language without having also provided a satisfactory means by which connections to other representational formats can be made. Language has the feel of a first-generation computing device—a breakthrough that is very exciting, potentially enormously useful, but expensive, cumbersome, slow and difficult to operate, limited in its application, vulnerable to misuse, and bearing significant risks. It is powerful enough, even in its present primitive form, to drive out other systems, but is perhaps destined to be replaced soon (in the evolutionary order) by better designed and more effective symbolic representational modes.

In the context of psychoanalytic theory, the patient's difficulty in verbalizing emotional experience has been understood as "resistance"—motivated, consciously or unconsciously, to avoid contents that have been warded off. As we can now see, the limitations of the referential process constitute fundamental difficulties in emotional expression, independent of specific factors of resistance or warding off. Language has significant limitations as well as considerable power in facilitating the integration of systems with which psychoanalysis is fundamentally concerned.

The child takes a giant step forward in her cognitive development when she discovers, during the second year of life, that things have names. In the development of emotional communication, with which we are concerned here, there are potentially both gains and losses associated with this advance. On the positive side, the acquisition of language gives the child new ways to understand her world and herself, new entry into the knowledge and meanings of her culture, new ways to share her experience with others, new levels on which to relate. Now the child can tell what she is afraid of or what she wants, to the extent that she is willing to do so, and to the extent that she knows; can listen to someone explain that it is not necessary to be afraid; and can reason with herself as well.

On a deeper level, Dore (discussed in Stern, 1985) has speculated that language functions as a transitional phenomenon, in the sense of Winnicott (1971). The word is given to the child from the outside, but the thought or knowledge to which it will be attached already exists in the child's mind. As Stern says:

> In this sense the word, as a transitional phenomenon . . . occupies a midway position between the infant's subjectivity and the mother's objectivity. . . . It is in this deeper sense that language is a union experience, permitting a new level of mental relatedness through shared meaning. (1985, p. 172)

Unfortunately, language frequently does not work for the sharing of emotional meanings in this way. While language provides a vast new universe in which to relate to others, it also provides an equally vast and fundamentally uncharted universe in which to be alone, *by default or by intent.* As the child will learn, there are many representations of crucial importance in mental, and particularly in emotional, life for which words cannot be found. However, it is not only failure by default—the intrinsic difficulty of expressing subsymbolic experience in words—but also failure by intent, which interferes with verbal communication of emotion. Language is the medium that humans invented and over which we have the most intentional control; it is also the medium most vulnerable to intentional misuse. Language can be used to disguise and distort feelings as well as to communicate them. No other species has developed a communicative mode that can be used in the service of deliberate obfuscation and dissociation in this way.

The redeeming feature of this problematic psychic organization is that the inclusion of language gives the human information processor the power to redesign itself. The postulated Designer–Controller of the system was apparently aware of this power, as indicated by His/Her several attempts to limit language and its spread:

> Now listen: all the earth uses one tongue, one and the same words. Watch: they journey from the east, arrive at a valley in the land of Sumer, settle there.
>
> "We can bring ourselves together," they said, "like stone on stone, use brick for stone: bake it until hard." For mortar they heated bitumen.
>
> "If we bring ourselves together," they said, "we can build a city and tower, its top touching the sky—to arrive at fame. Without a name we're unbound, scattered over the face of the earth."
>
> Yahweh came down to watch the city and tower the sons of man were bound to build. "They are one people, with the same tongue," said Yahweh. "They conceive this between them, and it leads up until no boundary exists to what they will touch. Between us, let's descend, baffle their tongue until each is scatterbrain to his friend."
>
> From there Yahweh scattered them over the whole face of earth; the city there came unbound. (Rosenberg & Bloom, 1990, p. 73)

The metaphor of speech as performing binding functions, which is pervasive in this passage, is retained explicitly in the psychoanalytic account of the secondary process. In Vygotsky's (1934) seminal formulation, the binding of thought and speech is represented in the psychological construct of "word meaning"; in our extension of this formulation, we have introduced the construct of "emotional meaning," the linking of emotion, thought, and word. The danger that development of one's own language will loosen the control of another's authority—past or present, external or internalized—exists alongside of the powerful potential of language for collaborative therapeutic work, facilitating connection to the other and contributing to organization of oneself. The analyst, in contrast to the pathological parent, needs to endure and foster his patient's separation, connectedness, and growth.

2. The Dead Man's Tale

Remember that what you are told is really three-fold; shaped
by the teller, reshaped by the listener, concealed from both by
the dead man of the tale.
  —VLADIMIR NABOKOV *(The Real Life of Sebastian Knight)*

In pathology, the dreaded affect is dissociated from the symbols that evoke
it, then may be covered over with new symbols in a failed attempt at repair.
Dead men are materially inert but, like other symbols, have enormous
power, beyond what is intended. Symbols can be the subject of a tale, can
express a meaning, or can conceal one. The dead man of the tale has
different meanings at different times and for different people. These
meanings, while shifting, are real nonetheless.

The tales that have been concealed are told in the free association.
They are shaped by the teller through mapping of the emotion schemas—
including failed and dissociated schemas—onto language. In contrast to
Schafer's (1980) position, the shape of the narratives is strictly constrained. The dreaded happenings, forbidden desires, and conflicting
expectations, which are verbalized in the free association, are prototypes
(traces or ghosts) of the repeated episodes of the patient's life, as these
are registered in the emotion schemas. They are represented in the
organized formats of the subsymbolic and symbolic systems, to varying
degrees, prior to their telling, but may not yet have been acknowledged
in verbal form.

In treatment, the tales are reshaped by the listener and the teller
together. Reconstruction in both senses—retrieval and rebuilding—can

occur. The patient can then arrive at an emotional insight that is at the same time something he "never thought of before"—and something he "knew all along." He may indeed have "known it all along"—but in the nonverbal system only. It becomes a new tale when the referential connections have been built.

The development of the referential process proceeds interactively with the change in the emotion structures themselves. Emotion categories and emotion prototypes develop initially, in the first relationships of life, without intervention by language. To bring about change in the emotion schemas, new symbols and new connections are required. Psychoanalysis provides a *second chance* to symbolize one's emotion structures in the context of a relationship, to reshape one's schemas and one's tales, and to claim them as one's own. In contrast to feelings, and in contrast to external events, symbols are what humans are able to control and direct.

Psychoanalysis is about the building of autonomy. In psychoanalysis, the one who brings the tale, and shares it, then owns the symbol in a special way. The owning of the symbol, rather than being haunted by it, is the only genuine autonomy one can achieve. Optimally, in psychoanalysis, the tale is told rather than concealed; through telling and listening, the tale comes alive and takes a new form.

References

Abraham, A., & Mathai, K. V. (1983). The effect of right temporal lobe lesions on matching smells. *Neuropsychologia, 21,* 277–281.

Albiniak, B. A., & Powell, D. A. (1981). Peripheral autonomic mechanisms and Pavlovian conditioning in the rabbit (*Oryctolagus cuniculis*). *Journal of Comparative Physiology and Psychology, 94,* 1101–1113.

Anderson, J. R. (1978). Arguments concerning representations for mental imagery. *Psychological Review, 85,* 249–277.

Anderson, J. R. (1983). *The architecture of cognition.* Cambridge, MA: Harvard University Press.

Antrobus, J. (1991). Dreaming: Cognitive processes during cortical activation and high afferent thresholds. *Psychological Review, 98,* 96–121.

Arlow, J. A. (1953). Masturbation and symptom formation. *Journal of the American Psychoanalytic Association, 1,* 45–58.

Arlow, J. A. (1955). Notes on oral symbolism. *Psychoanalytic Quarterly, 24,* 63–74.

Arlow, J. A. (1969). Unconscious fantasy and disturbances of conscious experience. *Psychoanalytic Quarterly, 38,* 1–27.

Arlow, J. A. (1975). The structural hypothesis: Theoretical considerations. *Psychoanalytic Quarterly, 44,* 509–525.

Arlow, J. A. (1979). The genesis of interpretation. *Journal of the American Psychoanalytic Association, 27,* 193–206.

Arlow, J. A., & Brenner, C. (1964). *Psychoanalytic concepts and the structural theory.* New York: International Universities Press.

Aserinsky, E., & Kleitman, N. (1953). Regularly occurring periods of ocular motility and concomitant phenomena during sleep. *Science, 118,* 361–375.

Baars, B. (1986). *The cognitive revolution in psychology.* New York: Guilford Press.

Bachevalier, J., & Mishkin, M. (1984). An early and a late developing system for learning and retention in infant monkeys. *Behavioral Neuroscience, 98,* 770–778.

Baddeley, A. D. (1986). *Working memory.* Oxford, UK: Clarendon Press.

Baerson, A. (1993, December). *The effect of the patient's referential activity on the analyst's intervention.* Paper presented at the meeting of the American Psychoanalytic Association, New York.

Bargh, J. A. (1989). Conditional automaticity: Varieties of automatic influence in social perception and cognition. In J. S. Uleman & J. A. Bargh (Eds.), *Unintended thought* (pp. 3–51). New York: Guilford Press.

Bartlett, F. C. (1932). *Remembering: A study in social psychology.* Cambridge, UK: Cambridge University Press.

Baudelaire, C. (1857). *Les fleurs du mal* (R. Howard, Trans.). Boston: David R. Godine, 1982.

Bauer, R. M. (1984). Autonomic recognition of names and faces in prosopagnosia: A neuropsychological application of the guilty knowledge test. *Neuropsychologia, 22,* 457–469.

Beebe, B., & Lachmann, F. (1988). The contribution of mother–infant mutual influence to the origins of self and object representations. *Psychoanalytic Psychology, 5,* 305–337.

Beres, D. (1962). The unconscious fantasy. *Psychoanalytic Quarterly, 31,* 309–328.

Bergin, A. E., & Strupp, H. H. (1972). *Changing frontiers in the science of psychotherapy.* Chicago: Aldine–Atherton.

Berlin, B., & Kay, P. (1969). *Basic color terms: Their universality and evolution.* Berkeley: University of California Press.

Biederman, I., & Cooper, E. (1992). Size invariance in visual object priming. *Journal of Experimental Psychology: Human Perception and Performance, 18,* 121–133.

Bisiach, E., & Luzzatti, C. (1978). Unilateral neglect of representational space. *Cortex, 14,* 129–133.

Bogen, J. E. (1969). The other side of the brain: II. An appositional mind. *Bulletin of the Los Angeles Neurological Societies, 34*(3), 135–162.

Bornstein, M. (1979). Perceptual development: Stability and change in feature perception. In M. Bornstein & W. Kessen (Eds.), *Psychological development from infancy: Image to intention* (pp. 37–81). Hillsdale, NJ: Erlbaum.

Bornstein, M. (1985). Infant into adult: Unity to diversity in the development of visual categorization. In J. Mehler & R. Fox (Eds.), *Neonate cognition* (pp. 115–138). Hillsdale, NJ: Erlbaum.

Bowen, J. (1988). The relationship between imagery and referential activity (Doctoral dissertation, Adelphi University, 1987). *Dissertation Abstracts International, 48*(9B), 2776.

Bower, G. H. (1981). Mood and memory. *American Psychologist, 36,* 129–148.

Bransford, J. D., & Franks, J. J. (1971). The abstraction of linguistic ideas. *Cognitive Psychology, 2,* 331–350.

Brenner, C. (1953). An addendum to Freud's theory of anxiety. *International Journal of Psycho-Analysis, 34,* 18–24.

Brenner, C. (1980). Metapsychology and psychoanalytic theory. *Psychoanalytic Quarterly, 49,* 189–214.

Brenner, C. (1992). The structural theory and clinical practice. *Journal of Clinical Psychoanalysis, 1,* 369–380.

Broadbent, D. E. (1958). *Perception and communication.* New York: Pergamon Press.

Brodal, A. (1982). *Neurological anatomy.* New York: Oxford University Press.

Brooks, D. N., & Baddeley, A. D. (1976). What can amnesic patients learn? *Neuropsychologia, 14,* 111–122.

Brooks, L. R. (1970). An extension of the conflict between visualization and reading. *Quarterly Journal of Experimental Psychology, 22,* 91–96.

Brown, R., & McNeill, D. (1966). The tip of the tongue phenomenon. *Journal of Verbal Learning and Verbal Behavior, 5,* 325–337.

Brugman, C. M. (1988). *The story of over: Polysemy, semantics, and the structure of the lexicon.* New York: Garland.

Bruner, J. S. (1966). On cognitive growth. In J. S. Bruner, R. S. Oliver, & P. M. Greenfield (Eds.), *Studies in cognitive growth* (pp. 1–67). New York: Wiley.

Bucci, W. (1984). Linking words and things: Basic processes and individual variation. *Cognition, 17,* 137–153.

Bucci, W. (1985). Dual coding: A cognitive model for psychoanalytic research. *Journal of the American Psychoanalytic Association, 33,* 571–607.

Bucci, W. (1988). Converging evidence for emotion structures: Theory and method. In H. Dahl, H. Kaechele, & H. Thomae (Eds.), *Psychoanalytic process research strategies* (pp. 29–50). New York: Springer-Verlag.

Bucci, W. (1989). A reconstruction of Freud's tally argument: A program for psychoanalytic research. *Psychoanalytic Inquiry, 9,* 249–281.

Bucci, W. (1993). The development of emotional meaning in free association. In A. Wilson & J. E. Gedo (Eds.), *Hierarchical concepts in psychoanalysis: Theory, research, and clinical practice* (pp. 3–47). New York: Guilford Press.

Bucci, W. (1995). The power of the narrative: A multiple code account. In J. W. Pennebaker (Ed.), *Emotion, disclosure and health* (pp. 71–92). Washington, DC: American Psychological Association.

Bucci, W. (1997). Empirical studies of "good" and troubled hours: A multiple code interpretation. *Journal of the American Psychoanalytic Association, 45,* 1–34.

Bucci, W. (in press). Emotion structures, narrative structures and the CCRT. In L. Luborsky, H. Kaechele, R. Dahlbender, & L. Diguer (Eds.), *The CCRT method and its discoveries.*

Bucci, W., & Freedman, N. (1978). Language and hand: The dimension of referential competence. *Journal of Personality, 46,* 594–622.

Bucci, W., & Freedman, N. (1981). The language of depression. *Bulletin of the Menninger Clinic, 45,* 334–358.

Bucci, W., Kabasakalian-McKay, R., & the RA Research Group. (1992). *Instructions for scoring referential activity (RA) in transcripts of spoken narrative texts.* Ulm, Germany: Ulmer Textbank.

Bucci, W., & Miller, N. (1993). Primary process analogue: The referential activity (RA) measure. In N. Miller, L. Luborsky, J. Barber, & J. Docherty (Eds.), *Psychodynamic treatment research* (pp. 387–406). New York: Basic Books.

Buck, R. (1988). *Human motivation and emotion.* New York: Wiley.

Burley, W. J. (1975). *Wycliffe and the pea-green boat.* London: Victor Gollancz.

Cahill, L., Prins, B., Weber, M., & McGaugh, J. L. (1994). Beta-adrenergic activation and memory for emotional events. *Nature, 371,* 702–704.

Cain, W. S., & Krause, R. J. (1979). Olfactory testing: Rules for odor identification. *Neurological Research, 1,* 1–9.

Campbell, I. M., & Gregson, R. A. M. (1972). Olfactory short-term memory in normal, schizophrenic and brain-damaged cases. *Australian Journal of Psychology, 24,* 179–185.

Campos, J., & Stenberg, C. (1980). Perception of appraisal and emotion: The onset of social referencing. In M. E. Lamb & L. Sherrod (Eds.), *Infant social cognition.* Hillsdale, NJ: Erlbaum.

Cannon, W. B. (1927). The James–Lange theory of emotions: A critical examination and an alternative theory. *American Journal of Psychology, 39,* 106–124.

Chase, W. G., & Clark, H. H. (1972). Mental operations in the comparison of sentences and pictures. In L. W. Gregg (Ed.), *Cognition in learning and memory* (pp. 205–232). New York: Wiley.

Chomsky, N. (1957). *Syntactic structures.* The Hague: Mouton & Co.

Chomsky, N. (1965). *Aspects of the theory of syntax.* Cambridge, MA: MIT Press.

Claparède, E. (1911). Reconnaissance et moiité [Recognition and me-ness]. In D. Rapaport (Ed.), *Organization and pathology of thought* (pp. 58–75). New York: Columbia University Press, 1951. (Reprinted from *Archives de Psychologie, 11,* 79–90)

Clark, E. V. (1977). Strategies and the mapping problem in first language acquisition. In J. Macnamara (Ed.), *Language learning and thought* (pp. 147–168). San Diego, CA: Academic Press.

Cohen, N. J. (1984). Preserved learning capacity in amnesia: Evidence for multiple memory systems. In L. R. Squire & N. Butters (Eds.), *Neuropsychology of memory* (pp. 83–103). New York: Guilford Press.

Cohen, N. J., & Squire, L. R. (1980). Preserved learning and retention of pattern-analyzing skill in amnesia: Dissociation of knowing how and knowing that. *Science, 210,* 207–209.

Cooper, L. A., Schacter, D. L., Ballestros, S., & Moore, C. (1992). Priming and recognition of transformed three-dimensional objects: Effects of size and reflection. *Journal of Experimental Psychology: Learning, Memory and Cognition, 18,* 43–57.

Corballis, M. C. (1989). Laterality and human evolution. *Psychological Review, 96,* 492–505.

Dahl, H. (1978). A new psychoanalytic model of motivation: Emotions as appetites and messages. *Psychoanalysis and Contemporary Thought, 1,* 373–408.

Dahl, H. (1988). Frames of mind. In H. Dahl, H. Kaechele, & H. Thomae (Eds.), *Psychoanalytic process research strategies* (pp. 51–66). New York: Springer-Verlag.

Dahl, H., Kaechele, H., & Thomae, H. (Eds.). (1988). *Psychoanalytic process research strategies.* New York: Springer-Verlag.

Davidson, R. J. (1984). Affect, cognition and hemispheric specialization. In C. E. Izard, J. Kagan, & R. Zajonc (Eds.), *Emotions, cognition and behavior* (pp. 320–365). Cambridge, UK: Cambridge University Press.

Davidson, R. J., & Schwartz, G. E. (1977). Brain mechanisms subserving self-generated imagery: Electrophysiological specificity and patterning. *Psychophysiology, 14,* 598–601.

DeCasper, A., & Carstens, A. (1980). Contingencies of stimulation: Effects on learning and emotion in neonates. *Infant Behavior and Development, 4,* 19–36.

DeCasper, A., & Fifer, W. (1980). Of human bonding: Newborns prefer their mothers' voices. *Science, 208,* 1174.

DeCasper, A., & Spence, M. (1986). Prenatal maternal speech influences newborns' perceptions of speech sounds. *Infant Behavior and Development, 9,* 133–150.

Deleval, J., De Mol, J., & Noterman, J. (1983). La perte des images souvenirs. *Acta Neurologica Belgica, 83,* 61–79.

Denis, M. (1975). *Représentation imagée et activité de mémorisation.* Paris: Editions du CNRS.

Derogatis, L. R. (1983). *SCL-90: Administration, scoring and procedures manual for the revised version.* Baltimore: Clinical Psychometric Research.

Descartes, R. (1650). *Philosophical works* (E. S. Haldane & G. R. T. Pross, Trans.). Cambridge, UK: Cambridge University Press, 1931.

Desimone, R., Albright, T. D., Gross, C. G., & Bruce, C. J. (1984). Stimulus-selective properties of inferior temporal neurons in the macaque. *Journal of Neuroscience, 4,* 2051–2062.

Dodd, M., & Bucci, W. (1987). The relation of cognition and affect in the orientation process. *Cognition, 27,* 53–71.

Dove, K., & Bucci, W. (1997). *Timing and contents of analytic intervention in the referential cycle.* Paper presented at the meeting of the Society for Psychotherapy Research, Geilo, Norway.

Downer, J. D. C. (1961). Changes in visual gnostic function and emotional behavior following unilateral temporal lobe damage in the split-brain monkey. *Nature, 191,* 50–51.

Dyer, M. (1988). The promise and problems of connectionism. *Behavioral and Brain Sciences, 11,* 32–33.

Eagle, M. N. (1984). *Recent developments in psychoanalysis: A critical evaluation.* New York: McGraw-Hill.

Edelman, G. M. (1989). *The remembered present: A biological theory of consciousness.* New York: Basic Books.

Edelson, M. (1983). Is testing psychoanalytic hypotheses in the psychoanalytic situation really impossible? *Psychoanalytic Study of the Child, 38,* 61–109.

Eimas, P. D. (1975). Speech perception in early infancy. In L. B. Cohen & P. Salapatek (Eds.), *Infant perception: From sensation to cognition* (Vol. 2, pp. 193–231). New York: Academic Press.

Eimas, P. D., Siqueland, E. R., Jusczyk, P., & Vigorito, J. (1971). Speech perception in infants. *Science, 171,* 303–306.

Eisenstein, S., Levy, N. A., & Marmor, J. (1994). *The dyadic transaction: An investigation into the nature of the psychotherapeutic process.* New Brunswick, NJ: Transaction.

Ekman, P. (1984). Expression and the nature of emotion. In K. R. Scherer & P. Ekman (Eds.), *Approaches to emotion* (pp. 319–343). Hillsdale, NJ: Erlbaum.

Ellsworth, P. C. (1994). William James and emotion: Is a century of fame worth a century of misunderstanding? *Psychological Review, 101,* 222–229.

Emde, R. N. (1983, March). *The affective core.* Paper presented at the Second World Congress of Infant Psychiatry, Cannes, France.

Emde, R. N., Klingman, D. H., Reich, J. H., & Wade, J. D. (1978). Emotional expression in infancy: I. Initial studies of social signaling and an emergent model. In M. Lewis & L. Rosenblum (Eds.), *The development of affect* (pp. 125–148). New York: Plenum Press.

Engelkamp, J. (1986). Motor programs as part of the meaning of verbal items. In I. Kurcz, G. W. Shugar, & J. H. Danks (Eds.), *Knowledge and language* (pp. 115–138). Amsterdam: North-Holland.

Engen, T. (1982). *The perception of odors.* New York: Academic Press.

Engen, T. (1987). Remembering odors and their names. *American Scientist, 75,* 497–503.

Engen, T., Kuisma, J. E., & Eimas, P. D. (1973). Short-term memory of odors. *Journal of Experimental Psychology, 99,* 222–225.

Erdelyi, M. H. (1985). *Psychoanalysis: Freud's cognitive psychology.* New York: Freeman.

Erikson, E. H. (1954). The dream specimen of psychoanalysis. *Journal of the American Psychoanalytic Association, 2,* 5–56.

Eskanazi, B., Cain, W. S., Novelly, R. A., & Mattson, R. (1986). Odor perception in temporal lobe epilepsy patients with and without temporal lobectomy. *Neuropsychologia, 24,* 553–562.

Fagan, J. F. (1974). Infant recognition memory: The effects of length of familiarization and type of discrimination task. *Child Development, 45,* 351–356.

Fairbairn, W. R. D. (1954). *An object-relations theory of the personality.* New York: Basic Books.

Fantz, R. L. (1964). Visual experience in infants: Decreased attention to familiar patterns relative to novel ones. *Science, 146,* 668–670.

Fantz, R., Fagan, J., & Miranda, S. (1975). Early visual selectivity. In I. Cohen & P. Salapatek (Eds.), *Infant perception: From sensation to cognition* (Vol. 1, pp. 249–346). New York: Academic Press.

Farah, M. J. (1984). The neurological basis of mental imagery: A componential analysis. *Cognition, 18,* 245–272.

Farah, M. J. (1988). Is visual imagery really visual? Overlooked evidence from neuropsychology. *Psychological Review, 95,* 307–317.

Farah, M. J. (1991). Patterns of co-occurrence among the associative agnosias: Implications for visual object representation. *Cognitive Neuropsychology, 8,* 1–19.

Feigl, H. (1956). Some major issues and developments in the philosophy of science of logical empiricism. In H. Feigl & M. Scriven (Eds.), *The foundations of science and the concepts of psychology and psychoanalysis* (pp. 3–37). Minneapolis: University of Minnesota Press.

Fenichel, O. (1945). *The psychoanalytic theory of neurosis.* New York: Norton.

Finke, R. A., & Kosslyn, S. M. (1980). Mental imagery acuity in the peripheral visual field. *Journal of Experimental Psychology: Human Perception and Performance, 6,* 126–139.

Finke, R. A., & Schmidt, M. J. (1978). The quantitative measure of pattern representation in images using orientation-specific color aftereffects. *Perception and Psychophysics, 23,* 515–520.

Fodor, J. A. (1983). *Modularity of mind.* Cambridge, MA: MIT Press.

Fodor, J. A., & Pylyshyn, Z. W. (1988). Connectionism and cognitive architecture: A critical analysis. *Cognition, 28,* 3–71.

Foley, R. (1987). Hominid species and stone-tool assemblages. *Antiquity, 61,* 380–392.

Fonagy, P., & Moran, G. (1993). Selecting single case research designs for clinicians. In N. E. Miller, L. Luborsky, J. P. Barber, & J. P. Docherty (Eds.), *Psychodynamic treatment research: A handbook for clinical practice* (pp. 62–95). New York: Basic Books.

Franco, L., & Sperry, R. W. (1977). Hemisphere lateralization for cognitive processing of geometry. *Neuropsychologia, 15,* 107–114.

Fretter, P., Bucci, W., Broitman, J., Silberschatz, G., & Curtis, J. (1994). How the patient's plan relates to the concept of transference. *Psychotherapy Research, 4,* 56–70.

Freud, S. (1895a). Project for a scientific psychology. *Standard Edition, 1,* 295–391. London: Hogarth Press, 1966.

Freud, S. (1895b). Studies on hysteria. *Standard Edition, 2,* 3–305. London, Hogarth Press, 1955.

Freud, S. (1900). The interpretation of dreams. *Standard Edition, 4 & 5.* London: Hogarth Press, 1953.

Freud, S. (1912). The dynamics of the transference. *Standard Edition, 12,* 99–108. London: Hogarth Press, 1958.

Freud, S. (1915). The unconscious. *Standard Edition, 14,* 166–215. London: Hogarth Press, 1957.

Freud, S. (1916–1917). Introductory lectures on psycho-analysis. *Standard Edition, 15 & 16.* London: Hogarth Press, 1963.

Freud, S. (1923). The ego and the id. *Standard Edition, 18,* 12–66. London: Hogarth Press, 1961.

Freud, S. (1932). Preface to the third (revised) English edition of *The interpretation of dreams. Standard Edition, 4,* xxvii–xxviii. London: Hogarth Press, 1953.

Freud, S. (1933). New introductory lectures on psycho-analysis. *Standard Edition, 22,* 1–182. London: Hogarth Press, 1964.

Freud, S. (1937a). Analysis terminable and interminable. *Standard Edition, 23,* 216–253. London: Hogarth Press, 1964.

Freud, S. (1937b). Constructions in analysis. *Standard Edition, 23,* 255–269. London: Hogarth Press, 1964.

Freud, S. (1940). An outline of psycho-analysis. *Standard Edition, 23,* 144–207. London: Hogarth Press, 1964.

Freud, S. (1954). *The origins of psycho-analysis: Letters to Wilhelm Fliess, drafts and notes: 1887–1902* (M. Bonaparte, A. Freud, & E. Kris, Eds.). New York: Basic Books.

Friedman, R., Udoff, A., & Bucci, W. (1994, May). *Maternalism: A new view of female sexuality.* Paper presented at the annual meeting of the American Academy of Psychoanalysis, Philadelphia.

Galin, D. (1974). Implications for psychiatry of left and right cerebral specialization: A neurophysiological context for unconscious processes. *Archives of General Psychiatry, 30,* 572–583.

Gardner, H. (1983). *Frames of mind: The theory of multiple intelligences.* New York: Basic Books.

Gardner, R. A., & Gardner, B. T. (1969). Teaching sign language to a chimpanzee. *Science, 165,* 664–672.

Gazzaniga, M. S. (1983). Right-hemisphere language following brain bisection: A 20-year perspective. *American Psychologist, 38,* 525–537.

Gazzaniga, M. S. (1985). *The social brain.* New York: Basic Books.

Gazzaniga, M. S. (1988). The dynamics of cerebral specialization and modular interactions. In L. Weiskrantz (Ed.), *Thought without language* (pp. 430–450). Oxford, UK: Clarendon Press.

Gazzaniga, M. S., & LeDoux, J. E. (1978). *The integrated mind.* New York: Plenum Press.

Gazzaniga, M. S., & Smylie, C. S. (1984). Dissociation of language and cognition: A psychological profile of two disconnected right hemispheres. *Brain, 107,* 145–153.

Gedo, J. E. (1995). Working through as metaphor and as a modality of treatment. *Journal of the American Psychoanalytic Association, 43,* 339–356.

Gesteland, R. C. (1986). Speculations on receptor cells as analyzers and filters. *Experientia, 42,* 287–291.

Gill, M. M. (1967). The primary process. In R. R. Holt (Ed.), *Motives and thought: Psychoanalytic essays in honor of David Rapaport* (pp. 259–298). New York: International Universities Press.

Gill, M. M. (1976). Metapsychology is not psychology. In M. M. Gill & P. S. Holzman (Eds.), Psychology versus metapsychology: Psychoanalytic essays in memory of George S. Klein. *Psychological Issues, 9*(Monograph No. 36), 71–105.

Gill, M. M., & Holzman, P. S. (Eds.). (1976). *Psychology versus metapsychology.* New York: International Universities Press.

Goldberger, M. (1995). Commentary [to Gedo, J. (1995), Working through as metaphor and as a modality of treatment]. *Journal of the American Psychoanalytic Association, 43,* 360–365.

Goldenberg, G., Podreka, I., Steiner, M., & Willmes, K. (1987). Patterns of regional cortical blood flow related to memorizing of high and low imagery words: An emission computer tomography study. *Neuropsychologia, 25,* 473–486.

Greco, C., Hayne, H., & Rovee-Collier, C. (1990). Roles of function, reminding, and variability in categorization by 3-month-old infants. *Journal of Experimental Psychology: Learning, Memory, and Cognition, 16,* 617–633.

Grossi, D., Orsini, A., & Modafferi, A. (1986). Visuoimaginal constructional apraxia: On a case of selective deficit of imagery. *Brain and Cognition, 5,* 255–267.

Grossman, W. I., & Stewart, W. A. (1976). Penis envy: From childhood wish to developmental metaphor. *Journal of the American Psychoanalytic Association, 24,* 193–212.

Grünbaum, A. (1984). *The foundations of psychoanalysis.* Berkeley: University of California Press.

Hadamard, J. (1949). *An essay on the psychology of invention in the mathematical field.* Princeton, NJ: Princeton University Press.

Halgren, E. (1976). Activity of human hippocampal formation and amygdala neurons during olfaction, memory, movement, and other behaviors (Doctoral dissertation, UCLA). *Dissertation Abstracts International, 37,* 1956B. (University Microfilms No. 76-22, 194)

Hartmann, H. (1950). Comments on the psychoanalytic theory of the ego. *Psychoanalytic Study of the Child, 5,* 74–96.

Hawking, S. W. (1988). *A brief history of time: From the big bang to black holes.* New York: Bantam Books.

Henke, P. G. (1982). Telencephalic limbic system and experimental gastric pathology: A review. *Neuroscience and Biobehavior Reviews, 6,* 381–390.

Henning, H. (1916). *Der Geruch [Smell]* (rev. ed.). Leipzig, Germany: Barth.

Hewett, C. (1977). Viewing control structures as patterns of passing messages. *The Artificial Intelligence Journal, 8,* 232–264.

Hillerman, T. (1989). *Talking God.* New York: Harper & Row.

Hillis, D. (1985). *The connection machine.* Cambridge, MA: MIT Press.

Hinton, G. E. (1984). Parallel computations for controlling an arm. *Journal of Motor Behavior, 16,* 171–194.

Hirsch, R. (1974). The hippocampus and contextual retrieval of information from memory. *Behavioral Biology, 12,* 421–444.

Hirsch, R. (1980). The hippocampus, conditional operations, and cognition. *Physiological Psychology, 8,* 175–182.

Hirsch, R., & Krajden, J. (1982). The hippocampus and the expression of knowledge. In R. L. Isaacson & N. E. Spear (Eds.), *The expression of knowledge* (pp. 213–241). New York: Plenum Press.

Hobson, J. A. (1988). *The dreaming brain.* New York: Basic Books.

Hobson, J. A., Lydic, R., & Baghdoyan, H. A. (1986). Evolving concepts of sleep cycle generation: From brain centers to neuronal populations. *Behavioral and Brain Sciences, 9,* 371–448.

Hobson, J. A., & McCarley, R. W. (1977). The brain as a dream state generator: An activation-synthesis hypothesis of the dream process. *American Journal of Psychiatry, 134,* 1335–1348.

Hoffman, I. Z., & Gill, M. M. (1988). A scheme for coding the patient's experience of the relationship with the therapist (PERT): Some applications, extensions, and comparisons. In H. Dahl, H. Kaechele, & H. Thomae (Eds.), *Psychoanalytic process research strategies* (pp. 67–98). New York: Springer-Verlag.

Holt, R. R. (1962). A critical examination of Freud's concept of bound versus free cathexis. In R. R. Holt, *Freud reappraised: A fresh look at psychoanalytic theory* (pp. 71–113). New York: Guilford Press, 1989.

Holt, R. R. (1965). A review of some of Freud's biological assumptions and their influence on his theories. In R. R. Holt, *Freud reappraised: A fresh look at psychoanalytic theory* (pp. 114–140). New York: Guilford Press, 1989.

Holt, R. R. (1966). Measuring libidinal and aggressive motives and their controls by means of the Rorschach test. In D. Levine (Ed.), *Nebraska Symposium on Motivation* (Vol. 14, pp. 1–47). Lincoln: University of Nebraska Press.

Holt, R. R. (1967a). Beyond vitalism and mechanism: Freud's concept of psychic energy. In R. R. Holt, *Freud reappraised: A fresh look at psychoanalytic theory* (pp. 141–168). New York: Guilford Press, 1989.

Holt, R. R. (1967b). The development of the primary process: A structural view. In R. R. Holt, *Freud reappraised: A fresh look at psychoanalytic theory* (pp. 253–279). New York: Guilford Press, 1989.

Holt, R. R. (1976a). Drive or wish? A reconsideration of the psychoanalytic theory of motivation. In M. M. Gill & P. S. Holzman (Eds.), Psychology versus metapsychology: Psychoanalytic essays in memory of George S. Klein. *Psychological Issues, 9*(Monograph No. 36), 158–197.

Holt, R. R. (1976b). The present status of Freud's theory of the primary process. In R. R. Holt, *Freud reappraised: A fresh look at psychoanalytic theory* (pp. 280–301). New York: Guilford Press, 1989.

Holt, R. R. (1985). The current status of psychoanalytic theory. In R. R. Holt, *Freud reappraised: A fresh look at psychoanalytic theory* (pp. 324–344). New York: Guilford Press, 1989.

Holt, R. R. (1989). *Freud reappraised: A fresh look at psychoanalytic theory.* New York: Guilford Press.

Holtzman, J. D., Sidtis, J. J., Volpe, B. T., Wilson, D. H., & Gazzaniga, M. S. (1981). Dissociation of spatial information for stimulus localization and the control of attention. *Brain, 104,* 861–862.

Home, J. J. (1966). The concept of mind. *International Journal of Psycho-Analysis, 47,* 42–49.

Honig, W. K. (1978). Studies of working memory in the pigeon. In S. H. Hulse, H. Fowler, & W. K. Honig (Eds.), *Cognitive processes in animal behavior* (pp. 211–248). Hillsdale, NJ: Erlbaum.

Hoppe, K. D. (1977). Split brains and psychoanalysis. *Psychoanalytic Quarterly, 46,* 220–244.

Horel, J. A., & Keating, E. G. (1969). Partial Klüver–Bucy syndrome produced by cortical disconnection. *Brain Research, 16,* 281–284.

Horowitz, M. J., Marmar, C., Krupnick, J., Wilner, N., Kaltreider, N., & Wallerstein, R. (1984). *Personality styles and brief psychotherapy.* New York: Basic Books.

Horowitz, M. J., Stinson, C., Curtis, D., Ewert, M., Redington, D., Singer, J., Bucci, W., Mergenthaler, E., Milbrath, C., & Hartley, D. (1993). Topics and signs: Defensive control of emotional expression. *Journal of Consulting and Clinical Psychology, 61,* 421–430.

Hull, C. L. (1943). *Principles of behavior.* New York: Appleton-Century-Crofts.

Hull, J. (1990). *Attunement and the rhythm of dialogue in psychotherapy: I. Empirical findings.* Paper presented at annual conference of the Society for Psychotherapy Research, Wintergreen, WV.

Inhelder, B., & Piaget, J. (1958). *The growth of logical thinking.* New York: Basic Books.

Isakower, O. (1938). A contribution to the patho-psychology of phenomena associated with falling asleep. *International Journal of Psycho-Analysis, 19,* 331–447.

Iwata, J., LeDoux, J. E., Meeley, M. P., & Arneric, J. (1986). Intrinsic neurons in the amygdaloid field projected to by the medial geniculate body mediate emotional responses conditioned to acoustic stimuli. *Brain Research, 383*(1–2), 195–214.

Izard, C. (1977). *Human emotions.* New York: Plenum Press.

Jacobs, W. J., & Nadel, L. (1985). Stress induced recovery of fears and phobias. *Psychological Review, 92,* 512–531.

Jacobson, E. (1964). *The self and the object world.* New York: International Universities Press.

Jaffe, J., & Feldstein, S. (1970). *Rhythms of dialogue.* New York: Academic Press.

James, W. (1884). What is emotion? *Mind, 19,* 188–205.

James, W. (1890). *The principles of psychology.* New York: Dover, 1950.

James, W. (1894). The physical basis of emotion. *Psychological Review, 1,* 516–529. (Reprinted in *Psychological Review, 101,* 205–210)

Johnson, M. (1983). A multiple-entry, modular memory system. In G. H. Bower (Ed.), *The psychology of learning and motivation* (Vol. 17, pp. 81–123). New York: Academic Press.

Johnson, M. (1987). *The body in the mind: The bodily basis of meaning, imagination, and reasoning.* Chicago: University of Chicago Press.

Johnson-Laird, P. N. (1989). Mental models. In M. I. Posner (Ed.), *Foundations of cognitive science* (pp. 469–499). Cambridge, MA: MIT Press.

Johnston, J. R. (1988). Children's verbal representation of spatial location. In J. Stiles-Davis, M. Kritchevsky, & U. Bellugi (Eds.), *Spatial cognition: Brain bases and development* (pp. 195–205). Hillsdale, NJ: Erlbaum.

Jones, E. (1953). *The life and works of Sigmund Freud* (Vol. 1). New York: Basic Books.

Jones, E. E. (1995). How will psychoanalysis study itself? In T. Shapiro & R. Emde (Eds.), *Research in psychoanalysis: Process, development, outcome* (pp. 91–108). New York: International Universities Press.

Jones, E. E., & Windholz, M. (1990). The psychoanalytic case study: Toward a method for systematic inquiry. *Journal of the American Psychoanalytic Association, 38,* 985–1015.

Kalmykova, K., Mergenthaler, E., & Bucci, W. (1997). *Relationship episodes and computer referential activity.* Paper presented at the meeting of the Society for Psychotherapy Research, Geilo, Norway.

Kapp, B. S., Pascoe, J. P., & Bixler, M. A. (1984). The amygdala: A neuroanatomical systems approach to its contributions to aversive conditioning. In L. R. Squire & N. Butters (Eds.), *Neuropsychology of memory* (pp. 478–488). New York: Guilford Press.

Kay, S., Fiszbein, A., & Opler, L. (1987). The Positive and Negative Syndrome Scale (PANSS) for schizophrenia. *Schizophrenia Bulletin, 13,* 261-276.

Keller, H. (1908). *The world I live in.* New York: Century.

Kepecs, J. G., & Wolman, R. (1972). Preconscious perception of the transference. *Psychoanalytic Quarterly, 16,* 172-194.

Kernberg, O. F. (1984). *Severe personality disorders: Psychotherapeutic strategies.* New Haven, CT: Yale University Press.

Kernberg, O. F. (1990). New perspectives in psychoanalytic affect theory. In R. Plutchik & H. Kellerman (Eds.), *Emotion: Theory, research and experience* (pp. 115-131). New York: Academic Press.

Kernberg, O. F. (1995). Psychoanalytic object relations theories. In B. E. Moore (Ed.), *Psychoanalysis: The major concepts* (pp. 450-462). New Haven, CT: Yale University Press.

Kirk-Smith, M. D., Van Toller, C., & Dodd, G. H. (1983). Unconscious odour conditioning in human subjects. *Biological Psychology, 17,* 221-231.

Klein, G. S. (1970). *Perception, motives and personality.* New York: Knopf.

Klein, G. S. (1973). Is psychoanalysis relevant? *Psychoanalysis and Contemporary Science, 2,* 3-21.

Klein, G. S. (1976). *Psychoanalytic theory: An exploration of essentials.* New York: International Universities Press.

Klein, M. (1948). *Contributions to psychoanalysis, 1921-1945.* London: Hogarth Press.

Klein, M. H., Mathieu, P. L., Gendlin, E. T., & Kiesler, D. J. (1970). *The Experiencing Scale: A research and training manual.* Madison: Wisconsin Psychiatric Institute, Bureau of Audio Visual Instruction.

Kline, P. (1981). *Fact and fantasy in Freudian theory* (2nd ed.). New York: Methuen.

Klüver, H., & Bucy, P. C. (1937). Psychic blindness and other symptoms following bilateral temporal lobectomy in rhesus monkeys. *Journal of Physiology, 119,* 352-353.

Kohut, H. (1977). *The restoration of the self.* New York: International Universities Press.

Kosslyn, S. M. (1975). Information representation in visual images. *Cognitive Psychology, 7,* 341-370.

Kosslyn, S. M. (1983). *Ghosts in the mind's machine: Creating and using images in the brain.* New York: Norton.

Kosslyn, S. M. (1987). Seeing and imagining in the cerebral hemispheres: A computational approach. *Psychological Review, 94,* 148-175.

Kosslyn, S. M., Ball, T. M., & Reiser, B. J. (1978). Visual images preserve metric spatial information: Evidence from studies of image scanning. *Journal of Experimental Psychology: Human Perception and Performance, 4,* 47-60.

Kris, E. (1936). The psychology of caricature. *International Journal of Psycho-Analysis, 17,* 285-303.

Kris, E. (1952). *Psychoanalytic explorations in art.* New York: International Universities Press.

Kris, E. (1956). On some vicissitudes of insight in psychoanalysis. *International Journal of Psycho-Analysis, 37,* 445-455.

Krystal, H. (1988). *Integration and self-healing: Affect, trauma, alexithymia.* Hillsdale, NJ: Analytic Press.

Kuhl, P. K., & Miller, J. D. (1975). Speech perception by the chinchilla: Voiced-voiceless distinction in alveolar plosive consonants. *Science, 190,* 69–72.

Kuhl, P. K., & Miller, J. D. (1976). Speech perception by the chinchilla: Identification functions for synthetic VOT stimuli. *Journal of the Acoustical Society of America, 60,* 581.

Lakoff, G. (1987). *Women, fire, and dangerous things: What categories reveal about the mind.* Chicago: University of Chicago Press.

Lang, P. J. (1994). The varieties of emotional experience: A meditation on James–Lange Theory. *Psychological Review, 101,* 211–221.

Langacker, R. (1987). *Foundations of cognitive grammar* (Vol. 1). Stanford, CA: Stanford University Press.

Lange, C. (1885). *The emotions* (I. A. Haupt, Trans.). Baltimore: Williams & Wilkins, 1922.

Lawless, H. T. (1978). Recognition of common odors, pictures, and simple shapes. *Perception and Psychophysics, 24,* 493–495.

Lawless, H. T., & Engen, T. (1977). Associations to odors: Interference, mnemonics, and verbal labeling. *Journal of Experimental Psychology: Human Learning and Memory, 3,* 52–59.

Lazarus, R. S. (1984). Thoughts on the relations between emotion and cognition. In K. R. Scherer & P. Ekman (Eds.), *Approaches to emotion* (pp. 247–270). Hillsdale, NJ: Erlbaum.

LeDoux, J. E. (1986). Sensory systems and emotion: A model of affective processing. *Integrative Psychiatry, 4,* 237–248.

LeDoux, J. E. (1989). Cognitive–emotional interactions in the brain. *Cognition and Emotion, 3,* 267–289.

LeDoux, J. E., Sakaguchi, A., Iwata, J., & Reis, D. J. (1986). Interruption of projections from the medial geniculate body to an archi-neostriatal field disrupts the classical conditioning of emotional responses to acoustic stimuli in the rat. *Neuroscience, 17,* 615–627.

LeDoux, J. E., Sakaguchi, A., & Reis, D. J. (1984). Subcortical efferent projections of the medial geniculate nucleus mediate emotional responses conditioned by acoustic stimuli. *Journal Neuroscience, 4,* 683–698.

Leslie, A. M. (1982). The perception of causality in infants. *Perception, 11,* 173–186.

Leslie, A. (1988). The necessity of illusion: Perception and thought in infancy. In L. Weiskrantz (Ed.), *Thought without language* (pp. 185–210). Oxford, UK: Clarendon.

Leventhal, H. (1984). A perceptual-motor theory of emotion. In K. R. Scherer & P. Ekman (Eds.), *Approaches to emotion* (pp. 271–291). Hillsdale, NJ: Erlbaum.

Levine, D. N., Warach, J., & Farah, M. J. (1985). Two visual systems in mental imagery: Dissociation of "what" and "where" in imagery disorders due to bilateral posterior cerebral lesions. *Neurology, 35,* 1010–1018.

Levy, J. (1970). Information processing and higher psychological functions in the disconnected hemispheres of commissurotomy patients (Doctoral dissertation, California Institute of Technology, 1970). *Dissertation Abstracts International, 31,* 1542B. (University Microfilms No. 70-14, 844)

Levy, J. (1983). Language, cognition, and the right hemisphere: A response to Gazzaniga. *American Psychologist, 38,* 542–546.

Levy, J., Trevarthen, C., Sperry, R. (1972). Perception of bilateral chimeric figures following hemispheric deconnexion. *Brain, 95,* 61–78.

Lewin, B. D. (1946). Sleep, the mouth, and the dream screen. *Psychoanalytic Quarterly, 15,* 419–434.

Lewin, B. D. (1948). Inferences from the dream screen. *International Journal of Psycho-Analysis 29,* 224–231.

Lewis, M., & Brooks, J. (1975). Infant's social perception: A constructivist view. In L. Cohen & P. Salapatek (Eds.), *Infant perception: From sensation to cognition* (Vol. 2, pp. 102–148). New York: Academic Press.

Liberman, A. M., Cooper, F. S., Shankweiler, D. P., & Studdert-Kennedy, M. (1967). Perception of the speech code. *Psychological Review, 74,* 431–461.

Loewald, H. W. (1978). Primary process, secondary process and language. In J. H. Smith (Ed.), *Psychiatry and the humanities: Psychoanalysis and language* (Vol. 3, pp. 235–270). New Haven, CT: Yale University Press.

Luborsky, L. (1988). A comparison of three transference related measures applied to the specimen hour. In H. Dahl, H. Kaechele, & H. Thomae (Eds.), *Psychoanalytic process research strategies* (pp. 109–115). New York: Springer-Verlag.

Luborsky, L., Barber, J. P., Binder, J., Curtis, J., Dahl, H., Horowitz, L. M., Horowitz, M., Perry, J. C., & Schacht, T. (1993). Transference-related measures: A new class based on psychotherapy sessions. In N. Miller, L. Luborsky, J. Barber & J. Docherty, (Eds.), *Psychodynamic treatment research* (pp. 326–341). New York: Basic Books.

Luborsky, L., & Crits-Cristoph, P. (1988). The assessment of transference by the CCRT method. In H. Dahl, H. Kaechele, & H. Thomae (Eds.), *Psychoanalytic process research strategies* (pp. 99–108). New York: Springer-Verlag.

Luborsky, L., & Crits-Cristoph, P. (1990). *Understanding transference: The CCRT method.* New York: Basic Books.

Luborsky, L., Popp, C., Barber, J. P., & Shapiro, D. (Eds.). (1994). *Psychotherapy Research, 4*(3 & 4), 151–290. [Special Issue]

Luborsky, L., Stuart, J., Friedman, S., Seligman, D. A., Bucci, W., Pulver, S., & Woody, G. (1996). *A collection of completely tape-recorded psychoanalyses as a research resource.* Paper presented at the midwinter meetings of the American Psychoanalytic Association, New York City.

Lyman, B. J., & McDaniel, M. A. (1986). Effects on encoding strategy on long-term memory for odours. *Quarterly Journal of Experimental Psychology, 38,* 753–765.

Lynch, G., & Baudry, M. (1988). Structure–function relationships in the organization of memory. In M. S. Gazzaniga (Ed.), *Perspectives in memory research* (pp. 23–91). Cambridge, MA: MIT Press.

MacLean, P. D. (1949). Psychosomatic disease and the "visceral brain": Recent developments bearing on the Papez theory of emotion. *Psychosomatic Medicine, 11,* 338–353.

MacLean, P. D. (1952). Some psychiatric implications of physiological studies on fronto-temporal portion of limbic system (visceral brain). *Electroencephalography and Clinical Neurophysiology, 4,* 407–418.

Mahler, M. S. (1968). *On human symbiosis and the vicissitudes of individuation.* New York: International Universities Press.

Mahler, M. S., Pine, F., & Bergman, A. (1975). *The psychological birth of the human infant: Symbiosis and individuation.* New York: Basic Books.

Mahut, H. (1985). Dissociation of two behavioral functions in the monkey after early hippocampal ablations. In B. E. Will, P. Schmitt, & J. C. Dalrymple-Alford (Eds.), *Brain plasticity, learning, and memory* (pp. 353–362). New York: Plenum Press.

Malamut, B. L., Saunders, R. C., & Mishkin, M. (1984). Monkeys with combined amygdalo-hippocampal lesions succeed in object discrimination learning despite 24-hour intertrial intervals. *Behavioral Neuroscience, 98,* 759–769.

Mandler, G. (1975). *Mind and emotion.* New York: Wiley.

Mandler, G. (1984). *Mind and body.* New York: Norton.

Mandler, J. (1991). Prelinguistic primitives. In L. A. Sutton & C. Johnson (Eds.), *Proceedings of the seventeenth annual meeting of the Berkeley Linguistics Society* (pp. 414–425). Berkeley, CA: Berkeley Linguistics Society.

Mandler, J. (1992). How to build a baby: II. Conceptual primitives. *Psychological Review, 99,* 587–604.

Margenau, H. (1950). *The nature of physical reality.* New York: McGraw-Hill.

Marr, D., & Poggio, T. (1976). Cooperative computation of stereo disparity. *Science, 194,* 283–287.

Martindale, C. (1975). *Romantic progression: The psychology of literary history.* Washington, DC: Hemisphere.

Marty, P., & de M'Uzan, M. (1963). La pensée opératoire. *Revue Française de Psychanalyse, 27*(Suppl.), 345–356.

McClelland, J. L., Rumelhart, D. E., & Hinton, G. E. (1989). The appeal of parallel distributed processing. In D. E. Rumelhart, J. L. McClelland, & the PDP Research Group, *Parallel distributed processing: Explorations in the microstructure of cognition* (Vol. 1, pp. 3–44). Cambridge: MIT Press.

McCollough, C. (1965). Color adaptation of edge-detectors in the human visual system. *Science, 149,* 1115–1116.

McDougall, J. (1989). *Theaters of the body: A psychoanalytic approach to psychosomatic illness.* New York: Norton.

McLaughlin, J. (1978). Primary and secondary process in the context of cerebral hemispheric specialization. *Psychoanalytic Quarterly, 47,* 237–266.

Meltzoff, A. N. (1988). Infant imitation and memory: Nine-month-olds in immediate and deferred tests. *Child Development, 59,* 217–225.

Mergenthaler, E. (1985). *Textbank systems: Computer science applied in the field of psychoanalysis.* Heidelberg: Springer-Verlag.

Mergenthaler, E. (1992). *Emotion/Abstractness as indicators of "hot spots" in psychotherapy transcripts.* Paper presented at the 23rd Annual International Meeting of the Society for Psychotherapy Research, Berkeley, CA.

Mergenthaler, E. (1996). Emotion-abstraction patterns in verbatim protocols: A new way of describing psychotherapeutic processes. *Journal of Consulting and Clinical Psychology, 64,* 1306–1315.

Mergenthaler, E., & Bucci, W. (1993). *Computer-assisted procedures for analyzing verbal data in psychotherapy research.* Paper presented at the 24th Annual International Meeting of the Society for Psychotherapy Research, Pittsburgh, PA.

Mergenthaler, E., & Stinson, C. H. (1992). Psychotherapy transcription standards. *Psychotherapy Research, 2,* 58–75.

Miller, N. E., Luborsky, L., Barber, J. P., & Docherty, J. P. (Eds.). (1993). *Psychodynamic treatment research: A handbook for clinical practice.* New York: Basic Books.

Miller, S. (1994). The waking nightmare (Doctoral dissertation, Adelphi University, 1994). *Dissertation Abstracts International, 55*(2B), 600B.

Milner, B. (1962). Les troubles de la memoire accompagnant des lésions hippocampiques bilatérales [Disorders of memory accompanying bilateral hippocampal lesions]. In P. Passovant (Ed.), *Physiologie de l'hippocampe* (pp. 257–272). Paris: Centre National de la Recherche Scientifique.

Milner, B. (1974). Hemispheric specialization: Scope and limits. In F. O. Schimdt & F. G. Worden (Eds.), *The neurosciences: Third study program* (pp. 75–89). Cambridge, MA: MIT Press.

Milner, B., Corkin, S., & Teuber, H. L. (1968). Further analysis of the hippocampal amnesic syndrome: 14-year follow-up study of H. M. *Neuropsychologia, 6,* 215–234.

Minsky, M. (1975). A framework for representing knowledge. In P. H. Winston (Ed.), *The psychology of computer vision* (pp. 211–277). New York: McGraw-Hill.

Mishkin, M., Malamut, B., & Bachevalier, J. (1984). Memories and habits: Two neural systems. In G. Lynch, J. L. McGaugh, & N. M. Weinberger (Eds.), *Neurobiology of learning and memory* (pp. 65–77). New York: Guilford Press.

Mishkin, M., & Petri, H. L. (1984). Memories and habits: Some implications for the analysis of learning and retention. In L. R. Squire & N. Butters (Eds.), *Neuropsychology of memory* (pp. 287–296). New York: Guilford Press.

Mishkin, M., Ungerleider, L. G., & Macko, K. A. (1983). Object vision and spatial vision: Two cortical pathways. *Trends in Neurosciences, 6,* 414–417.

Monk, R. (1990). *Ludwig Wittgenstein: The duty of genius.* New York: Penguin Books.

Moore, K. (1992). An application of linguistic narrative analysis to psychoanalytic process research (Doctoral dissertation, University of Detroit, 1992). *Dissertation Abstracts International, 53*(2B), 1070.

Morey, J. (1992). Towards empirically based theory of mind in schizophrenia: Cognitive processes, symptomatology, and referential activity (Doctoral dissertation, Adelphi Universitiy, 1989). *Dissertation Abstracts International, 53*(5B), 2550.

Morse, P. A., & Snowdon, C. T. (1975). An investigation of categorical speech discrimination by rhesus monkeys. *Perception and Psychophysics, 17,* 9–16.

Nabokov, V. (1992). *The real life of Sebastian Knight.* New York: Random House.

Nachman, P., & Stern, D. N. (1983). *Recall memory for emotional experience in pre-linguistic infants.* Paper presented at the National Clinical Infancy Fellows Conference, Yale University, New Haven, CT.

Nebes, R. D. (1972). Dominance of the minor hemisphere in commissurotomized man in a test of figural unification. *Brain, 95,* 633–638.

Nebes, R. D. (1973). Perception of spatial relationships by the right and left hemispheres in commissurotomized man. *Neuropsychologia, 3,* 285–289.

Neisser, U. (1967). *Cognitive psychology.* New York: Appleton-Century-Crofts.

Nemiah, J. C., & Sifneos, P. E. (1970a). Affect and fantasy in patients with psychosomatic disorders. In O. W. Hill (Ed.), *Modern trends in psychosomatic medicine* (Vol. 2, pp. 430–439). London: Butterworths.

Nemiah, J. C., & Sifneos, P. E. (1970b). Psychosomatic illness: A problem of communication. *Psychotherapy and Psychosomatics, 18,* 154–160.

Nissen, M. J., & Bullemer, P. (1987). Attentional requirements of learning: Evidence from performance measures. *Cognitive Psychology, 19,* 1–32.

Nissen, M. J., Knopman, D. S., & Schacter, D. L. (1987). Neurochemical dissociation of memory systems. *Neurology, 37,* 789–794.

Norman, D. A. (Ed.). (1981). *Perspectives on cognitive science.* Norwood, NJ: Ablex.

Norman, D. A. (1986). Reflections on cognition and parallel distributed processing. In D. E. Rumelhart, J. L. McClelland, & the PDP Research Group, *Parallel distributed processing: Explorations in the microstructure of cognition* (Vol. 2, pp. 531–546). Cambridge, MA: MIT Press.

Noy, P. (1969). A revision of the psychoanalytic theory of the primary process. *International Journal of Psycho-Analysis, 50,* 155–170.

Noy, P. (1973). Symbolism and mental representation. *Annual of Psychoanalysis, 1,* 125–158.

Noy, P. (1979). The psychoanalytic theory of cognitive development. *Psychoanalytic Study of the Child, 34,* 169–215.

Oakley, D. A. (1983). The varieties of memory: A phylogenetic approach. In A. Mayes (Ed.), *Memory in animals and humans* (pp. 20–82). Cambridge, UK: Van Nostrand Reinhold.

O'Keefe, J., & Nadel, L. (1978). *The hippocampus as a cognitive map.* Oxford, UK: Clarendon Press.

Okie, J. E. (1992). Action, somatization and language in borderline inpatients (Doctoral dissertation, Adelphi University, 1991). *Dissertation Abstracts International, 53,* 759–760.

Olds, J. (1958). Self-stimulation of the brain. *Science, 127,* 315–324.

Olton, D. S., Becker, J. T., & Handelmann, G. E. (1979). Hippocampus, space, and memory. *Behavioral and Brain Sciences, 2,* 313–365.

Ornstein, R. (1972). *The psychology of consciousness.* San Francisco: Freeman.

Paivio, A. (1966). Latency of verbal associations and imagery to noun stimuli as a function of abstractness and generality. *Canadian Journal of Psychology, 20,* 378–387.

Paivio, A. (1971). *Imagery and verbal processes.* New York: Holt, Rinehart & Winston.

Paivio, A. (1986). *Mental representations: A dual coding approach.* New York: Oxford University Press.

Paivio, A., Clark, J. M., Digdon, N., & Bons, T. (1989). Referential processing: Reciprocity and correlates of naming and imaging. *Memory and Cognition, 16*, 163–174.

Panksepp, J. (1982). Towards a general psychobiological theory of emotions. *Behavioral and Brain Sciences, 5*, 407–467.

Papez, J. W. (1937). A proposed mechanism of emotion. *Archives of Neurology and Psychiatry, 38*, 725–743.

Parker, R. M., Jr. (1990). *Burgundy: A comprehensive guide to the producers, appelations, and wines.* New York: Simon & Schuster.

Perry, J. C. (1993). Defenses and their effects. In N. E. Miller, L. Luborsky, J. P. Barber, & J. P. Docherty (Eds.), *Psychodynamic treatment research: A handbook for clinical practice* (pp. 274–306). New York: Basic Books.

Petersen, S. E., Fox, P. T., Posner, M. I., Mintun, M., & Raichle, M. E. (1988). Positron emission tomographic studies of the cortical anatomy of single word processing. *Nature, 331*, 585–589.

Peterson, M. J. (1975). The retention of imagined and seen spatial matrices. *Cognitive Psychology, 7*, 181–193.

Piaget, J. (1950). *The psychology of intelligence.* London: Routledge & Kegan Paul.

Pinker, S. (1989). *Learnability and cognition: The acquisition of argument structure.* Cambridge, MA: MIT Press.

Plutchik, R. (1980). *The emotions: A psycho-evolutionary synthesis.* New York: Harper & Row.

Podgorny, P., & Shepard, R. N. (1978). Functional representations common to visual perception and imagination. *Journal of Experimental Psychology: Human Perception and Performance, 4*, 21–35.

Poincaré, H. (1956). Mathematical creation. In J. R. Newman (Ed.), *The world of mathematics* (pp. 2041–2050). New York: Simon & Schuster.

Posner, M. I., & Rothbart, M. K. (1989). Intentional chapters on unintended thoughts. In J. S. Uleman & J. A. Bargh (Eds.), *Unintended thought* (pp. 450–469). New York: Guilford Press.

Posner, M. I., & Snyder, C. R. R. (1975). Attention and cognitive control. In R. Solso (Ed.), *Information processing and cognition: The Loyola Symposium* (pp. 55–85). Hillsdale, NJ: Erlbaum.

Premack, D., & Premack, A. J. (1983). *The mind of an ape.* New York: Norton.

Pribram, K. H. (1984). Emotion: A neurobehavioral analysis. In K. R. Scherer & P. Ekman (Eds.), *Approaches to emotion* (pp. 13–38). Hillsdale, NJ: Erlbaum.

Pribram, K. H., & Gill, M. M. (1976). *Freud's project reassessed.* London: Hutchinson.

Pylyshyn, Z. W. (1973). What the mind's eye tells the mind's brain: A critique of mental imagery. *Psychological Bulletin, 80*, 1–24.

Radna, R. J., & MacLean, P. D. (1981). Vagal elicitation of respiratory-type and other unit responses in basal limbic structures of squirrel monkeys. *Brain Research, 213*, 45–61.

Rapaport, D. (1960). The structure of psychoanalytic theory: A systematizing attempt. *Psychological Issues, 2*(2, Monograph No. 6).

Rapaport, D., Gill, M. M., & Schafer, R. (1968). *Diagnostic psychological testing.* New York: International Universities Press.

Rasmussen, T., & Milner, B. (1977). The role of early brain damage in determining the lateralization of cerebral speech functions. In S. Simond & D. Blizard (Eds.), *Evolution and lateralization of the brain* (pp. 355–369). New York: New York Academy of Science.

Rausch, R., Serafetinides, E. A., & Crandall, P. H. (1977). Olfactory memory in patients with anterior temporal lobectomy. *Cortex, 13,* 445–452.

Reiser, M. F. (1985). Converging sectors of psychoanalysis and neurobiology: Mutual challenge and opportunity. *Journal of the American Psychoanalytic Association, 33,* 11–34.

Richardson, J. T. E., & Zucco, G. M. (1989). Cognition and olfaction: A review. *Psychological Bulletin, 105,* 352–360.

Rickert, E. J., Bennett, T. L., Lane, P. L., & French, J. (1978). Hippocampectomy and the attenuation of blocking. *Behavioral Biology, 22,* 147–160.

Ricoeur, P. (1977). The question of proof in Freud's psychoanalytic writings. *Journal of the American Psychoanalytic Association, 25,* 835–871.

Riddoch, M. J., & Humphreys, G. W. (1987). A case of integrative visual agnosia. *Brain, 110,* 1431–1462.

Rilke, R. M. (1983). *The notebooks of Malte Laurids Brigge* (S. Mitchell, Trans.). New York: Random House.

Roediger, H. L., III, & Blaxton, T. A. (1987). Retrieval modes produce dissociations in memory for surface information. In D. S. Gorfein & R. R. Hoffman (Eds.), *Memory and learning: The Ebbinghaus Centennial Conference* (pp. 349–379). Hillsdale, NJ: Erlbaum.

Roland, P. E., & Friberg, L. (1985). Localization of cortical areas activated by thinking. *Journal of Neurophysiology, 53,* 1219–1243.

Rosch, E. (1975). Cognitive representations of semantic categories. *Journal of Experimental Psychology: General, 104,* 192–233.

Rosch, E. (1978). Principles of categorization. In E. Rosch & B. B. Lloyd (Eds.), *Cognition and categorization* (pp. 27–48). Hillsdale, NJ: Erlbaum.

Rosenberg, D., & Bloom, H. (1990). *The book of J* (D. Rosenberg, Trans.). New York: Random House.

Rosenberg, S., & Simon, H. A. (1977). Modeling semantic memory: Effects of presenting semantic information in different modalities. *Cognitive Psychology, 9,* 293–325.

Rozin, P., & Schull, J. (1989). The adaptive–evolutionary point of view in experimental psychology. In R. C. Atkinson, R. J. Herrnstein, G. Lindzey, & R. D. Luce (Eds.), *Handbook of experimental psychology* (pp. 503–546). New York: Wiley–Interscience.

Rubin, D. C., Groth, E., & Goldsmith, D. J. (1984). Olfactory cuing of autobiographical memory. *American Journal of Psychology, 97,* 493–507.

Rubinstein, B. B. (1965). Psychoanalytic theory and the mind–body problem. In N. S. Greenfield & W. C. Lewis (Eds.), *Psychoanalysis and current biological thought* (pp. 35–56). Madison: University of Wisconsin Press.

Rubinstein, B. B. (1976). On the possibility of a strictly clinical psychoanalytic theory: An essay in the philosophy of psychoanalysis. In M. M. Gill & P. S. Holzman (Eds.), Psychology versus metapsychology: Psychoanalytic essays in memory of George S. Klein. *Psychological Issues, 9*(Monograph No. 36), 229-364.

Ruggiero, F. T., & Flagg, S. F. (1976). Do animals have memory? In D. L. Medin, W. A. Roberts, & R. T. Davis (Eds.), *Processes of animal memory* (pp. 1-19). Hillsdale, NJ: Erlbaum.

Rumelhart, D. E. (1980). Schemata: The building blocks of cognition. In R. Spiro, B. Bruce, & W. Brewer (Eds.), *Theoretical issues in reading comprehension* (pp. 33-58). Hillsdale, NJ: Erlbaum.

Rumelhart, D. E., McClelland, J. L., & the PDP Research Group. (1986). *Parallel distributed processing: Explorations in the microstructure of cognition.* Cambridge, MA: MIT Press.

Rumelhart, D. E., & Norman, D. A. (1982). Simulating a skilled typist: A study of skilled cognitive–motor performance. *Cognitive Science, 6,* 1-36.

Rycroft, C. (1968). *Imagination and reality.* New York: International Universities Press.

Sacks, O., & Wasserman, R. (1987, November 19). The case of the color-blind painter. *New York Review of Books,* pp. 25-34.

Samstag, N. (1996). A meta-analysis of Referential Activity (Doctoral dissertation, Adelphi University, 1996). *Dissertation Abstracts International.*

Sandler, J. (1987). *From safety to superego: Selected papers of Joseph Sandler.* New York: Guilford Press.

Schab, F. R. (1991). Odor memory: Taking stock. *Psychological Bulletin, 109,* 242-251.

Schacht, T., Binder, J., & Strupp, H. (1984). The dynamic focus. In H. Strupp & J. Binder (Eds.), *Psychotherapy in a new key: A guide to time-limited dynamic psychotherapy* (pp. 65-109). New York: Basic Books.

Schachter, S. (1959). *The psychology of affiliation.* Stanford, CA: Stanford University Press.

Schachter, S., & Singer, T. E. (1962). Cognitive, social and physiological determinants of emotional state. *Psychological Review, 69,* 379-397.

Schacter, D. L. (1987). Implicit memory: History and current status. *Journal of Experimental Psychology: Learning, Memory and Cognition, 13,* 501-518.

Schacter, D. L. (1989). Memory. In M. A. Posner (Ed.), *Foundations of cognitive science* (pp. 683-725). Cambridge, MA: MIT Press.

Schacter, D. L., Cooper, L. A., & Delaney, S. M. (1990). Implicit memory for unfamiliar objects depends on access to structural descriptions. *Journal of Experimental Psychology: Learning, Memory and Cognition, 119,* 5-24.

Schacter, D. L., & Moscovitch, M. (1984). Infants, amnesics, and dissociable memory systems. In M. Moscovitch (Ed.), *Infant memory* (pp. 173-216). New York: Plenum Press.

Schafer, R. (1976). *A new language for psychoanalysis.* New Haven, CT: Yale University Press.

Schafer, R. (1980). Action and narration in psychoanalysis. *New Literary History, 12,* 61-85.

Schank, R. C., & Abelson, R. P. (1977). *Scripts, plans, goals, and understanding.* Hillsdale, NJ: Erlbaum.

Scherer, K. R. (1984). On the nature and function of emotion: A component process approach. In K. R. Scherer & P. Ekman (Eds.), *Approaches to emotion* (pp. 293–317). Hillsdale, NJ: Erlbaum.

Schneider, W. (1988). Structure and controlling subsymbolic processing. *Behavioral and Brain Sciences, 11,* 51–52.

Segal, S. J. (1972). Assimiliation of a stimulus in the construction of an image: The Perky effect revisited. In P. W. Sheehan (Ed.), *The function and nature of imagery* (pp. 203–301). New York: Academic Press.

Segal, S. J., & Fusella, V. (1970). Influence of imaged pictures and sounds on detection of visual and auditory signals. *Journal of Experimental Psychology, 83,* 458–464.

Shallice, T. (1982). Specific impairments of planning. *Philosophical Transactions of the Royal Society of London, Series B. Biological Sciences, 298,* 199–209.

Shepard, R. N. (1975). Form, formation, and transformation of internal representation. In R. Solso (Ed.), *Information processing and cognition: The Loyola Symposium* (pp. 87–122). Hillsdale, NJ: Erlbaum.

Shepard, R. N., & Cooper, L. A. (1982). *Mental images and their transformations.* Cambridge, MA: MIT Press.

Shepard, R. N., & Metzler, J. (1971). Mental rotation of three-dimensional objects. *Science, 171,* 701–703.

Sherry, D. F., & Schacter, D. L. (1987). The evolution of multiple memory systems. *Psychological Review, 94*(4), 439–454.

Shettleworth, S. J. (1983). Function and mechanism in learning. In M. D. Zeiler & P. Harzem (Eds.), *Advances in the analysis of behavior* (Vol. 3, pp. 1–39). New York: Wiley.

Shevrin, H. (1974). Brain wave correlates of subliminal stimulation, unconscious attention, primary- and secondary-process thinking and repressiveness. In M. Mayman (Ed.), Psychoanalytic research: Three approaches to experimental study of subliminal processes. *Psychological Issues, 8*(Monograph No. 30), 56–87.

Shevrin, H. (1995). Is psychoanalysis one science, two sciences, or no science at all? A discourse among friendly antagonists. *Journal of the American Psychoanalytic Association, 43,* 1–24.

Sidtis, J. J., Volpe, B. T., Wilson, D. H., Rayport, M., & Gazzaniga, M. S. (1981). Variability in right-hemisphere language function: Evidence for a continuum of generative capacity. *Journal of Neuroscience, 1,* 323–331.

Simon, H. A. (1967). Motivational and emotional controls of cognition. *Psychological Review, 74,* 29–39.

Simon, H. A., & Kaplan, C. A. (1989). Foundations of cognitive science. In M. I. Posner (Ed.), *Foundations of cognitive science,* (pp. 1–47). Cambridge, MA: MIT Press.

Smith, H., & McDougall, W. (1920). Some experiments in learning and retention. *British Journal of Psychology, 10,* 198–209.

Solomon, G. F. (1987). Psychoneuroimmunology: Interactions between central nervous system and immune system. *Journal of Neuroscience Research, 18,* 1–9.

Solomon, P. R. (1977). The role of hippocampus in blocking and conditioned inhibition of the rabbit's nictitating membrane response. *Journal of Comparative Physiology and Psychology, 91,* 407–417.

Spelke, E. S. (1985). Perception of unity, persistence, and identity: Thoughts on infants' conceptions of objects. In J. Mehler & R. Fox (Eds.), *Neonate cognition: Beyond the blooming buzzing confusion* (pp. 89–113). Hillsdale, NJ: Erlbaum.

Spence, D. P. (1982). *Narrative truth and historical truth: Meaning and interpretation in psychoanalysis.* New York: Norton.

Spence, D. P., Dahl, H., & Jones, E. (1993). Impact of interpretation on associative freedom. *Journal of Clinical and Consulting Psychology, 61,* 395–402.

Squire, L. R. (1982). The neuropsychology of human memory. *Annual Review of Neuroscience, 5,* 241–273.

Squire, L. R. (1992). Memory and the hippocampus: A synthesis from findings with rats, monkeys, and humans. *Psychological Review, 99,* 195–231.

Squire, L. R., & Cohen, N. J. (1984). Human memory and amnesia. In G. Lynch, J. McGaugh, & N. Weinberger (Eds.), *Neurobiology of learning and memory* (pp. 3–64). New York: Guilford Press.

Steele, R. S. (1979). Psychoanalysis and hermeneutics. *International Review of Psycho-Analysis, 6,* 389–411.

Stern, D. N. (1985). *The interpersonal world of the infant.* New York: Basic Books.

Stern, W. (1914). *Psychologie der fruehen Kindheit.* Leipzig: Quelle and Meyer.

Stone, P. J., Dunphy, D. C., Smith, M. S., & Ogilvie, D. M. (1966). *The general inquirer: A computer approach to content analysis.* Cambridge, MA: MIT Press.

Strachey, J. (1934). The nature of the therapeutic action of psycho-analysis. In L. Paul (Ed.), *Psychoanalytic clinical interpretation* (pp. 362–378). New York: Free Press, 1963.

Strauss, M. S. (1979). Abstractions of proto-typical information by adults and 10-month-old infants. *Journal of Experimental Psychology: Human Learning and Memory, 5,* 618–632.

Strupp, H. H., & Binder, J. L. (Eds.). (1984). *Psychotherapy in a new key.* New York: Basic Books.

Sullivan, H. S. (1953). *The interpersonal theory of psychiatry.* New York: Norton.

Sumner, D. (1962). On testing the sense of smell. *Lancet, 2*(7262), 895–897.

Swanson, L. W. (1983). In W. Seifert (Ed.), *Neurobiology of the hippocampus* (pp. 3–19). London: Academic Press.

Sweetser, E. (1990). *From etymology to pragmatics: Metaphorical and cultural aspects of semantic structure.* Cambridge, UK: Cambridge University Press.

Talmy, L. (1988). Force dynamics in language and cognition. *Cognitive Science, 12,* 49–100.

Teller, V., & Dahl, H. (1986). The microstructure of free association. *Journal of the American Psychoanalytic Association, 34,* 763–798.

Thomae, H., & Kaechele, H. (1987). *Psychoanalytic practice: Vol. 1. Principles.* Berlin: Springer-Verlag.

Thomae, H., & Kaechele, H. (1992). *Psychoanalytic practice: Vol. 2. Clinical studies.* Berlin: Springer-Verlag.

Thomas, G. J., & Spafford, P. S. (1984). Deficits for representational memory induced by septal and cortical lesions (singly and combined) in rats. *Behavioral Neuroscience, 98,* 394–404.

Titchener, E. B. (1910). *A textbook of psychology.* New York: Macmillan.

Tolstoy, L. (1939). *Anna Karenina.* New York: Random House.

Tomkins, S. S. (1962). *Affect, imagery, consciousness: Vol. 1. The positive affects.* New York: Springer.

Tomkins, S. S. (1984). Affect theory. In K. R. Scherer & P. Ekman (Eds.), *Approaches to emotion* (pp. 163–195). Hillsdale, NJ: Erlbaum.

Tomkins, S. S., & McCarter, R. (1964). What and where are the primary affects? Some evidence for a theory. *Perceptual and Motor Skills, 18,* 119–158.

Tranel, D., & Damasio, A. R. (1985). Knowledge without awareness: An autonomic index of facial recognition by prosopagnosics. *Science, 228,* 1453–1454.

Tronick, E. (1989). Emotions and emotional communication in infants. *American Psychologist, 44,* 112–119.

Tronick, E. Z., & Cohn, J. F. (1989). Infant–mother face-to-face interaction: Age and gender differences in coordination and the occurrence of miscoordination. *Child Development, 60,* 85–92.

Tulving, E. (1972). Episodic and semantic memory. In E. Tulving & W. Donaldson (Eds.), *Organization of memory* (pp. 381–403). New York: Academic Press.

Tulving, E. (1983). *Elements of episodic memory.* Oxford, UK: Clarendon Press.

Tulving, E. (1985). How many memory systems are there? *American Psychologist, 40,* 385–398.

Udoff, A. (1996). Maternalism in psychoanalysis: An empirical study (Doctoral dissertation, Adelphi University, 1995). *Dissertation Abstracts International, 56*(6), 3468B.

Ungerleider, L. G., & Mishkin, M. (1982). Two cortical visual systems. In D. J. Ingle, M. A. Goodale, & R. J. W. Mansfield (Eds.), *Analysis of visual behavior* (pp. 549–586). Cambridge, MA: MIT Press.

Van Essen, D. C. (1985). Functional organization of primate visual cortex. In A. Peters & E. G. Jones (Eds.), *Cerebral cortex* (Vol. 3, pp. 259–329). New York: Plenum Press.

von Bertalanffy, L. (1950). The theory of open systems in physics and psychology. *Science, 3,* 23–29.

Vygotsky, L. (1934). *Thought and language.* Cambridge, MA: MIT Press, 1986.

Wallerstein, R. S. (1988). One psychoanalysis or many? *International Journal of Psycho-Analysis, 69,* 5–21.

Wallerstein, R. S. (1993). The effectiveness of psychotherapy and psychoanalysis: Conceptual issues and empirical work. In T. Shapiro & R. N. Emde (Eds.), *Research in psychoanalysis: Process, development, outcome* (pp. 299–312). Madison, CT: International Universities Press.

Warrington, E. K., & Weiskrantz, L. (1968). New method of testing long-term retention with special reference to amnesic patients. *Nature, 217,* 972–974.

Warrington, E. K., & Weiskrantz, L. (1974). The effect of prior learning on subsequent retention in amnesic patients. *Neuropsychologia, 12,* 419–428.

Warrington, E. K., & Weiskrantz, L. (1982). Amnesia: A disconnection syndrome? *Neuropsychologia, 20,* 233–248.

Waters, R. S., & Wilson, W. A. (1976). Speech perception by rhesus monkeys: The voicing distinction in synthesized labial and velar stop consonants. *Perception and Psychophysics, 19,* 285–289.

Watson, J. B. (1913). Psychology as the behaviorist views it. *Psychological Review, 20,* 158–177.

Waugh, N. C., & Norman, D. A. (1965). Primary memory. *Psychological Review, 72,* 89–104.

Wechsler, D. (1981). *Wechsler Adult Intelligence Scale–Revised.* San Antonio, TX: Psychological Corporation.

Wegman, C. (1985). *Psychoanalysis and cognitive psychology: A formalization of Freud's theory.* New York: Academic Press.

Weir, C. (1976). Auditory frequency sensitivity in the neonate: A signal detection analysis. *Journal of Experimental Child Psychology, 21,* 219–225.

Weiskrantz, L. (1956). Behavioral changes associated with ablation of the amygdaloid complex in monkeys. *Journal of Comparative and Physiological Psychology, 49,* 381–391.

Weiskrantz, L. (1986). *Blindsight: A case study and implications.* New York: Oxford University Press.

Weiss, J. (1993). Empirical studies of the psychoanalytic process. In T. Shapiro & R. N. Emde (Eds.), *Research in psychoanalysis: Process, development, outcome* (pp. 7–29). Madison, CT: International Universities Press.

Weiss, J., Sampson, H., & the Mount Zion Psychotherapy Research Group. (1986). *The psychoanalytic process: Theory, clinical observation, and empirical research.* New York: Guilford Press.

Werner, H., & Kaplan, B. (1984). *Symbol formation.* Hillsdale, NJ: Erlbaum.

Whorf, B. L. (1950). *Four articles on metalinguistics.* Washington, DC: Foreign Service Institute.

Whorf, B. L. (1964). *Language, thought and reality.* Cambridge, MA: MIT Press.

Widlocher, D. (1990). Neurobiologie et psychanalyse: Les opérateurs de commutation. *Revue Internationale de Psychopathologie, 2,* 335–356.

Winnicott, D. W. (1971). *Playing and reality.* New York: Basic Books.

Winograd, T. (1975). Frame representations and the declarative-procedural controversy. In D. G. Bobrow & A. M. Collins (Eds.), *Representation and understanding: Studies in cognitive science* (pp. 185–210). New York: Academic Press.

Wundt, W. (1912). *An introduction to psychology* (R. Pintner, Trans.). London: George Allen. (Reprinted by Arno Press, New York, 1973)

Yuille, J. C. (1986). The futility of a purely experimental psychology of cognition: Imagery as a case study. In D. F. Marks (Ed.), *Theories of image formation* (pp. 197–224). Bronx, NY: Brandon House.

Zaidel, E. (1983). A response to Gazzaniga: Language in the right hemisphere: Convergent perspectives. *American Psychologist, 38,* 542–546.

Zajonc, R. B. (1980). Feeling and thinking: Preferences need no inferences. *American Psychologist, 35,* 151–175.

Zajonc, R. B. (1984a). The interaction of affect and cognition. In K. R. Scherer & P. Ekman (Eds.), *Approaches to emotion* (pp. 239–246). Hillsdale, NJ: Erlbaum.

Zajonc, R. B. (1984b). On primacy of affect. In K. R. Scherer & P. Ekman (Eds.), *Approaches to emotion* (pp. 259–270). Hillsdale, NJ: Erlbaum.

Zbrodoff, N. J., & Logan, G. D. (1986). On the autonomy of mental processes: A case study of arithmetic. *Journal of Experimental Psychology: General, 115,* 118–130.

Index

CPSIA information can be obtained at www.ICGtesting.com
Printed in the USA
235618LV00002B/45/P